Complete Book *of*

Alternative

Nutrition

The

Complete Book *of*

Alternative

Nutrition

Powerful
New Ways
to Use Foods,
Supplements,
Herbs and
Special Diets to
Prevent and Cure Disease

by Selene Y. Craig, Jennifer Haigh,
Sarí Harrar and the Editors of
PREVENTION. Magazine Health Books

BERKLEY BOOKS,
NEW YORK

This book is intended as a reference volume only, not as a medical manual. Keep in mind that nutritional needs vary from person to person, depending on age, sex, health status and total diet. The information here is designed to help you make informed decisions about your health. It is not intended as a substitute for any treatment that may have been prescribed by your doctor. If you suspect that you have a medical problem, we urge you to seek competent medical help.

THE COMPLETE BOOK OF ALTERNATIVE NUTRITION

A Berkley Book / published by arrangement with
Rodale Press

PRINTING HISTORY
Rodale Press edition published 1997
Berkley trade paperback edition / October 1998

The Complete Book of Alternative Nutrition Editorial Staff

Senior Managing Editor: **Edward Claflin**
Staff Writers: **Selene Y. Craig, Jennifer Haigh, Sarí Harrar**
Head Researcher: **Michelle Szulborski Zenie**
Researchers and Fact Checkers: **Valerie Edwards, Jane Unger Hahn, Joely Johnson**
Senior Copy Editor: **Jane Sherman**
Art Director: **Jane Colby Knutila**
Associate Art Director: **Faith Hague**
Cover and Interior Designer: **Elizabeth Youngblood**
Photo Editor: **Susan Pollack**
Cover Photographer: **Jeremy Wolff**
Interior Photographer: **John Herr**
Studio Manager: **Stefano Carbini**
Technical Artists: **David Q. Pryor, Karen Lomax**
Manufacturing Coordinator: **Melinda B. Rizzo**
Office Staff: **Roberta Mulliner, Julie Kehs, Bernadette Sauerwine, Mary Lou Stephen**

Rodale Health and Fitness Books
Vice-President and Editorial Director: **Debora T. Yost**
Design and Production Director: **Michael Ward**
Research Manager: **Ann Gossy Yermish**
Copy Manager: **Lisa D. Andruscavage**
Book Manufacturing Director: **Helen Clogston**

General Adviser

Elson Haas, M.D., medical director of the Preventive Medical Center of Marin in San Rafael, California, and author of *Staying Healthy with Nutrition*

Specialty Advisers

Ancestral Nutrition: Loren Cordain, Ph.D., director of the Colorado State University Human Performance Research Center in Fort Collins and a researcher in the field of ancestral nutrition

Ayurveda: Virender Sodhi, M.D. (Ayurvedic), N.D., a naturopathic physician and director of the American School of Ayurvedic Sciences in Bellevue, Washington

Chinese Nutrition: Maoshing Ni, Ph.D., co-founder and vice-president of Yo San University of Traditional Chinese Medicine in Santa Monica, California, and co-author of *The Tao of Nutrition*

Macrobiotics: Chris Akbar, personal assistant to Michio Kushi at the Kushi Institute in Becket, Massachusetts

The Longevity Diet: Roy L. Walford, M.D., professor of pathology at the University of California, Los Angeles, UCLA School of Medicine and a researcher in the field of longevity

The Ornish Program: Lee Lipsenthal, M.D., medical director of the Preventive Medicine Research Institute in Sausalito, California; Helen Roe, R.D., nutritionist at the Preventive Medicine Research Institute in Sausalito, California

The Raw Foods Diet: Morgan Martin, N.D., a naturopathic physician and professor of nutrition at Bastyr University in Seattle

Vegetarianism: Michael Klaper, M.D., a nutritional medicine specialist in private practice

An Explanation of Alternative Medicine Degrees

While gathering research for *The Complete Book of Alternative Nutrition*, we called on scores of specialists and practitioners in a wide range of different areas. Many, including medical doctors, researchers, nutritionists and other experts from universities and research institutions throughout the United States, do come from a background of "conventional" medicine. After their names, you'll find familiar degrees—M.D. for a medical degree and Ph.D. for a doctorate.

But many of the degrees earned by experts in alternative health are not as familiar. They're granted by a wide variety of boards, schools and associations of alternative medicine. And while the degrees are recognized by practitioners and specialists, they're not well-known to most of us.

To help guide you, here are definitions of some of the less familiar degrees that you'll find in this book.

B.A.M.S. (Bachelor of Ayurvedic Medicine and Surgery)

Granted by schools in India, this college degree is the equivalent of a Western M.D., but it's given in Ayurvedic medicine. Anyone with a B.A.M.S. must have four years of graduate studies. In the United States there are no state-recognized certification exams or titles for practitioners of Ayurvedic medicine: Most practitioners in the United States have either an N.D. or an M.D. degree and practice under one of those titles.

D.C. (Doctor of Chiropractic)

Chiropractic is a system of diagnosing and treating disease based on the theory that health depends on the normal function of the nervous system. Chiropractors generally treat disease by manipulating various parts of the spinal column. Practitioners with D.C. degrees are licensed to practice in 44 states and the District of Columbia, but they are forbidden by law to write prescriptions for medication.

D.O. (Doctor of Osteopathy)

Osteopathy is based on the theory that the body can protect itself against disease when all of the bones and organs have a normal structural relationship, the environment is favorable and nutrition is adequate. Osteopaths use conventional medical treatments, but they emphasize the importance of normal body mechanics and may use manipulation of the body to help correct a condition. A member of the American Osteopathic Association must have a total of 150 hours of continuing education every year.

L.Ac. (Licensed Acupuncturist)

This degree means that the acupuncturist has a state license or a diploma from a European school.

M.A.Sc. (Master of Ayurvedic Science)

In India this is a college degree that requires three years of postgraduate studies, including an internship of two years. It's the next step beyond a B.A.M.S., which takes four years, so the practitioner with an M.A.Sc. has a total of seven years of Ayurvedic study.

N.D. (Doctor of Naturopathy)

N.D. licensure laws require a resident premed course of at least four years and 4,000 hours of study at a college recognized by the state examining board. N.D.'s are considered the general practitioners of the natural healing world.

O.M.D. (Oriental Medical Doctor)

This degree generally indicates some additional training beyond getting a state license to practice acupuncture. It's also used by some Chinese M.D.'s who are licensed medical doctors in China but not in the United States and by U.S. practitioners who complete O.M.D. degree programs at foreign schools.

Contents

Part

From Ancient to Alternative: Special Diets for Better Health

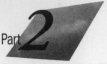

Part 2

The Alternative Pharmacy

Part 3

The New Nutrition for Healing

Part **4**

Your Guide to Healing with Alternative Nutrition

Introduction

"Let food be thy medicine, and medicine thy food," said Hippocrates, the student and teacher of anatomy who is commonly regarded as the Father of Medicine, in about 400 B.C.

Now, 2,400 years later, Hippocrates' words remain a potent reminder that food heals our bodies and keeps us well.

But doctors have not always heeded those words. For decades in this century, the mainstream medical community was skeptical about any suggestion that arthritis, heart disease, cancer and numerous other ailments could be prevented or treated through nutrition. Not so long ago, doctors who espoused alternative approaches ran the risk of being labeled health hucksters or food faddists.

Today, in the face of overwhelming evidence, the pendulum has swung the other way, and many in the mainstream medical community are hailing the healing power of food. Many scientists studying the field of alternative nutrition are discovering—and in some cases rediscovering—therapies that have proven effective against many diseases.

Sometimes new research simply confirms what sages have been saying since the dawn of time. In other cases, we're learning surprising new things about the foods that our ancestors ate as well as about the brand-new food products that appear on supermarket shelves.

In this book we're not trying to map out the absolute right way for everyone to eat, because it may be different for each person. Instead we're exploring many different ways of eating healthfully. Depending on your health concerns, lifestyle and food preferences, one of these nutrition strategies may be just right for you. On the other hand, you may choose to combine elements of more than one of these approaches.

But whatever you eat now, and wherever you shop for food, if you're really motivated to take control of your health, you can—and this book can act as a guide. Here's how.

Discover Diets for Better Health

Look in part 1 for a wide range of alternative diets, including many from other cultures and traditions that may be very unfamiliar. Among these diets are vegetarianism, with its many benefits for weight control and arterial health; ancestral nutrition, a diet that's rich in nuts, seeds, berries, root vegetables and wild game; and macrobiotics, an alternative diet that first came into vogue in the 1960s.

Some of the diets that are described in this section, such as Dr. Dean Ornish's Reversal Diet and the Pritikin Eating Plan, have been tested by scientific research that involved thousands of participants. Others, such as Dr. Roy Walford's Longevity Diet, which was given its first trial run in the experimental Biosphere in the Arizona desert, seem to have great benefits for health and longevity but have yet to stand the test of time.

In part 1 you'll also discover some of the most ancient diets on Earth, such as the raw foods diet, religion-based nutrition, Ayurvedic nutrition and Chinese nutrition, plus the power of a diet that is better described as no diet—fasting. For centuries, people of every faith have practiced fasting from time to time, and now researchers have discovered that, for many people, fasting has some very beneficial effects on health.

Explore the Alternative Pharmacy

In part 2, "The Alternative Pharmacy," you'll find an array of space-age, New Age and age-old concoctions and healing herbs. Some, like garlic, are familiar. Others, like shark cartilage or coenzyme Q_{10}, may seem more foreign: If you've heard anything at all about these strange new discoveries, it's probably just enough to leave you wondering what they do and whether the claims of their power will hold up under closer scrutiny.

If you were to believe the claims of advertisers, marketers and nutritional supplement zealots, you might think that the newest of these concoctions can do everything—cure cancer, prevent heart disease, even wipe out the common cold. So many sound so promising! But we know that much-touted cures often fizzle under the magnifying glass of scientific research. How are you supposed to know the difference between what works and what doesn't?

In part 2, we'll bring you up-to-date on the latest research. Some of the alternative herbs and supplements actually can help prevent and fight disease. Some of them are safe, effective alternatives to prescription medications with unpronounceable names and a long list of side effects. Others, however, do nothing at all. A few may even be harmful (so heed the warnings you'll find in this section).

Target Health Problems—And Prevent Them

You *can* . . . Cure diabetes! . . . Relieve arthritis pain! . . . End consti-pation! . . . Reverse heart disease!

Strangely enough, many of us are likely to believe these claims if they come from a drug company, a doctor or an advertiser. But what if such claims were posted in the fruit-and-vegetable section of your local super-market or emblazoned across every whole-grain product you buy?

When it comes to addressing specific health problems, many of us are more likely to rely on pills prescribed by a white-coated doctor and pro-cured from the local pharmacy than to trust the powerful healing foods that are no farther away than the local grocery store. The fact is, many of us are missing out on healing powers that no drug can duplicate.

Medical experts now know that eating well can be a powerful antidote to disease, reducing your risk for medical problems such as Type II diabetes, high cholesterol, high blood pressure and even cancer. And if you already have a medical condition, food can often be an aid. Although often overlooked by doctors, the right food can help you get the most from medical treatment, possibly even reducing or eliminating your need for medication.

In "The New Nutrition for Healing," part 3 of this book, you'll discover the latest news from the cutting edge of nutrition research—from the doctors, nutritionists and food researchers on the front lines.

And in part 4 you'll find a detailed chart showing the diets, herbs and supplements in this book that can help prevent or reverse specific conditions or diseases. In fact, if you already have a health condition that concerns you, this part of the book may be a good place to begin.

Finding Your Way

Of course, we still don't know the whole story about using nutrition as an alternative to conventional medicine. We need to keep in mind that our understanding of nutrition is really a work in progress. Every month brings new discoveries in the quest to understand the health-promoting power of food.

In this book, we've drawn from the wisdom of the ages as well as from the more recent explosion in knowledge about nutrition. If you're interested in using the food on your plate for optimal health, this book will give you a complete, authoritative overview of the complete range of choices. And everywhere you turn, you'll find information to help you discover more alternatives and make new diet and food discoveries on the path to better health.

Edward Claflin
Senior Managing Editor
Rodale Health and Fitness Books

Part

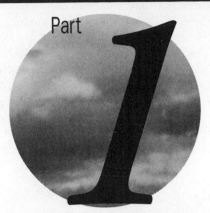

1

**From Ancient to Alternative:
Special Diets for Better Health**

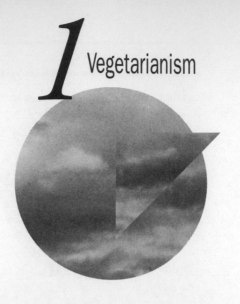

1 Vegetarianism

The Once and Future Diet

Revolutions begin in the oddest places. Your grocery store, for example: If you've taken a leisurely walk down the frozen foods aisle lately, you may have noticed that burgers ain't what they used to be.

What they used to be was beef—the high-fat, high-cholesterol favorite that's as dear to American hearts as it is hazardous to American arteries.

What they're turning into, increasingly, is veggie burgers, meatless patties that look like meat and cook like meat but are made of plant-based ingredients such as soybeans, oats, rice, mushrooms, onions and other vegetables.

Like daffodils in early spring or the first golden leaves of autumn, veggie burgers are a sign of the times—a tip-off that change is in the wind. Their popularity signals a profound shift in American eating habits: A survey by the National Restaurant Association found that more than half of us are eating less red meat than we used to. And a record number of Americans—12.4 million—now call themselves vegetarians.

A Diet for All Reasons

While vegetarianism is clearly on the increase, meatless diets are nothing new. Throughout history, people around the world have followed vegetarian diets not by choice but out of necessity. "In many developing

A Better Burger

As more and more people investigate the meatless life, food companies are responding with an ever-widening variety of new products, from meatless burgers to a whole new breed of quick, convenient entrées that would look right at home in your hot dog bun or next to your scrambled eggs. Along with vegetarian burgers, meatless hot dogs and sausages have become increasingly popular in recent years.

The nutritional content of "veggie meat" varies widely from brand to brand, but most stack up quite favorably next to beef.

One of the most popular veggie burgers, the gardenburger (made by Wholesome and Hearty Foods) has 140 calories, 2.5 grams of fat and a substantial 5 grams of fiber per 2.8-ounce patty.

Compare that to a beef hamburger, with 245 calories and 18 grams of fat, and it's easy to see why vegetarian burgers are catching on, even with people who aren't vegetarians.

"They're good transition foods for new vegetarians who still get an occasional craving for meat," says Suzanne Havala, R.D., a nutritionist in Charlotte, North Carolina, and nutritional adviser to the Vegetarian Resource Group.

Veggie meats can also help vegetarians fit into social situations where meatless fare isn't available, she adds. "Vegetarians can take them to outdoor picnics, and they're good to give to kids who just want to eat what everyone else is eating."

But while veggie meats are certainly better for you than hot dogs or hamburgers, they're still processed foods and shouldn't be a mainstay of your diet, says Havala. "As with any processed food, the more of these products people eat, the less room they have in their diets for more nutritious foods like vegetables, legumes and whole grains."

---

countries, people live long, healthy lives on traditional diets that are totally vegetarian. They do just fine with no meat, dairy, eggs or other animal products," notes Michael Klaper, M.D., a nutritional medicine specialist in private practice.

Vegetarianism is also part of the spiritual lives of many people around the world. All five of the world's major religions—Christianity, Judaism, Islam, Hinduism and Buddhism—have traditionally restricted meat consumption to one degree or another. And many modern-day Buddhists and Seventh-Day Adventists follow a vegetarian diet as an expression of religious belief.

Vegetarianism has also been associated with the environmental movement. Many vegetarians are deeply concerned with world hunger and feel that if more people ate "lower on the food chain," the earth's resources could be used more effectively to feed more people. "For every 16 pounds of grain and soy fed to beef cattle in the United States, we get only 1 pound back in meat on our plates," observes Frances Moore Lappé in *Diet for a Small Planet*, one of the most influential books on vegetarianism ever written.

Then there's the environmental cost of raising huge numbers of animals for slaughter, including the razing of thousands of acres of tropical rain forest to provide grazing lands for cattle. Environmentalists charge that the Western meat-eating habit wastes water and fuel, depletes topsoil and pollutes groundwater. "Essentially, the argument is that an animal-based agricultural system wastes resources that are in limited supply and creates pollution and contamination at a rate that we can't undo," says Suzanne Havala, R.D., a nutritionist in Charlotte, North Carolina, and nutrition adviser to the Vegetarian Resource Group.

Veg Inroads

Despite the venerable age of the vegetarian movement, the idea of restricting meat intake for health reasons is recent. In the 1830s, health reformer Sylvester Graham (inventor of the graham cracker) railed against the evils of a meat-based, highly refined modern diet. By the turn of the century, John Harvey Kellogg was treating patients with a vegetarian diet at his famous Battle Creek Sanitarium in Michigan and had begun manufacturing a line of meat substitutes and breakfast cereals. Around the same time, Upton Sinclair wrote *The Jungle*, a scathing exposé of the meat-packing industry, which made eating meat seem like dangerous business indeed.

Vegetarianism made headlines again in the 1960s and 1970s, when environmentally conscious young people gave up meat for a variety of spiritual, political and health reasons.

But now good health is a prime motivator, and the appeal of vegetarianism has less to do with ideology than with feeling well. Surveys show that most vegetarians say health is their primary concern. And their approach is well-supported by research showing that people who eat a plant-based diet have a much lower risk of developing "diseases of civilization" such as heart disease, diabetes and certain types of cancer.

No longer seen as a countercultural movement, vegetarianism is now mainstream. And the veggie lifestyle isn't the property of just the young. In fact, a study by the National Restaurant Association showed that diners over 65 are more likely than any other age group to seek out vegetarian menu items.

A Wide Net

With so many people identifying themselves as vegetarian, just about everyone knows at least one person who follows a meatless or mostly meatless diet. You may do so yourself. But ask a handful of these folks what they ate for dinner last night, and the range of answers may surprise you.

"The word *vegetarian* means different things to different people," says Havala. Some self-declared vegetarians subsist on sprouts and tofu. Others dine on fast-food chicken nuggets and consider themselves vegetarians because they avoid red meat. Some vegetarians favor exotic meatless cuisines from around the world. Others just substitute beans for beef in the family meat loaf.

At one end of the spectrum are true vegetarians, or vegans, who avoid all foods of animal origin, including meat, fish, poultry, eggs and dairy products. Vegans account for just 4 percent of vegetarians, says Havala—and many turn to veganism for ethical reasons.

"I'm a vegan because I don't want to cause another living being to suffer because of my diet," says Heidi Prescott, national director of the Fund for Animals in Silver Spring, Maryland, a nonprofit organization dedicated to promoting the humane treatment of animals, who's been a strict vegan for eight years.

"I don't believe animals were put on Earth for humans to use and abuse—I don't believe we have the right to do it," she says. As for animal products like milk, says Prescott, "all other species are weaned after infancy. That's the natural progression. We're the only ones who turn to the milk of another species, and it isn't natural or necessary."

While most vegans adopt the diet for ethical reasons, veganism also offers significant health benefits: Vegans tend to have less body fat, lower blood pressure and lower cholesterol than vegetarians who aren't as strict.

The Frugal Vegetarian

"It's amazing how many people tell me they can't afford to become vegetarian," says Suzanne Havala, R.D., a nutritionist in Charlotte, North Carolina, and nutritional adviser to the Vegetarian Resource Group. "But after people make the switch, they wonder how they could ever afford to eat meat.

"It's true that fresh produce can be kind of expensive, but if people substitute plant foods for meat, fish and poultry, they inevitably end up saving money," she says.

Of course, some vegetarians spend more money on food than others. Here are a few ways to make sure your diet is as healthy for your bank account as it is for your body.

Eat in season. "Buying fruits and vegetables in season is one way to keep costs down, and since they tend to be fresher than produce imported from Mexico or South America, they might even be healthier," says Havala.

Avoid processed foods. The less that's been done to your food before you buy it, the cheaper it will be: Dried beans are one of the best deals in the supermarket, while canned beans are more expensive, notes Havala.

Make it yourself. Using convenience food—whether it's a can of vegetarian chili, a frozen entrée or a jar of meatless spaghetti sauce—is usually more expensive than cooking from scratch. To save time on hectic days, try making a big pot of soup or a vegetarian casserole over the weekend and freeze it for later in the week.

At the same time, because vegans consume a limited number of different foods, they're more vulnerable to nutritional deficiencies than vegetarians who eat some animal products, says Connie Weaver, Ph.D., professor of foods and nutrition at Purdue University in West Lafayette, Indiana. "It takes a bit more education to put together an adequate vegan diet," she says.

But for the other 96 percent of vegetarians, the chosen diet isn't an all-or-nothing proposition: In fact, many vegetarians consume at least some animal products. Ovo-vegetarians eat a vegan diet plus eggs, lacto-vegetarians allow themselves dairy products, and ovo-lacto-vegetarians eat both. Then there are pollo-vegetarians, who eat chicken, and pesco-vegetarians, who eat fish. And some people who call themselves vegetarians or semi-vegetarians actually eat a little bit of everything, including a token amount of meat.

Heart Disease: Lessons from China

Whichever vegetarian diet you choose, you won't be alone. Every kind of vegetarian diet has thousands or millions of adherents around the world. And as scientists study these populations, they're learning powerful lessons about the health benefits of a plant-based diet.

When it comes to studying the relationship between diet and health, China is an epidemiologist's dream. The most populous country on Earth, China is teeming with examples of how very different lifestyles affect health and longevity. Chinese from different regions live, work and eat differently. They also die differently: Some live long, healthy lives, while others die prematurely of heart disease—the same condition that kills more Americans than any other disease.

In 1983, an international team of scientists began the overwhelming task of investigating how the diets and lifestyles in different parts of China affect the risks of death from killer diseases. By 1988, the China Project on Nutrition, Health and Environment had uncovered some compelling evidence that a vegetarian lifestyle offered unsurpassed protection against chronic illnesses.

Among other things, the scientists discovered that rural Chinese who eat a traditional diet of grains, vegetables and fruits have very low rates of heart disease. They also have cholesterol readings of 150 mg/dl (milligrams per deciliter) or lower—well below the level that Western health authorities advise us to strive for. Diabetes, obesity and most types of cancer are also rare in the rural Chinese.

The situation is quite different in large Chinese cities, where people eat a diet that's closer to the way Americans eat, complete with meat, poultry, eggs and dairy products as well as foods high in sugar. And they also eat more refined foods like baked goods made with white flour. As they have switched to our Western diet, these urban Chinese have begun to experience serious Western-style health problems.

Clearly, the rural Chinese are doing something right. In fact, they're doing many things right, according to T. Colin Campbell, Ph.D., professor of nutritional biochemistry at Cornell University in Ithaca, New York, and one of the architects of the China Project.

Pieces of the Puzzle

While the China Project has renewed interest in the health benefits of vegetarian eating, many of the lessons it provides aren't new ones, says Dr. Campbell.

Scientists have long known that vegetarians are less vulnerable to atherosclerosis, the clogging of the arteries that's a major component of heart disease. Some Western doctors are even using vegetarian-based diets to lessen atherosclerosis in heart attack patients whose arteries are clogged from years of eating a high-fat, meat-based Western diet. (Among the foremost proponents of this diet plan is Dean Ornish, M.D., director of the Preventive Medicine Research Center in Sausalito, California, and author of *Dr. Dean Ornish's Program for Reversing Heart Disease*, whose program is described in chapter 7.)

Studies also show that vegetarian diets help control high blood pressure, a major risk factor for heart disease. For African-Americans, who seem to be genetically predisposed to high blood pressure, a long-term commitment to a vegetarian lifestyle could be a safe and inexpensive way to keep blood pressure in check without drugs.

Vegetarians also have lower levels of fibrinogen, a blood protein that's necessary for clotting. Elevated fibrinogen levels are a proven risk factor for heart attack and stroke.

The Chinese diet is also high in fiber. The average Chinese eats 34 grams of fiber per day, compared with only 10 grams of fiber for the average American.

The net results: With reduced fat, lower cholesterol, lower blood pressure and less clotting potential, your risk of heart disease takes a tumble. With every bite of vegetarian fare, you're helping yourself build a bridge toward a healthier heart. And studies show that a diet that's rich in fruits and vegetables also decreases the risk of stroke.

Chock-Full of Protection

Investigators are also studying the role of antioxidant nutrients in vegetarian fare, the amount and types of protein in the diet and the role of dietary fiber. All of these contributing factors may help explain why a vegetarian diet is such a powerful weapon against heart disease.

"There are probably hundreds of thousands of protein forms, hundreds of thousands of different antioxidant nutrients that we know virtually nothing about," says Dr. Campbell. "Science has barely touched the tip of the iceberg on this one."

Dr. Campbell's experiences have led him to embrace vegetarianism personally: He's been eating a plant-based diet for the past 20 years. Most recently, his work on the China Project convinced him to eliminate milk and eggs from his diet, and he's been a complete vegan since the late 1980s. "I'm convinced that if a person consciously wants to maintain good health, this has got to be part of his daily living," he says.

Whether you're trying to shed pounds, lower your blood pressure or bring down your cholesterol, Dr. Klaper says, the more you can eliminate animal products from your diet, the more dramatic the results will be. If you have high cholesterol and are eating a standard American diet, simply eliminating meat will probably bring down the cholesterol numbers that foretell troubled heart problems. But if you adopt a vegan diet, the drop will be much greater. "The best way to lower cholesterol is to stop eating it, and if you eliminate all animal products, your cholesterol intake will be zero," says Dr. Klaper.

"What we do know is that heart disease is rare in countries where the diet is plant-based, and it has reached epidemic proportions in countries with the highest consumption of meat and other animal products," he says. "We can wait another 20 years for science to figure out all the mechanisms involved, or we can take sensible action now that will most likely result in a longer life free of disease."

"There's no risk involved with eating a plant-based diet, no downside," says Dr. Campbell. "Only good can come from it. We can't see into the future, but we do know that in the end, we're going to be better off."

Other doctors add that a plant-based diet must be well-balanced, especially with high-protein foods. But as long as that's happening, they agree that there are many pluses to a vegetarian diet.

Meat: A Prime Cancer Suspect

The vegetarian diet is also a powerful weapon against cancer. A landmark British study of over 11,000 people found that vegetarians were 40 percent less likely to die of cancer than people who ate meat.

Just how a vegetarian diet fights off cancer is still a mystery, but scientists do know that dietary fat is part of the picture. Fat appears to play a role in the development of hormone-driven cancers, including breast, prostate and ovarian cancer. "The chemicals in animal foods are likely to play a role as well in increasing the risk of cancer," according to Elson Haas, M.D., medical director of the Preventive Medical Center of Marin in San Rafael, California, and author of *Staying Healthy with Nutrition*.

Particularly dangerous is saturated fat—the kind found in animal products such as meat, fish and dairy products. In the New York University Women's Health Study, a landmark study of 14,291 New York City women, those who ate the most red meat were nearly twice as likely to develop breast cancer within five years as those who ate the least.

But fat isn't the only substance in meat that's been linked to cancer. Researchers have also targeted a group of chemicals called heterocyclic amines (HAs), which appear to cause cancer in laboratory animals. HAs are by-products of the cooking process: Any time you grill a burger, stir-fry some chicken or broil a piece of fish, HAs are produced.

The Cancer-Fighting Nutrients

When it comes to the cancer-fighting benefits of a vegetarian diet, what you eat is at least as important as what you give up. Vegetarians, as a rule, eat more fruits and vegetables than omnivores do. And these foods combat cancer on several different fronts.

As children, the first thing we're taught about fruits and vegetables is that they're loaded with vitamins and minerals. Among the most important of those nutrients, says Dr. Klaper, are the antioxidant vitamins C and E and beta-carotene. They're called antioxidants because they prevent damage from a process known as oxidation. If left unchecked, oxidation results in all manner of cellular damage—wrinkled skin, cataracts, arterial plaque and, some researchers believe, certain types of cancer.

But vitamins and minerals are only one part of the story. Fruits and vegetables are loaded with thousands of different compounds known as phytochemicals, many of which have shown cancer-fighting potential in laboratory studies.

A vegetarian diet also supplies plenty of fiber—about 34 grams per day, compared to the 10 grams we get if we're eating a standard Western diet. Whole grains in particular are rich in insoluble fiber, a type that has been associated with reduced risk of colon cancer. And many fruits and vegetables have abundant soluble fiber, the kind that dissolves or forms a gel, as well as insoluble fiber. Both types help your body process food quickly and efficiently. And the faster undigested food passes through your intestines, the less you're exposed to cancer-causing chemicals found in that food.

Soy Soldiers

There's a reason that vegetarians tend to eat a wide variety of soy products, such as tofu. Besides providing fiber, protein, vitamins, minerals and fatty acids, soy foods are rich in chemicals called phytoestrogens, which are believed to play a role in warding off cancer.

These compounds seem to fight cancer in a couple of ways. Some cancers, such as breast and prostate cancer, are associated with elevated levels of male and female sex hormones. Since phytoestrogens help clear excess hormones from the blood, they sweep out the cancer-related substances. Also, in animal studies, phytoestrogens have been shown to inhibit the growth of breast tumors. Taken together, these two factors go a long way toward explaining why breast and prostate cancer rates are low in countries like Japan, where soy foods are part of the traditional diet.

Researchers have taken into account that it's not just meatless diets that separate vegetarians from other groups. Vegetarians tend to smoke less, weigh less and come from more affluent backgrounds than meat-eaters.

The Secret Life of Soy

Soy foods like tofu and soy milk are considered staples in many vegetarian kitchens, and for good reason: They're nutritious and versatile and make great stand-ins for meat, eggs and dairy products, according to Earl Mindell, Ph.D., professor of nutritional science at Pacific Western University in Los Angeles and author of *Earl Mindell's Soy Miracle*. What's more, regular consumption of soy seems to have a beneficial effect on cholesterol levels and has even been linked to lower rates of breast and prostate cancer.

Here are a few ways to reap the benefits of what might be nature's most perfect food, according to Dr. Mindell.

Soybeans. These beans are yellow, brown or black. To cook them, soak them in water for several hours and then simmer for two to three hours until they are soft enough to mash between your tongue and the roof of your mouth. They are a nutritious addition to soups, stews and casseroles.

Soy milk. You can use soy milk, which is extracted from soybeans through soaking and cooking, just as you use dairy milk: Drink it by itself, pour it over cereal or use it in creamy soups, sauces and puddings. Soy milk can also replace regular milk in baking.

Tofu. Made from soy milk, with the consistency of soft cheese, tofu is a bland, protein-rich food that takes on the flavor of whatever it's combined with. Use firm tofu as you would ground beef: Toss it into stews, chili or tacos Sliced and marinated, tofu can be grilled or sautéed and added to a sandwich. Silken tofu is delicious when blended into creamy desserts like puddings, custards and "cheesecakes." It can be found in the produce section of most large supermarkets.

Tempeh. This is an Indonesian favorite that's made of fermented soybeans and grain. The chewy bean cakes are often used in spicy dishes. Look for them in health food stores and Asian markets.

Soy flour. This flour is rich in a type of protein that's been shown to lower cholesterol. Use it to replace about a fifth of the flour in your favorite pancake, muffin or quickbread recipes. (You can't use it in regular bread recipes, since it interferes with the action of yeast.) It adds moistness and a mild nutty flavor. You can also use it to replace eggs in baking by substituting one tablespoon of soy flour plus one tablespoon of water for each egg.

Miso. A savory, spreadable mixture of fermented soybeans and rice or barley, miso is often used diluted in sauces, adding a salty, rich taste. It also makes a flavorful vegetarian soup base. Use a quarter-cup of miso paste per quart of water. Miso can be found in Asian markets and many health food stores.

These lifestyle differences must also be acknowledged before scientists can say how much protection is carried in the diet.

But even when bad habits like smoking and drinking are taken into account, a vegetarian diet may still offer some protection against cancer. The biggest risk factors for oral cancer, for example, are smoking or chewing tobacco and drinking alcohol. Yet some research shows that diet can also play a role. A study conducted in India found that vegetarian Indian men were nearly 40 percent less likely to develop oral cancer than men who ate meat—even if the vegetarians had other habits like smoking and drinking that put them in a high-risk category.

A Strong Infrastructure

All of the evidence isn't in yet, but some experts believe that a vegetarian diet may also help prevent osteoporosis, the brittle-bone disease that affects up to 20 million American women.

Experts agree that getting enough calcium is essential for building and maintaining strong bones throughout our lives. For most people—including lacto-vegetarians—that means drinking milk and eating yogurt and cheese, rich sources of calcium that's easily absorbed by the body.

But some studies suggest that in spite of its high calcium content, a diet loaded with dairy products may not be the best strategy for preventing osteoporosis.

"Epidemiological studies consistently show that countries where people eat the most dairy products also have the highest rates of osteoporosis," says Dr. Campbell. "And the more dairy products a population eats, the more osteoporosis there is."

Scientists still aren't sure why diets rich in dairy might increase the rate of osteoporosis, but some think the high protein content of milk products might have something to do with it. Data from the China Project shows that Chinese women whose diets included the most meat, fish and dairy products excreted significantly more calcium than those who consumed a strictly plant-based diet.

"Osteoporosis isn't a disease of calcium deficiency—it's far more a disease of calcium loss," says Dr. Klaper. "Osteoporosis results from calcium leaving the bones and going out in the urine. Dairy products are rich in calcium, but they also contain a lot of protein, and a high-protein diet has been shown to increase the excretion of calcium."

So while strict vegetarians generally get less calcium than milk drinkers do, their lower-protein diets may mean they do a better job of holding on to the calcium they get. Vegetarians also tend to exercise more, eat less sugar and salt and avoid cigarettes and alcohol—and these healthy habits offer them extra protection against bone loss.

A lifetime of milk consumption may also affect a woman's hormone levels in a way that makes her more vulnerable to osteoporosis, adds Dr. Campbell. Young girls raised on dairy products may have more body fat, and they reach puberty earlier. In China, for example, girls typically go through puberty at around age 17, compared to 12 or 13 in more developed countries.

Girls raised on a Western diet don't just mature earlier, they also have higher hormone levels than girls who don't eat dairy foods, and those elevated levels are maintained through adulthood. When these women go through menopause, says Dr. Campbell, their hormone levels drop so sharply that they lose bone even faster than women whose hormone levels were lower to begin with, setting the stage for osteoporosis.

"This theory hasn't been well-investigated yet, but it could partly explain why dairy consumption is directly related to higher rates of osteoporosis," says Dr. Campbell.

Veggies for Joint Pain and Easier Breathing

Some studies show that a vegan diet may also be beneficial for people with rheumatoid arthritis, the kind that can begin to affect joints and cause pain at a young age. Norwegian researchers put 27 people with rheumatoid arthritis on a medically supervised fast, then instructed them to eat a vegetarian diet for a year. At the end of the year, the participants reported less joint pain, swelling and stiffness than another group who ate a traditional omnivorous diet.

In fact, so many of the patients on a vegetarian diet noticed an improvement that they stuck with the diet even after the study ended. When the researchers contacted them two years later, those who stayed on the vegetarian diet remained in better health than those who ate an ordinary diet.

Dr. Klaper's clinical experience bears out these findings. "Out of every hundred people I see with red, hot, swollen joints, 30 to 40 percent will see an improvement in their symptoms when they eliminate dairy products," he says. "Not everyone, of course, but there's a huge nutritional component to inflammatory conditions, and the proteins in dairy products are the most notorious offenders."

The same goes for asthma: If it runs in your family, a vegan diet can mean the difference between developing the condition and having a lifetime of easy breathing, according to Dr. Klaper. "There's a genetic component, but the other crucial thing we 'inherit' from our parents is our eating habits. If we grow up on a diet that's high in dairy products and eat that way all our lives, and asthma develops due to a dairy sensitivity, you can say it's partially genetic, but it's also a function of eating at the same table."

In the Garden of Better Health

With such an impressive body of research showing the benefits of a vegetarian diet, you might say, "Okay, but doesn't it take a long, long time to reap the benefits?" Actually, studies show that vegetarians don't have to wait around for 20 years to start experiencing the benefits of their healthy lifestyles. "Going vegetarian" offers plenty of tangible perks that you can start enjoying tomorrow.

One of the first changes new vegetarians notice is smoother, more efficient digestion. Vegetarians typically report fewer digestive problems, thanks in large part to the abundance of fiber in the average vegetarian diet.

That means less constipation and a much lower risk of developing diverticulosis, diverticulitis or hemorrhoids, says Havala.

Study after study shows that vegetarians enjoy better day-to-day health than omnivores do. In a survey of more than 27,000 Seventh-Day Adventists—some vegetarians, some not—those who ate meat reported more surgeries, x-rays and hospital stays than their vegetarian counterparts. They also had more allergies and more asthma and used twice as much medication as the vegetarians did.

Women may also notice a difference in their menstrual cycles after switching to a vegetarian diet. Research shows that vegetarian women have more regular cycles than women who eat meat, partly because vegetarians are less likely to go on very low calorie diets that can interfere with normal ovulation.

And the benefits don't end when menopause occurs. A *Prevention* magazine survey found that vegetarian women reported fewer menopausal symptoms like weight gain, hot flashes and problems sleeping.

A plant-based diet also offers special rewards for men: It helps control a number of risk factors for impotence, including high blood pressure, elevated cholesterol and atherosclerosis, says Irwin Goldstein, M.D., professor of urology at Boston University School of Medicine and author of *The Potent Male*. "Some studies show that being overweight is a risk factor for impotence, especially for men in their fifties. And since vegetarians are less likely to carry excess weight, that's another advantage," he adds.

Male or female, vegetarians also have a much lower risk of developing gallstones than omnivores do: One British study found that omnivorous women were twice as likely as vegetarian women to develop gallstones, possibly because of their much higher cholesterol intake.

Those concerned about staying mentally sharp well into old age have another powerful reason to consider a vegetarian diet. A study of 2,984 Seventh-Day Adventists found that those who ate meat, fish or poultry were more than twice as likely to become senile as their vegetarian counterparts. The role of diet in mental disorders is still poorly understood, but it looks as though a vegetarian diet may be as good for the mind as it is for the body.

Planning Your Protein

A well-planned vegetarian diet is nutritionally dense: low in fat, moderate in calories and high in vitamins, minerals and fiber, says Patricia Johnston, R.D., Dr.P.H., associate dean of the School of Public Health at Loma Linda University in California.

Many doctors and nutritionists say that a vegetarian diet provides adequate protein. "Protein really isn't something vegetarians have to worry about," says Dr. Johnston. "In the United States, unless you're living in extreme poverty and simply aren't getting enough food, protein deficiency is practically nonexistent."

In fact, she says, most Americans get far more protein than they need,

(continued on page 16)

A Duo-Diet Compromise

If you and your spouse both decide to go vegetarian, you don't necessarily have to switch to the same level of vegetarianism. If your spouse is an inveterate meat-eater, for instance, the best choice might be an ovo-lacto-vegetarian diet, in which eggs and dairy products are allowed. On the ovo-lacto diet, your spouse can still enjoy eggs for breakfast and easily substitute a cheese pizza for a roast beef sandwich at lunch. If you're on the strict vegan diet, on the other hand, you'll avoid all foods of animal origin, including eggs and dairy products, but you can easily make a vegan dinner that will please both of you.

Here's how you can make the duo-diet work, according to Suzanne Havala, R.D., a nutritionist in Charlotte, North Carolina, and nutrition adviser to the Vegetarian Resource Group.

For breakfast, your spouse might have French toast or waffles, minus the bacon, while you have cereal with soy milk. (A hint: If you've never tasted soy milk before, you may be pleasantly surprised by its creamy, full-bodied flavor. The vanilla-flavored varieties taste best on cereal, and you'll give your bones some help if you choose soy milk fortified with calcium. Rice milk is a lighter-tasting alternative that also comes in flavored and fortified varieties.)

Workday lunches are usually more difficult for the vegan. Most restaurants have at least one meatless dish on the menu, so your ovo-lacto spouse can get an egg salad sandwich, spaghetti with cheese and tomato sauce or pizza. For the vegan, however, finding something without eggs or dairy products can be a chore. If you go into a nonvegetarian restaurant and ask waiters if the pasta contains eggs or if there is butter in the sauce, you're likely to be met with a blank stare. The quickest solution is to try a Chinese restaurant, where you can get many stir-fried vegetable dishes.

When you're cooking at home, try some vegan dishes that will please your ovo-lacto spouse as well. If your spouse likes hearty meals, for instance, a typical main dish might be linguine with pesto-and-sun-dried-tomato sauce—and you can share the meal if you use eggless pasta and omit the Romano cheese from the sauce.

For the two-diet household, says Havala, here's a week's worth of basic meals that you can supplement with any side dishes of fruit, vegetables, grains or legumes.

Sunday   Breakfast—*Both:* eggless blueberry bran muffins
Lunch—*Ovo-lacto:* egg salad on whole-wheat toast with tomatoes and alfalfa sprouts
—*Vegan:* eggless egg salad sandwich made with chopped tofu, yellow mustard and soy mayonnaise
Dinner—*Ovo-lacto:* pasta with fresh tomatoes, basil and Romano cheese, with mango sorbet
—*Vegan:* pasta with marinara sauce, with fresh mango

Monday Breakfast—*Both:* Cantaloupe
—*Ovo-lacto:* French toast
—*Vegan:* cereal with soy milk
Lunch—*Ovo-lacto:* cheese pizza
—*Vegan:* pita sandwich with broccoli, cauliflower, carrots and peppers, with vinaigrette dressing
Dinner—*Both:* spinach salad with orange slices and raspberry vinaigrette dressing, with linguine in cheeseless pesto sauce with sun-dried tomatoes

Tuesday Breakfast—*Both:* Fresh fruit
—*Ovo-lacto:* buttermilk pancakes
—*Vegan:* oat bran bagel with fruit spread
Lunch—*Ovo-lacto:* meatless chef salad with eggs and cheese
—*Vegan:* green salad and whole-wheat crackers with hummus (mashed chick-pea spread)
Dinner—*Both:* stir-fried vegetables with tofu over brown rice

Wednesday Breakfast—*Ovo-lacto:* scrambled eggs and whole-wheat toast
—*Vegan:* cereal with sliced banana and soy milk
Lunch—*Ovo-lacto:* tomato-rice soup and grilled cheese sandwich
—*Vegan:* peanut butter sandwich on whole-wheat bread, with raw vegetables and black bean dip
Dinner—*Both:* yellow rice and black bean casserole

Thursday Breakfast—*Ovo-lacto:* cheese omelet with whole-wheat toast
—*Vegan:* cooked whole-grain cereal prepared with soy milk and maple syrup
Lunch—*Both:* Buddha's delight (stir-fried carrots, peppers, broccoli, bok choy and water chestnuts over rice)
Dinner—*Both:* vegetarian chili with kidney and pinto beans

Friday Breakfast—*Ovo-lacto:* shredded wheat and blueberries with milk
—*Vegan:* oatmeal with raisins and soy milk
Lunch—*Ovo-lacto:* cheese pizza
—*Vegan:* leftover vegetarian chili
Dinner—*Both:* grilled vegetarian burgers on whole-wheat English muffins, with tabbouleh salad with olives and tomatoes

Saturday Breakfast—*Both:* eggless waffles with fresh strawberry topping
Lunch—*Both:* Pasta salad with capers, broccoli, snow peas, corn, onions and peppers with whole-wheat garlic toast and watermelon
Dinner—*Both:* Chick-peas in curry sauce over couscous, with grilled squash, tomatoes and eggplant

especially men, who often get more than 100 grams a day instead of the recommended 50 to 55 grams. And eating too much protein has been implicated in a number of chronic illnesses, including osteoporosis and kidney disease. But other doctors find that people on vegetarian diets may end up with some deficiencies. "Most vegetarians need to pay attention to protein," notes Dr. Haas. And one of the best ways to get that needed protein is with soybeans and soybean products like tofu and tempeh.

A generation ago, some nutritionists believed that following a vegetarian diet meant paying special attention to the combinations of foods you ate at every meal. Some advocated "protein combining," a system of eating two or more "incomplete" protein sources such as wheat, beans or rice. They believed that the amino acids in these foods would add up to a "complete" protein that would contain all the amino acids found in animal proteins such as meat, eggs or milk.

Today, this theory has been largely discredited, says Dr. Johnston. "All foods contain amino acids: It doesn't matter whether they're plant foods or animal foods," she explains. "Today, we know that it doesn't really matter whether you're getting these different amino acids in the same meal or just in the same day: Your body can still utilize them. All you really need to do is eat a good variety of foods."

Where's the Iron?

Other nutrients that might be partially lacking in a vegetarian diet are iron and, to a lesser extent, zinc. Research shows that vegetarians generally have lower blood levels of iron than their meat-eating counterparts.

It's not that vegetarians don't consume enough iron: Plant sources are abundant, and most cereals are fortified with iron. But the iron found in plant foods is much harder for the body to absorb than the iron in meat. A study of Chinese Buddhist vegetarians found that their iron levels were about half those of meat-eaters, even though the vegetarian women actually consumed more iron than the meat-eating women.

As it turns out, though, getting less iron may not be such a bad thing. Iron was once considered so important that breads, cereals and noodles were fortified with it, but newer research suggests that many Americans are getting too much. Those who eat meat daily are getting large amounts of easily absorbable iron, which is stored in the body. And too much iron has been associated with free radical damage, a cellular process that contributes to atherosclerosis, or hardening of the arteries.

Of course, we do need a certain amount of iron, but a vegetarian diet that includes plenty of beans, whole grains, leafy green vegetables and dried fruits is unlikely to be deficient, says Dr. Klaper.

The Daily Value (DV) for iron is 18 milligrams. Some good vegetarian sources include cooked fresh spinach (6 milligrams per cup), cashews (4 milligrams per half-cup), lima beans (6 milligrams per cup), pinto beans (5 milligrams per cup) and dried figs (4 milligrams per ten figs). Many cereals are also fortified with iron. Some, like Grape-Nuts and Raisin Bran, have between 4 and 5 milligrams of iron per cup.

To help your body absorb as much iron as possible from these foods, be sure to eat them along with a fruit or vegetable high in vitamin C or take a vitamin C supplement to help with absorption. Research shows that consuming 75 milligrams of vitamin C—about the amount found in a kiwifruit, a glass of orange juice or a cup of cauliflower—at each meal can triple or quadruple the amount of iron that you absorb from your food. Peppers, broccoli, strawberries and brussels sprouts are also good sources of vitamin C. If you opt for a vegetable, eat it raw or very lightly steamed, says Dr. Weaver, since vitamin C can be destroyed in cooking. "The vitamin C makes all the difference," she says.

As for zinc, good sources are toasted wheat germ and miso. If you're on a vegetarian diet and not taking a supplement that has zinc, you might want to add these two foods to your daily menu.

The Calcium Connection

When it comes to calcium, lacto-vegetarians have it easy. If you can manage cereal and milk for breakfast, a cheese sandwich for lunch, a green salad at dinner and frozen yogurt for dessert, you've met or surpassed the Daily Value for this essential mineral, which is 1,000 milligrams for most adults and 1,500 milligrams for postmenopausal women. But if you follow a vegan diet, you'll have to be a little more creative in sneaking calcium into your meals, says Dr. Weaver.

The best sources of calcium in the vegan diet are leafy green vegetables such as kale and mustard greens. But while the calcium in most plant foods is relatively easy for the body to absorb, you would have to eat an awful lot of greens to meet the daily requirement for calcium, says Dr. Weaver. For instance, you'd have to eat 2½ cups of broccoli or nearly 3 cups of almonds to get the amount of calcium contained in a single glass of milk.

"It's theoretically possible to get enough calcium from plant foods, but it's not practical for most people," says Dr. Weaver. She recommends eating calcium-rich greens and nuts each day and making up the difference with calcium supplements. Cooking your greens and chewing them thoroughly allows the calcium to be more readily absorbed by the body, says Dr. Klaper. Some vegans may prefer to get the bulk of their calcium from fortified drinks like soy milk (available in health food stores) or calcium-fortified orange juice (now in most grocery stores). An eight-ounce glass of either beverage has as much calcium as the same size glass of milk.

On the other hand, vegans (as well as other vegetarians) may not need the DV of calcium recommended for the average American who is on a high-protein diet, Dr. Haas says. There is evidence that people on low-protein diets retain more of the calcium that's in their food. (For more details, see chapter 26.)

Be Aware of B$_{12}$

Six micrograms—that's the DV of vitamin B$_{12}$ needed by a healthy adult, and it's an infinitesimal amount. But what little B$_{12}$ your body needs, it *really* needs: B$_{12}$ is essential for building red blood cells and maintaining healthy nerve tissue. The very worst case: An ongoing B$_{12}$ deficiency can lead to severe anemia—a breakdown of the blood's ability to do its job—which can be fatal. "In my view, 25 to 50 micrograms of B$_{12}$ a day is a good level," says Dr. Haas.

For ovo-lacto-vegetarians, getting enough B$_{12}$ is as easy as eating breakfast: Pour skim milk over a bowl of fortified cereal, such as Cheerios or Raisin Bran, and you have half your DV before you're out of your pajamas.

But since B$_{12}$ is found almost exclusively in foods of animal origin, total vegetarians need to rely on supplements or fortified foods to get enough B$_{12}$.

It's not that the vegan diet is inadequate, says Dr. Klaper. The blame rests with modern technology: Back when people grew their own food and drank water from wells and streams, getting enough B$_{12}$ was easy. "Because B$_{12}$ is produced by bacteria in the soil and in the air, anyone who lives in contact with nature gets plenty of B$_{12}$," says Dr. Klaper. "The bacteria was present on the fresh fruits and vegetables our great-grandparents grew and in their drinking water, and there was a constant stream of B$_{12}$ moving through their digestive tracts."

Today, though, our chlorinated drinking water and well-scrubbed supermarket produce are free of B$_{12}$-producing bacteria, so most of the B$_{12}$ available to modern people is from animal products.

Getting Fortified

If you're a total vegetarian, you need supplements or fortified foods to get enough B$_{12}$, according to Dr. Klaper. Most breakfast cereals are fortified with B$_{12}$, and supplements are widely available. Many vegans also take B$_{12}$-fortified nutritional yeast or drink fortified soy milk, both of which are sold in health food stores. "If vegans get one of these B$_{12}$ sources a couple of times a week, they have nothing to worry about," says Dr. Klaper. Pregnant women on a vegan diet need a source of B$_{12}$ every day.

While some vegans object to taking supplements because they aren't "natural," Dr. Klaper urges them to be flexible. "Vegans need to understand that B$_{12}$ supplements don't come from animal sources, they come from bacteria, so they're a plant-derived food and an appropriate and necessary addition to the modern vegan diet.

"It's important that vegans have some source of vitamin B$_{12}$ in their diets a few times a week," he says. "It doesn't matter whether it's fortified cereal or fortified soy milk or vitamin tablets or nutritional yeast."

Some vegans get their B_{12} by eating lots of tempeh, a cake made of fermented soybeans and grain that's often fortified with B_{12}. They also take a multivitamin once a week.

Becoming Vegetarian

On the surface, going vegetarian seems simple enough: You just stop eating meat. But for most people, this is neither practical nor healthy, says Dr. Johnston.

"Instead of cutting out meat immediately, it's preferable to make some other changes in your diet first," she says.

Start by making an effort to eat more fruits, vegetables and whole grains. "Once you start focusing on those foods, meat tends to become less important," says Dr. Johnston. "If you're eating enough of these other foods, you might find that you don't have to make much of an effort to stop eating meat: It just gradually gets squeezed out of your diet."

This is also a good time to start weeding the "junk" out of your diet, if you haven't already. "Start thinking about what you're eating," says Dr. Johnston. "Before you put anything in your mouth, ask yourself if it's giving you the nutrients you need or if you're just filling yourself up with empty calories." If you learn to say no to sugary desserts, highly processed foods and nutritionally bankrupt snacks, you'll have more room in your diet for the nutritious foods your body craves.

Once your new, healthier eating habits are in place, it's pretty easy to plan one meatless dinner per week, whether it's pasta, bean burritos or even vegetable chow mein from the nearest Chinese take-out place, says Dr. Klaper. He also suggests making a big pot of vegetable soup or meatless chili and then reheating the leftovers for lunch the next day. "Suddenly, you're up to two or three vegetarian meals per week, and it couldn't be easier," he says.

Multiplying Your Meatless Choices

If you're making the transition to vegetarianism and you're not used to fixing meatless meals, invest in a good vegetarian cookbook or start out by borrowing one from the library. Variety is important. "Many people hit on two or three vegetarian meals that they like and eat them over and over again," says Dr. Johnston. "But the more you rely on a handful of favorite foods, the more likely you are to miss out on key nutrients, so it's important to keep trying new foods. And it makes your meals a lot more interesting!"

Remember, if you're going vegetarian, you've already limited your diet, so you don't want to restrict it any further. "When you declare certain foods off-limits, you become more vulnerable to nutritional deficiencies," says Dr. Johnston. "The more variety in your diet, the more insurance you have, nutritionally speaking."

A well-stocked pantry is essential, says Dr. Klaper. "I tell people to keep whole grains, pasta, lentils, beans and tomato sauces on hand," he says. "This way you'll always have the basic ingredients for a healthy meal. All you have to do is add plenty of fresh vegetables and some fruit."

Look Before You Eat

Before you dig into your meal, take a good look at what's on your plate, suggests Dr. Johnston. "You should see a variety of different colors and textures. If everything on your plate is soft and white—rice, macaroni, white bread—you're obviously eating an unbalanced meal." Liven things up with a little color—a baked sweet potato, a crunchy red pepper or some emerald-green broccoli—and your meal will be more appealing and a lot more nutritious.

You should also vary the way you prepare your food: If you steam your carrots one day, stir-fry them or eat them raw the next day. "Some cooking methods can destroy certain nutrients in foods," says Dr. Johnston. "It's not something vegetarians need to worry about unless they cook all their food the same way, day in and day out. That's when they risk missing out on important vitamins."

In general, the longer you cook vegetables, the more you deplete their nutrients, so choose quick methods like microwaving whenever possible. It's also a good idea to eat a few servings of raw fruits and vegetables each day, as single servings or in salads.

Above all, remember that true lifestyle changes take time. "It may take you six months to make the transition, but so what?" says Dr. Klaper. "It took you 30 or 40 years to develop your present eating habits. You don't have to change them overnight."

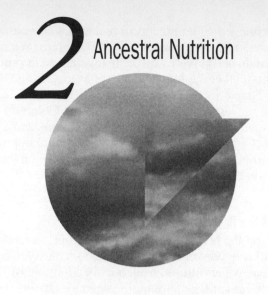

2 Ancestral Nutrition

Following in the Footsteps of Early Man

Before fast food and frozen entrécs. Before vitamin supplements and meal-replacement shakes. Before breakfast cereals—and even before bread—human beings got by.

For hundreds of thousands of years before the first crops were planted, our early ancestors fed themselves by hunting wild animals and gathering vegetables, seeds, nuts and fruits.

That this diet sustained our species for more than a million years is a matter of historical record. That it's still a viable way to eat—a way to get the fuel our bodies were designed to use—is a nutritional philosophy propounded by scientists like S. Boyd Eaton, M.D., an anthropologist and professor of radiology at Emory University in Atlanta and author of *The Paleolithic Prescription: A Program of Diet and Exercise and a Design for Living.*

The Hunter-Gatherer Diet

Unless you're an archaeologist or a student of anthropology, you might not realize that farming—that noblest of human pursuits that puts bread on your table and butter on your bread—is a pretty recent invention. Humans have been on the earth for well over 2 million years, and only in the last 10 or 12 thousand did we figure out how to till the soil. For most of our history, we bipeds flourished on a limited but nutritious diet of wild plants and freshly killed game.

Life has changed a lot in the most recent few thousand years, and we've invented a million new ways to feed ourselves. What hasn't changed much is the human body: We're still cruising around in pretty much the same classic model that our hunter-gatherer ancestors had.

"Genetic adaptation happens very slowly in terms of the human life span," says Loren Cordain, Ph.D., director of the Colorado State University Human Performance Research Center in Fort Collins and a researcher in the field of ancestral nutrition. "Our bodies haven't caught up with all of the changes in our diet. We're still programmed to thrive on the type of diet that our ancestors were eating 40,000 years ago," he says.

Peering at the Past

By studying the few remaining hunter-gatherer societies on Earth—people who still live very much as our ancestors must have lived—scientists know that the early diet differed from ours in a number of ways.

First, early humans ate a lot more vegetables, fruits, nuts and seeds than we do today. While modern folks struggle to eat the recommended five daily servings of produce, some contemporary hunter-gatherers eat as many as 20 different leafy vegetables, roots, stalks and seeds a day. They forage for seasonal fruit, berries, melons and flowers, which add even more bulk and nutrients to their diet.

The rest of the early human diet came from meat. Exactly how much animal food was eaten varied quite a bit according to the climate and geographic region. Meat made up 50 to 60 percent of the diet of modern Australian aborigines—and their ancestors—with the rest of their calories coming from plant foods. In traditional Eskimo communities, meat is the mainstay of the diet, with only about 10 percent plant foods.

The Have-Nots

Just as important as what our ancestors ate is what they didn't eat. Many of the foods we eat every day hadn't been discovered yet. These include grains like wheat, oats, rice and corn, and all foods made from them, such as breads, cereals and pasta. Also absent from the menu were dairy products, sweets (except honey), vegetable oils and alcohol.

By modern standards it's a pretty spartan diet. But archaeological records show that the hunter-gatherer diet was nutritious enough to produce a strapping, vigorous bunch of people. In fact, the average height of preagricultural people was around five feet five inches for women and five feet ten inches for men—just about the same as modern folk in affluent countries where kids are raised on the four food groups, observes Dr. Cordain.

The heartiness of early people isn't all that surprising when you consider the impressive nutrient density of their diets. Compared to the diet most of us eat today, the hunter-gatherer diet was richer in virtually every

Switching to Cave-Style Eating

If meat is something you've always enjoyed, but you're deterred by the fat, then the switch to an ancestral diet could be the start of a whole new game for you.

Provisions? Well, you'll probably have to contact a mail-order company that supplies game meat. If you don't go for rattlesnake, you can opt for pheasant breast, alligator tail or a few elk and buffalo steaks. You'll find that the meat is quite expensive, and you'll probably want to round out the diet with fish, free-range chicken and lots of fresh produce.

If you've never had elk steak for breakfast, you'll be surprised to discover that the meat is delicious. Alligator tail, on the other hand, is an acquired taste—what some describe as swampy—and it has a rubbery texture that could make you feel as if you're chewing on a balloon. For many people, the favorite is buffalo: You can marinate it overnight in some dry red wine with a few hunks of raw onion, then rub it down with a clove of garlic and just lightly sear it on both sides on the grill.

If you're used to eating your meat well-done, you may have to adjust your tastes a bit when you try wild game. Fat is what keeps meat tender, and game is so lean that a well-done elk or buffalo steak is dry and tough. Try it rare, though, and it tastes perfect.

If you don't like the idea of starting your day with game meat, the ancestral diet has alternatives. Fill up on fruit—whatever's in season. Or have a couple of handfuls of nuts mixed with raisins and other dried fruit.

At lunchtime you can reheat some leftover fish or meat in the microwave at work, along with some frozen vegetables. Finish your meal with a piece of fruit or a salad dressed with balsamic vinegar or lemon juice (no oil), and you'll probably feel perfectly satisfied. Best of all, with a meal like that, you may find that you don't lapse into the postprandial coma that hits most of us in midafternoon.

Many people feel hungry for much of the day when they try an ancestral diet. That's because most of us rely on starchy foods to fill us up. While meat itself is pretty filling, ancestral meals lean heavily toward fruit, salads and other green vegetables. You have to eat large quantities of those if you hope to feel satisfied on this diet.

---

important nutrient, according to Dr. Cordain.

The emphasis on fresh fruits and vegetables virtually guaranteed a good supply of vitamins and minerals—in some cases, many times the Daily Values used as standards of good nutrition by the U.S. Department of Health. In fact, computer analyses show that our ancestors' diet provided much more vitamin C and beta-carotene, more iron, potassium and magnesium and about twice as much calcium as most Americans are getting. And they got all this without the benefit of bread, milk, fortified cereals and vitamin supplements.

Going against the Grain

One of the most controversial areas in ancestral nutrition is the proper role of grains and dairy products—the "new foods"—in our diet.

Some proponents say that grains and dairy are foods our bodies weren't designed to eat and haven't "learned" to use effectively. "We're taught that grains and dairy are necessary for proper nutrition, but humanity did just fine without them for two million years," says Loren Cordain, Ph.D., director of the Colorado State University Human Performance Research Center in Fort Collins and a researcher in the field of ancestral nutrition.

Others say that whether you should eat grains and dairy foods depends partly on how your body reacts to them. "Milk causes problems for most of the adult population; lactose intolerance is the rule, not the exception," observes Ann Louise Gittleman, a clinical nutritionist in Bozeman, Montana, and author of *Your Body Knows Best: The Revolutionary Eating Plan That Helps You Achieve Your Optimal Weight and Energy Level for Life.*

If drinking milk gives you gas, constipation or abdominal cramps, you may be a prime candidate for eliminating dairy, according to Gittleman. Another option is to replace milk with fermented dairy products like yogurt or cheese, which are often easier to digest because they contain less lactose (the sugar that causes the problem) than milk does.

The same holds true for grains, says Gittleman. "As more and more people go to low-fat, high-carbohydrate diets that include huge quantities of whole grains, sensitivities are becoming more common," she says. "Most people with grain sensitivities don't know it: They have lots of bloating, fatigue and even some mineral deficiencies because they're overdoing foods that their bodies aren't adapted to."

If you suspect that you're sensitive to dairy or grains, try eliminating them for a week or two to see if your symptoms improve, suggests Gittleman. Then gradually reintroduce them, one food at a time, to see if your symptoms return.

"Some people can eat grains in moderation, with an occasional serving of yogurt, and others are better off without either one," explains Gittleman. "A diet that's optimal for one person doesn't necessarily work for somebody else."

Heart Disease: A Civilized Killer

"Nasty, brutish and short." That's how seventeenth-century essayist Thomas Hobbes described the life of early man: a brief, violent struggle ending in a painful death.

Well, there's no doubt that our primitive ancestors had it rough. They were vulnerable to animal predators and natural disasters—threats that we privileged citizens of modern developed countries don't have to face so frequently.

But before we start counting our blessings, we'd do well to note that many of our ancestors lived long, healthy lives without ever developing heart disease. The most notorious serial killer of the developed world, heart disease threatens the lives of more Americans than all other diseases combined.

Ancestral Health Insurance

What was it in the hunter-gatherer way of life that protected our ancestors from heart disease? Just about everything, says Dr. Eaton.

Because early people had a simple diet and an active lifestyle, it was nearly impossible to carry around excess weight—a well-documented risk factor for heart disease. "It would be incredibly difficult to get fat on a hunter-gatherer diet," says Dr. Cordain. He points out that most of the foods eaten by our roaming ancestors were low in calories. "You'd have to eat an unimaginable quantity of wild plants, and more meat than was actually available, in order to put on excess weight. It would probably be physically impossible, especially when you consider how active early people were," he says.

Ancestral diets are also low in fat, even in hunter-gatherer societies where meat consumption is highest. "It always amazes people that a diet can be low in fat even though you're getting as much as half your calories from meat," says Dr. Cordain. "But wild game meat is so much leaner than farm-raised meat that you can eat quite a bit of it and still consume very little fat." On average, wild game meat is about 4 percent fat, while many cuts of beef and pork are more than 35 percent fat.

Wild game isn't just leaner than commercial meat, it also contains a whole different type of fat. Commercial beef and pork, because the animals are raised on grain, are rich in the fatty acid known as omega-6, or linoleic acid, Dr. Cordain explains. And studies show that high levels of linoleic acid are associated with cardiovascular disease.

Hunting for Lower Cholesterol

There's another factor. The type of fat in wild meat is less likely to raise cholesterol levels than the kind found in commercial beef or pork. One study compared the cholesterol levels of men who ate a half-pound of beef a day with those of a control group who ate the same amount of Beefalo—meat from a breed of cattle that's a hybrid of beef and bison. (Beefalo contains more saturated fat than bison but significantly less than beef.)

After three months, the beef-eating men had a significant jump in harmful LDL (low-density lipoprotein) cholesterol—the kind that clogs up arteries and leads to heart disease. The Beefalo group saw no change even though they, too, were eating a half-pound of red meat every day.

Researchers concluded that wild game has just as much fat as our bodies need, and not much more. "Wild meat has the type of fat that our bodies are designed to consume," says Dr. Cordain.

Fish, too, supplies a type of fat that seems to be far less likely to lead

Forbidden Food in Your Family Tree

"Our ancestors didn't all eat the same way," says Ann Louise Gittleman, a clinical nutritionist in Bozeman, Montana, and author of *Your Body Knows Best: The Revolutionary Eating Plan That Helps You Achieve Your Optimal Weight and Energy Level for Life*. "They adapted to the types of food that were available to them and passed this genetic coding on to us."

In cultures with a long history of herding, for instance, people seem to be genetically adapted to a diet rich in dairy foods. Throughout their adult lives, they continue to produce the enzyme lactase, which allows them to digest milk efficiently—unlike adults from other ethnic groups, who typically experience gas and bloating after drinking milk. This explains why Chinese and African-American adults are usually lactose-intolerant, while most Scandinavians digest milk with no problem.

Lactose intolerance isn't the only such trait that's genetically based, says Gittleman. Your genetic background offers myriad clues about which foods you should be eating and which you're better off avoiding.

"Eating a diet that's really balanced to your chemistry and genetic requirements gives you the best insurance for long-term health," says Gittleman, whose interest in nutrition based on genetic background was sparked by the work of researchers and authors James D'Adamo, M.D., and Peter D'Adamo, M.D.

Tailoring the ancestral diet to your own genetic makeup isn't complicated, she adds. Knowing your ethnic background and blood type can help you discover what kind of diet your body is genetically programmed to follow.

In general, Gittleman recommends the meat-based hunter-gatherer diet for most Native Americans and people of Northern European descent, who often have Type O blood, and for the nearly 50 percent of African-Americans with Type O blood.

"O is the most ancient blood type, and people with Type O are best adapted to the very early human diet," she says. "Generally, they can tolerate a diet that has more fat and protein. They need animal protein, meat or fish, on a daily basis, as well as lots of leafy vegetables and root vegetables. They have the most problems digesting grains and seem to be better off without them."

---

to heart disease than the stuff that marbles your steak. Studies show that men who eat a diet rich in omega-3 fatty acids—found in tuna, salmon, clams and scallops, have lower heart-damaging triglycerides and higher HDL (high-density lipoprotein) cholesterol (the "good" kind) than men who eat little or no fish.

Fitter with Fiber

While our ancestors actually consumed more cholesterol than we do because of all the meat in their diet, they made up for it by getting an extra-

For people with Type A blood, Gittleman recommends a variation of the hunter-gatherer diet that emphasizes lean meats and fish and includes moderate servings of grains. About 42 percent of white Americans, including most people of Mediterranean descent, and about a quarter of African-Americans have Type A. "These people have less of the stomach acids needed to digest meat, so they do best on leaner meats or fish," she says. "And since they don't digest protein as easily, they tend to overdo grains and develop wheat or other grain allergies."

Those with Type A blood can handle grains in modest amounts—about two servings a day, Gittleman suggests. "It's also important that they control their fat intake by choosing fish or turkey over other meats." If you have Type A blood, she recommends eliminating or cutting way back on dairy products, especially if you have symptoms of lactose intolerance.

The other two blood types, B and AB, are considered new blood types because they seem to have evolved after the Agricultural Revolution, according to Gittleman. "They're the people who have adapted best to dairy products, especially fermented ones like cheese and yogurt," she says. These blood types are comparatively rare, making up about 14 percent of the white and 24 percent of the African-American populations. Many people of Jewish or Eastern European descent have Type B blood, while AB blood is most common in people of Romanian heritage.

If your blood is Type B or AB, aim for a balanced diet that includes plenty of fruits, vegetables, meat and fish and one or two servings of dairy foods each day, suggests Gittleman. Whenever possible, choose cheese or yogurt over milk, she adds. And be on the lookout for symptoms of lactose intolerance like bloating, constipation or gas. You can also eat grain products in moderation—once or twice a day—unless you're prone to fatigue, bloating or joint pain after eating grains.

"The most important thing is to listen to your body's signals and pay attention to how eating different foods makes you feel," says Gittleman. "If a food causes a bad reaction, the best advice is to cut back on it until your symptoms go away, even if that means eliminating it from your diet."

ordinary amount of fiber. Eating large quantities of fruits and vegetables every day provided loads of soluble fiber, the kind of fiber found in fruits, grains and some legumes. The benefit of this fiber is that it has been shown to lower cholesterol levels.

The mineral-rich hunter-gatherer diet also seems to be protective against high blood pressure, a major risk factor for heart disease. The diet is low in sodium and rich in potassium, a combination that seems to prevent high blood pressure.

Finally, our ancestors were free of two modern habits that have been proven to contribute to heart disease—smoking and consuming alcohol. Smoking contributes to artery-clogging atherosclerosis, and drinking alcohol has been linked to high blood pressure.

The Anti-cancer Diet

Next to worrying about how to avoid cancer—one of the most dreaded killers in the modern forest—outrunning mastodons and woolly mammoths must have been a walk in the park.

According to Dr. Cordain, everything we know about hunter-gatherer societies suggests that their simple diet provided unparalleled protection against cancer.

A growing body of research indicates that a diet rich in fruits and vegetables may be our best defense against many kinds of cancer. Fresh produce provides a complex mix of fiber, vitamins and minerals. Fruits and vegetables are also rich in phytochemicals, a group of compounds that appear to have anti-cancer properties. Researchers say that this unique combination may play a key role in fighting off cancer.

In the fiber department, modern hunter-gatherers get a mega-dose by eating 40 to 50 grams a day—two or three times what our highly refined Western diet contains. And some early societies, such as early Native American hunter-gatherers, probably ate as much as 130 grams of fiber a day.

The soluble fiber in fruits and vegetables helps us process our food faster, speeding up the elimination of harmful substances that could increase our risk of cancer. This may be one reason that fiber offers special protection against breast, colon and prostate cancer and possibly stomach, esophageal and oral cancer.

Hunter-gatherer diets are also loaded with vitamins and minerals. While many of these nutrients are being investigated for their cancer-fighting potential, scientists are particularly interested in a class of nutrients known as antioxidants. This group, which includes vitamins C and E, beta-carotene and selenium, is believed to protect human cells from free radical damage, a process that may play a role in the early development of cancer.

Besides being rich in nutrients, ancestral diets also tend to be low in fat. And whether it's on your steak or hanging over your belt, fat is a well-documented risk factor for cancer. Since our ancestors ate a lean diet and were themselves fit and trim, they were doubly protected.

Before Diabetes Was Invented

Another important benefit of ancestral nutrition, proponents say, is a decreased risk of developing Type II (non-insulin-dependent) diabetes, a serious metabolic disorder that affects over 12 million Americans. Unless properly controlled, diabetes can lead to life-threatening complications like cardiovascular disease, kidney problems, nerve degeneration and blindness.

In today's hunter-gatherer societies, diabetes is virtually nonexistent. But once these people abandon their traditional diets for a modern one high in processed foods, diabetes becomes a fact of life.

A century ago, diabetes was virtually unheard of among the Pima Indians of Arizona, who lived on a simple diet of beans, maize, squash and wild plants, with occasional fish or small game. But their original diet has now been replaced by a modern menu that's more likely to include white bread and chocolate bars than beans and maize. Today, the Pimas have the highest rate of adult diabetes in the world.

Part of the reason is the Pimas' inherited tendency to accumulate body fat and overproduce insulin, the hormone that converts food into energy. As long as they ate their traditional diet, which was low in fat and high in complex carbohydrates, the Pimas stayed slim and their blood sugar remained normal. But combine the Pimas' genetic makeup with a sedentary lifestyle and modern American diet—heavy on sugar, alcohol, white flour and other highly refined foods—and the result is a recipe for diabetes.

Of course, you don't have to be a Pima to develop diabetes: Being overweight and sedentary and eating a typical American diet is risky enough. At the same time, you don't have to be a Pima to benefit from their traditional lifestyle. Being more active and replacing sweets, alcohol and processed foods with fruits and vegetables are sensible steps that will help keep anybody's weight and blood sugar under control.

Bones like the Flintstones'

Ancestral diets also seem to prevent osteoporosis, the brittle-bone disease that affects an estimated 25 million Americans, mostly women.

Skeletons of early people show that men and women of all ages had strong, heavy bones, says Dr. Eaton. The health of their skeletons can be attributed to an active lifestyle and a balanced, calcium-rich diet.

Today, those at risk for osteoporosis are advised to either drink plenty of milk or take calcium supplements. So how did early people maintain strong bones long before either of these options existed?

First of all, even without dairy products, the hunter-gatherer diet is exceptionally rich in calcium, says Dr. Cordain.

Wild fruits and vegetables contain more calcium than modern cultivated varieties, according to Dr. Cordain, who has done computer analyses of modern hunter-gatherer diets. He believes it's quite possible to get enough calcium from the leafy greens available in today's markets.

"You can get between 800 and 1,000 milligrams of calcium per day, slightly higher than the current American average, which is between 600 and 800 milligrams," he says. And while those numbers are still lower than what's usually recommended for modern humans, our ancestors didn't need as much, notes Dr. Cordain. That's because salt intake doubles the amount of calcium we need, and salt was not part of the Paleolithic diet.

The high sodium content of the modern diet also makes us excrete much of the calcium we eat, he says. "Sodium and calcium compete in the kidney, and when you're getting high levels of sodium, the kidney has to excrete calcium. The epidemic of osteoporosis is related to high salt intake. When you consider that the average American woman eats four to ten grams of sodium per day, it's not surprising that osteoporosis has become a major problem."

Finally, because the hunter-gatherer diet is free of tobacco and caffeine, the risk of osteoporosis is also reduced.

A true hunter-gatherer diet that eliminates grains also improves your ability to absorb calcium, says Dr. Cordain. Whole-grain cereals are very high in lectins, protease inhibitors and phytic acid—all substances that bind up important minerals, including calcium, iron and zinc, he explains. "So if you're eating lots of high-calcium dairy products but eating a diet rich in whole grains, your bones probably aren't getting as much calcium as you think they are."

Another Bone Builder

Calcium isn't the only consideration if you're worried about osteoporosis, says Dr. Cordain. "In fact, the countries with the highest calcium consumption—the United States, Canada, Western Europe and Australia— also have the highest incidence of osteoporosis," he says.

To build strong bone, he says, it's important to balance calcium with magnesium, a mineral found in many fruits and vegetables. If you don't have the correct ratio, calcium and magnesium tend to cancel each other out, so if you're eating lots of calcium but almost no magnesium, some of that calcium is actually being washed out.

"In most Western countries, that's exactly what's happening," he adds. "The average American consumes about ten times as much calcium as magnesium, mostly because we don't eat enough fruits and vegetables." In the diet of hunter-gatherers, Dr. Cordain notes, the calcium-to-magnesium ratio is about one to one—one milligram of calcium for every milligram of magnesium. "So they actually retain more of the calcium they eat."

Eating the Ancestral Way

Following the ancestral diet isn't complicated, but it does require making a few changes in the way you plan meals and shop for groceries, says Lorrie Small, a Colorado school teacher, athlete and mother who has followed a hunter-gatherer diet for three years.

When you're shopping for groceries, plan to spend most of your time in the produce section. "It's amazing how many fruits and vegetables a family eats in one day on this diet," she says. At her house, they're part of every meal. "Usually, we have three vegetable dishes on the table at night, a huge bowl of fruit and a salad," says Small. She has also invested in two juicers and a food dehydrator, so fresh juices and dried fruit have become household staples.

The breakfast menu at Small's house is usually eggs or leftover meat plus some fruit. For lunches on Wednesday she usually takes vegetables and meat from home and heats them in the microwave at work. (Salad bars are also convenient on days when she's too busy to pack a lunch.) Dinner is the main meal of the day, with a main course of meat or fish and lots of vegetables.

For Small, who has meat at every meal, finding enough lean, high-quality meat is a challenge. "Wild game is the ideal, and we get it whenever we can," she says. "But unless somebody in the family is a hunter, it can be difficult to come by." In a pinch, there's always fish and free-range chicken, available at a local grocery store.

Many gourmet grocery stores and some farmers markets carry free-range poultry. Inquire at a butcher shop or in the meat department of your supermarket.

Hunting Hints

Once in a while, when game is in short supply, Small buys supermarket beef. She chooses the leanest cuts and limits the portions enough to keep her fat intake under control.

Adherents are quick to admit that eating meat three times a day can get pretty expensive. "Our grocery bills have definitely increased," says Bob Gotshall, a Colorado college professor who has been on the diet for several months. He often orders his meat from a local wild game distributor and tries to stick to ground meats rather than buying the pricier steaks. His favorite meats, elk and buffalo, also happen to be native to the Rocky Mountain region, so they are relatively easy to get and less expensive than other types of wild meat.

When it comes to cooking, grilling is the method of choice. But wild game might not need as much cooking time as other meats. "Wild meat is so lean that it can be tough if you overcook it," says Gotshall, who suggests turning off the grill when the meat is still pink in the middle. Small, another grilling fan, enjoys creating new marinades to help keep meat tender.

Eating in restaurants is surprisingly easy. "We've learned where to

Resources for Healing

Mail-Order Food Sources

Broken Arrow Ranch
P.O. Box 530
Ingram, TX 78025
1-800-962-4263

Colorado Mountain Game
825 Denver Avenue
Fort Lupton, CO 80621

Czimer Foods
13136 West 159th Street
Lockport, IL 60441

Game Sales International, Inc.
P.O. Box 7719
Loveland, CO 80537-0719
1-800-729-2090

The Native Game Company
2301 Nevada Avenue North
Minneapolis, MN 55427
1-800-952-6321

Wild Game, Inc.
2315 West Huron
Chicago, IL 60612

Try It for a Week

Ready to go for it? Here's a whole week of menus that resemble the first *Homo sapiens'* diet. While many of these foods are available at your supermarket, it's doubtful that you'll find a local source of alligator tail or elk steak. See "Resources for Healing" on page 31 for a list of suppliers.

Sunday Breakfast—Banana; 2 pears

Lunch—8-ounce grilled elk steak marinated in lemon juice and spices; peas

Dinner—Grilled pheasant breast; steamed broccoli, carrots and water chestnuts

Snack—Handful of raisins and walnuts

Monday Breakfast—Raisins and walnuts; grapefruit; calcium-fortified orange juice

Snack—Apple; apricot

Lunch—Leftover pheasant; 2 wedges cantaloupe; steamed green beans; vegetable juice cocktail

Snack—Papaya

Dinner—Grilled alligator tail; steamed asparagus; green salad with balsamic vinegar dressing (no oil)

Tuesday Breakfast—Dried apricots and a handful of walnuts; orange

Snack—Vegetable juice cocktail

Lunch—8 ounces grilled tuna steak; red peppers and snow pea pods; mango

Snack—Apple; raisins

Dinner—8-ounce grilled buffalo steak marinated in wine, onions and garlic; steamed asparagus; strawberries

---

go," Small explains. "At Italian restaurants, we'll have a meat or fish dish with a salad and a vegetable, and we leave the bread basket alone. At seafood restaurants we might order shrimp and a small steak to go with it, instead of eating all the other stuff." She does, however, avoid Mexican restaurants, since it's hard to order anything there that doesn't contain wheat or corn.

More Energy—And Better Looks

While proponents are enthusiastic about the long-term health benefits of ancestral nutrition, they're quick to point out that eating this way also makes them feel better in the short term. Both Small and Gotshall say that the diet has made a real difference in their energy levels.

"I don't have that slump at about one or two o'clock that I used to think was just part of life. Now I eat lunch and I go off feeling refreshed and rarin' to go," says Small. "And if one of the boys is sick and I have to be up during the

Wednesday	Breakfast—A handful each of raisins and mixed nuts; apricot; nectarine
	Lunch—8-ounce grilled swordfish steak; cauliflower; salad
	Snack—Grapes
	Dinner—Grilled free-range chicken breast marinated in lime juice and ginger; steamed kale; green salad
Thursday	Breakfast—Raisins and walnuts; calcium-fortified orange juice
	Snack—Red pepper strips
	Lunch—Leftover free-range chicken; green beans; watermelon
	Snack—Baby carrots; black olives
	Dinner—8-ounce elk steak; broccoli; vegetable juice cocktail; banana
Friday	Breakfast—Sunflower seeds; prunes; dried banana pieces; calcium-fortified orange juice
	Snack—Apple
	Lunch—Leftover elk steak; steamed peas and carrots
	Snack—Papaya
	Dinner—8-ounce mako shark steak; steamed asparagus; green salad with tomatoes and endive; 2 apricots
Saturday	Breakfast—Sunflower seeds; prunes; raisins; calcium-fortified orange juice
	Lunch—Leftover shark steak; tomato, zucchini and eggplant ratatouille; banana
	Snack—Mango; kiwifruit
	Dinner—8-ounce swordfish steak; ratatouille; steamed broccoli, carots and water chestnuts; honeydew melon

night with him, I recover from it a lot faster."

This new energy has carried over into her athletic performance. "I haven't been training the way I used to, but I notice that when I do go for a run, I feel really strong and I don't get tired, even if I haven't run in two weeks," she says. "I hardly even feel sore the next day, the way I used to whenever I took time off. I'm really anxious to get back to competing to see what this diet will do for me."

The ancestral diet also seems to have a beneficial effect on cholesterol levels. Small's husband has lowered his cholesterol reading from a slightly elevated 210 mg/dl (milligrams per deciliter) of total cholesterol to an exemplary 165 mg/dl.

Small, who follows a strict grainless, dairy-free diet, also noticed a difference in her skin and hair when she changed her diet.

"I used to have atopia—a skin condition that looked like tiny bumps on my arms and chest—but it's gone away. I've also noticed that most of my gray hair has gone away! Even my hairdresser noticed the difference. I'm only 37, but it runs in my family. I have five sisters who are all gray. What's weird is that if we're on vacation and I have a few days where I eat bread or pasta, I start noticing gray hairs again."

Both Small and Gotshall find that they eat a lot more on the ancestral diet, but all that extra food hasn't added up to weight gain. Quite the opposite.

At one point, Gotshall had to cut back on his exercise because of a knee injury. After six weeks without exercise, he expected to find that he had gained a few pounds. "That didn't happen, though," he says. "In fact, I think I lost a few pounds."

3 Macrobiotics

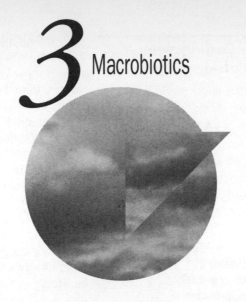

Traditional Eating for Modern Health

For most of us, breakfast means some combination of toast, cereal, bacon and eggs, coffee or similar, hearty all-American fare. But for Benjamin Spock, M.D., renowned author of *Dr. Spock's Baby and Child Care*, breakfast is composed of miso soup (made from fermented soybean paste), scrambled tofu, brown rice, pickles and bland, decaffeinated bancha twig tea. And although his morning fare may sound utterly inedible to lots of American eaters, Dr. Spock says it saved his life.

At 88 years of age, having suffered a heart attack, a subsequent stroke and severe bronchial infections, Dr. Spock faced a future in a wheelchair, with a grim prognosis for his health. At noon on September 6, 1991, with nothing left to lose, he started a macrobiotic diet—a highly structured and finely balanced vegetarian way of eating. Six weeks later, he was not only out of his wheelchair but was also swimming and doing yoga.

"It's amazing," says Dr. Spock, who now swears by the macrobiotic diet that gave him a second start. "People need to realize that a bad diet does damage to your body all through your life, but you don't do the dying from heart attacks, strokes and cancer until you reach late middle age. There's no doubt that a high-fat diet is lethal. I believe that people could live a much longer life, free of disease, by following a macrobiotic diet."

Barley Porridge Hot, Barley Porridge Cold . . .

Feeling a little under the weather? Start boiling your barley. Taking the advice of the father of Western medicine, Hippocrates, macrobiotics practitioners recommend eating nourishing, easy-to-digest barley porridge several times a day to help you get back on your feet. Here's a recipe that serves four.

....

> 1 **cup barley**
> **Pinch of sea salt**
> 4–5 **cups spring water**
> **Parsley sprigs**

In a 2-quart saucepan, combine the barley, salt and water. Bring to a boil, then reduce the heat, cover and cook 1¼ to 1½ hours, until creamy. Place in bowls and garnish with the parsley.

....

The Kitchen as Pharmacy

Macrobiotics—which sounds more like some New Age science than a diet—is actually not new at all, although it is a bit of a science. Based on traditional dietary practices from ancient times, its modern incarnation was developed in 1913 by a Japanese, Yukikazu Sakurazawa—later called George Ohsawa—who is said to have cured himself of tuberculosis with nothing but food.

Self-taught in Oriental medicine, Ohsawa believed wholeheartedly in the Asian principles of yin and yang—two opposite, complementary forces found in all of nature. By applying these principles, Ohsawa believed, people could live long, disease-free lives. The goal, he said, was to eat foods that were neither too yin (expansive) nor too yang (contractive). He believed that the ideal diet was based on grains. Eat no meat, eggs, dairy products, sugar, caffeine, alcohol or processed foods, he declared. By eliminating these foods, he believed that we would eat as our ancestors traditionally ate for thousands of years—and the way we were meant to eat.

To support his theories about grains and good health, Ohsawa pointed to Hippocrates, the father of Western medicine, who first used the term *macrobiotic*—then *makrobios*—to mean long (*macro-*) life (*-bios*). Hippocrates preached that people should understand how the body responds to eating different bread preparations—those made from pure flour, for instance, versus those made from winnowed or husked wheat. Unless we understood these differences, said Hippocrates, we couldn't possibly understand disease. Although that was more than 2,000 years ago, some of his food prescriptions for healing are still used in modern macrobiotics.

The New Macrobiotics

Embraced by the counterculture movement of the 1960s, one form of macrobiotics acquired a questionable reputation. When it was first in vogue, some of its advocates started following an extremely restrictive version called Zen macrobiotics, which espoused brown rice as the only perfect food. A few steadfast devotees ate nothing but brown rice and became ill. One even died. Although these ideas are not part of modern macrobiotics, they still haunt proponents.

"I've heard people call macrobiotics the killer diet, and I think that's ridiculous, especially since they're basing their judgments on a few extreme cases," says Terry Shintani, M.D., director of preventive medicine at the Waianae Coast Comprehensive Health Center in Hawaii and author of *Eat More, Weigh Less Diet*. "If you want a killer diet, try the American diet of hot dogs and apple pie. Nine hundred thousand people die as a result of that diet every year."

Although what was called Zen macrobiotics later went the way of bell-bottoms, macrobiotics is still regarded as a "hippie" diet by some. But it has been making a comeback, this time with high-profile advocates like Dr. Spock and *A-Team* star Dirk Benedict. Believing firmly in the principle of macrobiotics, these proponents have credited their diet with bringing about their remissions from heart disease and cancer.

Today, Michio Kushi—Ohsawa's favorite student—leads the world-wide macrobiotics community from his home in Brookline, Massachusetts. A political science and international law graduate of Tokyo University, Kushi brought the diet to America "as a healing response to the devastation of World War II."

Kushi and his wife, Aveline, have become magnets for macrobiotics practitioners in America. People with cancer or AIDS—or those who are just curious about macrobiotics—often come to their school, the Kushi Institute in Becket, Massachusetts, to stay and learn.

Macrobiotics is a bit different now than it was when it first hit the United States in the 1960s. Kushi has broadened the food choices and developed what is known as the standard macrobiotic diet, which is not a rigid diet but a basic food plan. On the standard macrobiotic diet, you're supposed to get 50 to 60 percent whole grains, 20 to 25 percent vegetables, 5 to 10 percent seaweeds and beans and 5 to 10 percent soups every day. If your condition permits, you can also have a small amount of white-fleshed fish and some fruit.

The Yin and Yang of Food

The crux of understanding the macrobiotic diet is understanding yin and yang. For a better picture of how these work, macrobiotics counselors recommend thinking of them in terms of natural rhythms, like inhaling and exhaling. When we inhale, our bodies expand and move outward—a yin force. When we exhale, our bodies contract and move inward—a yang force. According to macrobiotics practitioners, everything in the world, including food, can be classified in terms of its yin and yang energy.

Take a banana, for example. You may think of it as just a sweet breakfast treat. But in macrobiotics a banana is considered an extreme food that you should avoid because it's excessively yin.

(continued on page 40)

New Food Review

Developed by a Japanese-born man living on American soil, the standard macrobiotic diet is a melting pot of Asian and American foods, many of which may be unfamiliar to typical American cooks. The following glossary should help.

Go with the Grain

Macrobiotic eaters consider grains the perfect food and use a wide variety of both the common and the exotic. You can find these staple grains in natural food stores. They are generally soaked and boiled or pressure-cooked.

Barley. Light brown, with grains a little fatter than rice, barley is commonly sold as hulled barley. Soft, chewy and bland, it adds nice texture to soups.

Buckwheat. Sold either roasted or unroasted, these triangular-shaped kernels are good with vegetables. You can also use them in dumplings or pancakes.

Millet. Pale yellow, small and compact, millet grains fluff up when cooked and have a nutty flavor. They're good mixed with other grains or with beans.

Oats. Macrobiotic cooks recommend buying whole oats instead of the more processed Scotch or rolled oats. You can use them for stews, cookies and cereals.

Wheat. Wheat is used in many forms in macrobiotic cooking, from wheat flour to "wheat meat," or seitan—a salty, tender, simulated meat product made from wheat gluten, seaweed and soy sauce. Seitan can be toasted to make fu. Use the reddish-brown whole-wheat kernels, or wheat berries, in rice and bean dishes.

Roots and Shoots

Of all the vegetables used in macrobiotic cooking, the ones you're likely to find unfamiliar are the root vegetables and greens.

Bok choy. Rather bland on their own, the long white stalks of bok choy make a nice filler in vegetable dishes. You can also sauté it with fish or tofu.

Burdock. This long, thin, brown root vegetable has a firm texture and a strong, sweet, warm flavor. You can sauté, boil or deep-fry it.

Collard greens. Sweet and tender, these leafy greens, originally used in Native American and African-American cooking, are now popular in macrobiotics circles, where they're generally steamed or boiled.

Daikon. A favorite in Japan, this long white radish is sweet and spicy and goes well with rice and soups. It can be pickled or grated and used as a garnish. Boiled daikon greens are also used in macrobiotic cooking.

Kale. This, leafy green vegetable is often steamed before serving.

Lotus root. Hollow, rich and sweet, the lotus root is considered a precious vegetable in macrobiotic cooking. You can sauté it, boil it, stuff it and bake it or marinate it in rice vinegar and eat it raw.

Watercress. This leafy green vegetable has a bitter taste that macrobiotic cooks love to use to enhance salads in the spring. You can also boil or sauté it.

Dream Beans (and Bean Products)

Being largely vegetarian, people on macrobiotic diets depend on beans and bean products, such as tofu, for protein. If you want the best beans, buy dried, not canned, say the experts. Then soak and boil or pressure-cook them.

Adzuki beans. These are favorites of macrobiotic cooks. The shiny, reddish-purple beans are small and sweet and go with anything, especially grain dishes.

Natto. Strong-tasting and strong-smelling, this fermented soybean product is often eaten as a side dish.

Soybeans. Either yellow or black, soybeans are very sweet and go well with rice and casseroles. Yellow soybeans are best if cooked with kombu.

Tempeh. This fermented soybean product comes in a compacted cake of stuck-together beans. It has a mushroom-like aroma and is chewy and light.

Tofu. Processed soybeans shaped into a white cake and stored in cold water, tofu has very little taste of its own but readily absorbs other flavors.

Veggies from the Deep

Seaweeds—also called sea vegetables—are a staple in macrobiotic meals. They can be boiled or sautéed with other foods or toasted and crushed as a condiment for soups, salads and grains.

Arame. Resembling wiry black threads, arame is one of the milder sea vegetables. It makes a good side dish, especially when cooked with soybeans.

Dulse. Flat strips of dark red dulse are best prepared dry-roasted and crushed onto salads, soups and vegetables.

Hiziki. Shaped like black dried pine needles, hiziki is one of the sea vegetables with a strong ocean flavor. Generally sautéed in sesame oil, it's commonly eaten with onions and/or tofu.

Kombu. A type of kelp, the ubiquitous kombu is a popular accompaniment to grains, beans and root vegetables. It's also made into pickles, condiments and candy. It comes in dried sheets that are cut for cooking.

Nori. Like arame, nori is a mild sea vegetable. It comes in dried sheets that you can toast and crush onto salads, soups and grain dishes. Or you can use it to wrap around steamed fish or vegetables.

Wakame. Wakame is similar to kombu, but it's thinner and cooks more quickly.

The Seasons Change

Because macrobiotics proponents don't believe in using a lot of spices, they keep their food from being bland with an array of salty, sweet and sour seasonings. One of the most common is soy sauce.

Miso. This macrobiotic cornerstone is a salty paste made from fermented soybeans and grains. Miso paste is eaten daily in miso soup and can be added to almost any macrobiotic dish.

Sea salt. Early macrobiotic cooking was very salty. Although it's less so today, unrefined sea salt is still the central seasoning. Sea salt is sweeter than table salt and has more minerals.

Umeboshi plums. Indigenous to Japan, these apricot-like fruits are fermented in sea salt and enzymes to make a sour, salty treat or seasoning.

One Person's Yin Is Another Person's Yang

If you're familiar with Chinese medicine, you've probably noticed a discrepancy in yin/yang definitions. What macrobiotics practitioners consider yin and yang is sometimes completely opposite from what followers of Chinese medicine call yin and yang. Salt, for instance, is a yang food in macrobiotics circles, but it is called yin by Chinese medicine doctors.

That's because the founders of macrobiotics developed their own system of yin and yang that they thought Westerners would understand, explains Paul Pitchford, director of the Oriental Healing Arts Program at the Heartwood Institute in Garberville, California, and author of *Healing with Whole Foods*, who frequently lectures on macrobiotics. Although he would like to see the systems become uniform, Pitchford admits that it makes little difference, since both groups make similar nutritional recommendations despite using different yin and yang terminology.

As a general rule, foods that are cooling are considered yin, and foods that are warming are considered yang.

Yin foods tend to be light, juicy, sour, bitter, very sweet or hot and are plentiful in summer or in warm climates. Foods in the yin category also are likely to be cool in color, and they grow up out of the ground, like lettuce.

Yang foods, on the other hand, are generally heavy and dry, salty, slightly sweet or pungent and available in winter or in cooler climates. They tend to be warm in color, and they grow down into the earth, like carrots.

Of course, the categories aren't all that clear, and you really have to consult a macrobiotics expert to find out which foods fit into which category. But when in doubt, look for the food's dominant characteristics, say macrobiotics teachers. Grapefruit, for example, may have yang color, but since it is very sweet, light, juicy and cool and grows in a tropical climate—and that's the dominant feature—it is considered to be a highly yin food.

According to macrobiotics, disease can happen when you pile your plate with too much yin and not enough yang—or vice versa. Eat too much dense, fatty animal food, which is yang, and you'll get atherosclerosis, or contracting (yang) of the arteries. Too much alcohol, which is yin, leads to expansion (yin) of the cells and causes headache. Disease can also be a side effect of eating both extremes simultaneously—like high blood pressure from eating meat fat (extreme yang) and alcohol (extreme yin).

Although you can theoretically achieve balance by eating equal amounts of very yin and very yang foods, "it is best to eat foods that are neither too yin nor too yang, like brown rice," says Kushi.

Staying in the Zone

Kushi also recommends that people in America eat food grown only in the temperate zone, because tropical fruits and vegetables like grapefruit and tomatoes and other members of the nightshade family, including potatoes, eggplant and peppers, are too yin. The "arctic foods" like fatty meats are too yang. But if you're living in an area outside the temperate zone, you can make exceptions, says Kushi. In the tropics, for instance, people on a macrobiotic diet can eat more tropical fruits as well as spices, herbs and herbal teas, which cool the body, says Kushi. In polar regions, people who follow macrobiotics may eat warming, yang foods, like fish and other seafood.

Even if you live in a temperate zone like the United States, you should make minor adjustments to eat with the seasons, says Kushi. He recommends eating lighter, cooler foods in the spring and summer months and heavier, warmer foods in fall and winter.

Whole Foods, Flame-Broiled

Food selection is only part of determining yin or yang. How food is processed or cooked can also tilt the balance in either direction, say the experts.

The first rule to keep in mind when choosing foods is to keep them whole whenever possible. That is, eat corn instead of corn puffs and whole-grain cereal instead of doughnuts.

Whole food is the most nutritious, says Dr. Shintani. "Whole food has a certain amount of bulk, fiber, micronutrients and biochemicals," he says. "When we limit the parts of foods that we eat, we're relegated to a minimum

---

Rice Is Nice

If it's a macrobiotic meal, it must include a whole grain, and in terms of balance, brown rice is thought to be the perfect food. Here are some rice concoctions that you're sure to encounter as a new macrobiotic cook.

Rice balls. The perfect packing food, the rice ball is Japan's answer to the sandwich. At the center is a pickled apricot-like Japanese fruit called an umeboshi plum. Brown rice is packed into a firm ball around it, then wrapped with nori (seaweed).

Rice syrup. Most of the sweeteners used in macrobiotic cooking are made from rice or other grains. Rice syrup has a light, delicate flavor and is good for pies, cakes and other desserts. Other rice sweeteners include amasake, a white fermented liquid made from sweet rice, and mirin, cooking wine made from fermented sweet rice.

Mochi. Pounded Japanese sweet rice, mochi is usually sold in small cubes at natural food stores. You can eat it as a snack or for dessert.

Rice porridge. Like its barley cousin, rice porridge is a very popular dish for people who are sick or have weak digestion. It's just rice cooked with twice as much water as you would normally use, so the grains become soft and creamy.

The Standard Macrobiotic Diet

The road to good health is paved with foods that balance the contrasting forces of yin and yang, says Michio Kushi, father of modern macrobiotics and founder of the Kushi Institute in Becket, Massachusetts. This is the diet that he recommends.

Daily Foods (Temperate Climate)

Your daily diet should consist of the following combination of foods.

- 50 to 60 percent whole grains, especially brown rice, barley, millet, oats, rye, corn and buckwheat.
- 20 to 25 percent vegetables, especially green leafy vegetables like bok choy and kale, round vegetables like acorn squash and brussels sprouts and root vegetables like carrots and daikon.
- 5 to 10 percent cooked beans and sea vegetables, especially adzuki beans, chickpeas and lentils and the seaweeds nori, wakame and kombu.
- 5 to 10 percent soups, especially miso soup.

Beverages

These beverages are recommended.

- Roasted bancha twig or stem tea, a naturally bland, decaffeinated tea.
- Roasted barley or brown rice tea.
- Dandelion tea.
- Moderate amounts of spring or well water (not iced).

Occasional Foods

The following foods may be eaten two or three times a week, if your condition permits.

- Fresh, nonfat, white-meat fish, like cod, halibut and flounder.
- Fermented foods such as pickles, eaten daily to stimulate appetite and encourage digestion.
- Dried, cooked or fresh fruit, provided it isn't tropical, eaten one to three times a week.

---

amount of their nutrients. Processed food also contains a lot of flour and sugar that isn't good for you, and you have to eat more of it to fill you up, which leads to weight gain."

The second rule may be a bit harder for those who embrace our modern plug-in lifestyle. Advocates of macrobiotics say that you should ditch your microwave, unplug the electric stove and start cooking with fire. If you can't take it that far, at least start cooking with a gas range, which approximates traditional food preparation because you're cooking over a more natural flame.

"We believe that electric ranges and microwave ovens alter the natural structure of foods," says Gale Jack, macrobiotics counselor and cooking in-

- Lightly roasted nuts and seeds, such as pumpkin seeds, sesame seeds, pecans, walnuts, almonds and peanuts.
- Seasonings, such as rice syrup and barley malt as sweeteners and vinegars such as brown rice vinegar or umeboshi vinegar.

Foods to Avoid

The following foods are considered too yin, or stimulating, and should be avoided.

- Tropical fruits such as bananas, coconuts, figs, kiwifruits, mangoes and papayas.
- Tropical-origin and "nightshade" vegetables such as potatoes, tomatoes, eggplant, peppers, asparagus, spinach and avocado.
- Dairy foods such as butter, cheese, cream, ice cream, milk and yogurt.
- Sweeteners such as corn syrup, honey, molasses, saccharin, refined sugar, chocolate, molasses and foods containing these ingredients.
- Alcohol.
- Spices such as mustard, pepper and curry.

The following foods are considered too yang, or heavy, and should be avoided.
- Eggs.
- Meat and poultry.
- Red-meat fish and other seafood such as salmon, swordfish and tuna (although eaten infrequently).

Macrobiotics experts also recommend avoiding the following foods.
- Coffee, green tea, colored tea, black tea, stimulating herbal teas such as peppermint, and artificial beverages like soda.
- Mayonnaise and other oily dressings; tropical oils like coconut and palm oil.
- Artificially colored, preserved, sprayed or chemically treated foods.
- Refined and polished grains and flours and foods made from them.
- Mass-produced and processed foods such as canned, frozen and irradiated foods.

structor at the Kushi Institute and co-author of *Amber Waves of Grain: American Macrobiotic Cooking*. "You may as well not even eat macrobiotically if you cook with a microwave."

Making It a Macrobiotic World

To an advocate of macrobiotics, it appears as if modern eating habits have raised the risk of more disease. The need to get back to tradition is especially pressing as our cancer rates continue to rise, says Kushi.

In his view, "Our departure from traditional foods is why the cancer rate in this country has risen from one in eight people to one in three during the

Oodles of Noodles

In Japan, street vendors sell noodles in the same way that American vendors sell hot dogs. You can eat them plain, with soy sauce or in soups.

Here, while you can't get Japanese noodles at a ball game, you can get them at many natural food stores. When buying these noodles for macrobiotic dishes, make sure that they are whole-wheat or buckwheat without any artificial ingredients or preservatives.

Ramen. Ramen noodles are either udon or soba noodles that have been deep-fried.

Saifun. These are clear cellophane noodles made from small Asian beans called mung beans.

Soba. This type is made of buckwheat and whole-wheat flour. The higher the percentage of buckwheat, the higher the quality—and the price.

Somen. Somen are slender whole-wheat noodles half as thick as udon noodles.

Udon. These whole-wheat flour noodles are wider and thicker than soba noodles but are lighter in texture and flavor.

past 45 years." It's why heart disease continues to be the number one killer.

"Finally, people are doing epidemiological studies linking sickness to diet," adds Kushi, who believes that these studies vindicate the long-held beliefs of macrobiotics practitioners. "Macrobiotics is everywhere now. The Ornish heart disease diet, the new food pyramid—they're all based on macrobiotic principles."

The rewards of macrobiotic conversion are great, especially if you embrace a macrobiotic lifestyle as well as the diet, says Alex Jack, director of the One Peaceful World Society in Becket, Massachusetts, and author of *Let Food Be Thy Medicine*. "Macrobiotic living emphasizes exercise, positive thinking, drug-free living and spirituality. It leads to good health, long life and clarity. You discover your dreams so you can reach your potential. People have so much ability, but we get stuck in unhealthy ways that cloud our thinking and drag us down."

Macrobiotic Healing

Peruse the macrobiotics section of any bookstore and you'll see that advocates believe that their diet can actually do more than keep you healthy. They think it also can heal, although not necessarily cure, almost any ailment—including cancer, heart disease, arthritis, AIDS and depression.

Like the diet itself, macrobiotic theories on healing are based on the principles of yin and yang. Practitioners of macrobiotics tend to think of the entire body system in terms of these polarities. Your upper body is expansive and therefore yin. Your lower body is grounded and therefore yang. Hollow organs are yin, solid organs are yang. Intestines are yin but produce solids, which are yang.

Threats to the body also fall into these categories, experts say. Harmful viruses and bacteria are yin compared to the healthy cells of the body, which are dense, compact and yang.

According to macrobiotics advocates, illness is not something that happens to us. Germs are part of our natural order, and it is our responsibility to keep our body immune from them. It is also our responsibility to avoid diseases that develop over time, like heart disease, explains Kushi. "Continually eating too many yang foods, for example, will eventually cause excesses in your body, like high cholesterol, and lead to disease."

"Changing your diet works because you're giving your body the kind of food it needs to run," says Dr. Shintani, who also believes that the right diet can reverse chronic conditions like heart disease and dabetes. He sums up the macrobiotic view of these processes: "It's like having a car that takes unleaded gasoline, but you've been putting in diesel fuel for years, and it just hasn't been working right. Put in the right fuel, and it'll start running better. You don't need medicines for many diseases; you need to restore metabolism, and you do that through diet."

Tofu to Go

When you're following a diet without cheese, meat or eggs, you need something to fill the gaps. That "something" in macrobiotics is beans or bean products like tofu.

Practically tasteless on its own, tofu adds flavor-absorbing texture to literally hundreds of macrobiotic meals. Scramble it in the morning instead of eggs, stuff it into pasta instead of ricotta cheese or pile it on a sandwich instead of lunch meat. Tofu provides an instant protein boost, with eight grams packed in four ounces, or one-quarter of a block.

Studies show that tofu and other soy products also contain genistein, a compound that acts as an anti-estrogen in the body and may prove to be a potent cancer preventive.

Mending a Broken Heart

The expanding and contracting of the human heart as it beats is one of the most beautiful expressions of yin and yang, says Kushi. In his book *Diet for a Strong Heart*, written with Alex Jack, Kushi describes how you can treat heart disease nutritionally once you determine if the condition has been brought on by too much yin or too much yang, or both.

Heart diseases that involve enlargement and swelling of the heart and blood vessels, such as congestive heart failure, cardiomyopathy (any disease affecting the heart muscle) and certain other types, are primarily yin in origin, says Kushi. Those that involve constriction of the heart and blood vessels, such as atherosclerosis (hardening of the arteries), high blood pressure and coronary heart disease, are primarily yang.

To heal conditions that are yang-based, Kushi recommends following the standard macrobiotic diet, limiting consumption of fish and other seafood until the condition improves and totally eliminating meat, alcohol,

Ch-Ch-Changes: Six Weeks to Macrobiotic Eating

Want to get on the macrobiotics path but don't know where it begins? The following is a sample guideline for what you would have to give up and add to your diet week by week to make the transition from an all-American diet to a macrobiotic one.

	Stop Eating	Start Eating
Week One	Meat and meat products	Beans and bean products (like tofu) with grains
Week Two	Dairy products and eggs	Soy milk and tofu-based, imitation dairy products
Week Three	Sugar, sugary foods and very sweet fruits, like oranges	Rice syrup, lightly roasted nuts and seeds, and apples and berries
Week Four	Hot spices and aromatic herbs	Soy sauce, brown rice and umeboshi vinegars
Week Five	Tropical-origin vegetables like tomatoes, peppers, eggplant, spinach, potatoes and asparagus	Root vegetables like carrots and daikon, round vegetables like squash and cauliflower, leafy green vegetables like kale and scallions and sea vegetables like nori and wakame
Week Six	Coffee, alcohol and strong herbal teas	Bancha tea and brown rice tea

sugar and refined flour. For people with yin-based heart conditions, Kushi recommends the standard macrobiotic diet, allowing fish two to three times a week and limiting raw salads, fresh fruit and sweet desserts until the condition improves.

A Nod of Approval from Researchers

Although only a few studies have investigated the macrobiotics-cardiovascular relationship specifically, the past 30 years have produced an abundance of research on many elements of macrobiotics, such as low-fat, high-fiber foods and fresh vegetables and their impact on cardiovascular health.

"Where macrobiotics is really on solid ground is with its cholesterol- and blood pressure–lowering effects," explains epidemiologist William Castelli, M.D., former director of the Framingham Heart Study and currently medical director of the Framingham Cardiovascular Institute in Framingham, Massachusetts. "After all, the vegetarian societies in central China, which are close to macrobiotic, have no atherosclerosis, no high cholesterol and no blood pressure problems."

Echoing those sentiments is Robert Wissler, M.D., chairman of the Department of Pathology at the University of Chicago, Billings Hospital, who doesn't recommend following macrobiotics to the letter but agrees with most of its principles when it comes to preventing heart disease.

"Dairy, eggs and meat fat are out of the question if you want to avoid ather-osclerosis. The American Heart Association's recommendation to stay below 30 percent fat a day just isn't adequate." Dr. Wissler endorses the fat intake level of macrobiotics, which is less than 20 percent of your daily diet.

According to macrobiotics experts, you only have to look at Harvard Medical School research from the 1960s and 1970s to see that they are right.

Harvard Hails Macrobiotic Principles

More than 20 years ago, Harvard researchers declared that meat con-sumption would eventually take a toll on your ticker. In their first study, they found that eating meat was directly related to increases in blood pres-sure. For four months, they studied 210 men and women who were eating macrobiotic diets. They discovered that the people who ate no meat at all had average blood pressures of 110/61 for the men and 101/58 for the women. Those readings were at least two points lower than the blood pres-sure of men and women who ate even small amounts of meat.

In a related study, the researchers found similar correlations between eating meat and artery-clogging blood cholesterol. "When we took a group of 21 young macrobiotic men and women and had them eat roast beef and potatoes every night for a month, their cholesterol rose significantly—19 percent," says Dr. Castelli. "When they went back to their regular diet, it dropped again.

"This diet has got to be one of the healthiest in terms of longevity," he says. "Studies have shown that the Japanese fishermen who eat the old Jap-anese rural diet outlive everyone, and that's basically Michio Kushi's diet."

Just ask Dr. Spock, who shed 50 pounds and recovered from the ef-fects of a heart attack and stroke through macrobiotic eating. "I'm certainly skeptical about some of the things macrobiotics are opposed to, like eating tropical fruits," he says. "But the low-fat recommendations are right on the money. And my symptoms are gone, so I'm not going to start experimenting with the other aspects of the diet just to see whether or not they're correct."

Combating Cancer

Although major medical organizations like the National Cancer Institute concede that dietary measures may be helpful in the prevention of cancer, treating cancer with diet is not accepted in modern medical circles. In the macrobiotics community, however, it's another story.

While nobody is proclaiming that macrobiotics is the cure for cancer, people with personal stories of remissions have been enough to keep hope alive. Among them are a number of high-profile celebrities. Dirk Benedict, star of *Battlestar Galactica* and *The A-Team*, who wrote *Confessions of a Kamikaze Cowboy*, recounted his recovery from prostate cancer, attributing that recovery to macrobiotics. And although he died of cancer years later, Anthony Sattilaro, M.D., told his tale of remission from prostate cancer that had metastasized to his bones in his book *Recalled by Life*, which was a tribute to the macrobiotic diet he followed.

Try It for a Week

According to specialists in macrobiotics, you should make adjustments throughout the year to cook tasty, healthy meals for every season.

In summer, include more corn, long-grain rice, greens, summer fruits and bitter-tasting foods. The cooking time is shorter, and you should use less salt. In fall, include more round and root vegetables, short-grain rice, millet, autumn fruits such as apples, and pungent-tasting foods.

When winter comes along, you should include more root vegetables, buckwheat, rice and dried fruits. The cooking time is longer, and you should use more salt. Spring is a time for a few more greens, wheat, oats, barley and sour-tasting foods.

The following is a typical spring menu as prescribed at the Kushi Institute in Becket, Massachusetts. Beverages should be kept to a minimum, but roasted bancha tea, roasted brown rice tea, roasted barley tea, dandelion tea and spring or well water are preferred. If some of these foods are unfamiliar, see "New Food Review" on page 38 for descriptions.

Sunday Breakfast—Soft millet and onions; miso soup with leeks, corn and broccoli; steamed kale

Lunch—Rice balls; carrots and tops with toasted sesame seeds; Chinese cabbage pickles and daikon

Snack—Steamed sourdough bread with parsnip jam

Dinner—Rice with wheat berries; clear broth with tofu chunks and chives; chick-peas with umeboshi vinegar and squash; arame (a sea vegetable) with string beans, daikon and cauliflower; quick-sautéed dandelion greens; soy sauce and grated ginger for seasoning

Monday Breakfast—Soft rice with wheat berries; miso soup with daikon, shiitake mushrooms and toasted mochi; steamed cabbage

Lunch—Wheat bread slices with sweet-and-sour chick-pea puree

Snack—Carrot juice

Dinner—Rice and barley; udon noodles and summer squash in broth with soy sauce and shiitake mushrooms; natto with nori and scallions; sautéed burdock, carrots, onions and dried tofu; blanched collard greens with sauerkraut

Tuesday Breakfast—Soft rice and barley; miso soup with carrots, parsley, steamed Chinese cabbage and scallions

Lunch—Rice and barley salad with leftover sautéed vegetables

Snack—Boiled or steamed corn on the cob

"Cancer is challenging. Some people have remission; some feel better; some we can do nothing for," says Kushi. His own tragic experience taught him the unpredictability of cancer: He lost his daughter to cervical cancer, although he says she lived two years longer than her doctors expected.

Dinner—Rice; miso soup with scallions; pureed broccoli soup; adzuki beans with wheat berries and squash; dandelion greens and daikon; red cabbage and quick-pickled watercress

Wednesday Breakfast—Rice porridge with daikon, celery, watercress and miso; boiled cabbage and carrots

Lunch—Sushi; adzuki beans with squash and wheat berries; steamed watercress

Snack—Mochi (pounded sweet rice) with nori

Dinner—Rice and oats; split-pea soup with celery, carrots and onions; boiled daikon and squash; stewed tofu with fu (toasted wheat gluten), Chinese cabbage and shiitake mushrooms, with or without fish; raw salad; steamed green apple with rice syrup

Thursday Breakfast—Soft rice and whole oats; miso soup with cauliflower, leeks and dulse; steamed watercress

Lunch—Leftover tofu stew with udon noodles; leftover boiled vegetables; steamed celery

Snack—Blanched celery with tofu and umeboshi

Dinner—Rice and barley; lentils with leeks and corn, dried daikon and kombu; creamy onion soup, quick-sautéed Chinese cabbage with broccoli and celery; quick-pickled cucumbers, wakame and chives in umeboshi vinegar

Friday Breakfast—Soft rice and barley; miso soup with squash, onions and parsley; quick pickles

Lunch—Rice and barley with blanched vegetables; pureed lentils; dried daikon and kombu

Snack—Sweet vegetable drink

Dinner—Rice and chick-peas; millet soup with onions, parsnips and cabbage; boiled onions, cauliflower and carrots; quick-sautéed tempeh, cabbage, leeks and sauerkraut; turnips and turnip tops

Saturday Breakfast—Whole-oat porridge; steamed bread with parsnip jam; boiled salad with carrots and broccoli

Lunch—Rice and chick-pea balls; udon noodles in broth; leftover boiled vegetables; quick-pickled bok choy and carrots

Snack—Carrot juice and 1 slice steamed wheat bread

Dinner—Barley stew with corn, daikon, shiitake mushrooms and miso; tofu and scallions wrapped in nori; steamed kale with lemon juice and toasted sunflower seeds

Science Meets Yin—And Yang

Scientists still don't really know what causes cancer to appear in the body, much less what makes it go away. They do know that when cancer does occur, it's the result of a mutated cell that multiplies out of control, crowding out or taking over vital organs and causing them to fail.

The macrobiotic theory holds that cancer is a consequence of extremes, mostly dietary ones. Cancers that appear in deeper, lower, compact organs of the body such as the prostate are the result of too many yang foods like eggs, fish, meat, poultry, cheese and salty or hard baked foods, says Kushi. Cancers in more hollow, expanded organs such as the breast are from too many yin foods, like soft drinks, sugar, milk, citrus fruit, stimulants, chemicals, refined flour and foods containing artificial additives, he says.

In his book *The Cancer Prevention Diet*, Kushi categorizes common cancers as either yin or yang and then prescribes a diet accordingly. He says that yin cancers are those of the outer regions of the brain, the breast, esophagus, mouth, skin and stomach, as well as of the blood (leukemia) and lymph nodes (lymphomas). Yang cancers are those of the inner regions of the brain, the bones, colon, ovary, pancreas, prostate and rectum. And those caused by extremes of both include cancers of the bladder and kidney, liver, lung, spleen, lower stomach, tongue and uterus.

According to Kushi, people with yin-based cancers need to tilt their food selections to the yang side, possibly eating small amounts of fish once or twice a week, favoring cooked root vegetables and completely shunning fruits and extreme yin desserts. Those with yang-based cancers need more yin energy and may eat some dried or cooked fruits and lots of quick-cooked, crisp, green, leafy vegetables. For all cancers, Kushi advises strictly avoiding meat, eggs, poultry and dairy products, as well as oily, greasy foods and nuts and nut butters.

The Hormone Connection

Although there is almost no research on macrobiotics and cancer specifically, one lone (and very small) study has indicated that among people with certain cancers, a macrobiotic diet may make a difference.

The study was done at Tulane University in New Orleans, where researchers studied people with pancreatic and prostate cancer. They found that among 18 people with prostate cancer, which had spread to other organs, 9 who turned to macrobiotic diets lived an average of 14 years, compared with 7 years among those who made no dietary changes. Similarly, 23 people with pancreatic cancer who adopted a macrobiotic diet lived more than twice as long than those who did not.

Although he allows that the soy foods and vegetables in the macrobiotic diet may have had some anti-carcinogenic effects on the people in this study, lead researcher James P. Carter, M.D., professor of nutrition and chairman of the Nutrition Section in the Department of Applied Health Sciences at Tulane University School of Public Health and Tropical Medicine, believes it was the low-fat element of macrobiotics that really made the difference.

"This diet works in cancers that are responsive to hormones, like breast, prostate, ovarian and pancreas, because fat is a promoter of their progression. If you restrict daily fat intake to no more than 10 to 12 percent, it holds the cancer in check," says Dr. Carter.

One Woman's Story

Not surprisingly, some of the strongest advocates of macrobiotics are those who believe that the diet has been a crucial factor in the remission of their cancer. Elaine Nussbaum of New Jersey, author of *Recovery from Cancer*, was so elated after her recovery from body-wide cancer that she earned her master's degree in nutrition and became a macrobiotics teacher.

"I was diagnosed with uterine cancer back in 1980. It was a carcinosarcoma embedded in the lining of the uterus—a tumor that was too large to be removed. I was treated with radiation, chemotherapy and hormone medication before undergoing a radical hysterectomy. The doctors wanted me to stay on chemotherapy for two years after that. Before the end of the two years, the cancer spread to my bones and both lungs. My vertebrae were collapsing. I couldn't even stand. So we started again—more radiation, more chemotherapy. I was getting sicker and sicker. By the end of 1982, I was terminally ill," recalls Nussbaum.

"In February 1983, I stopped all medical treatments and began a macrobiotic approach. Within a year, I was free of the cancer," she says.

Under Pressure

Women in ancient China—probably tired of waiting around all day for their beans and rice to cook—used to boil their grains in massive cauldrons, placing stones on the lids to seal the steam inside. The trapped steam raised the temperature, so cooking in these pots produced moister, sweeter grains and legumes in less time than ordinary boiling.

While we may not have massive cast-iron cauldrons, we do have the equivalent—pressure cookers. Today's models are equipped with release valves and steam nozzles to make for safe, efficient cooking. A new pressure cooker comes with instructions from the manufacturer, which should be followed for safety. For best results, macrobiotic cooks recommend filling your pressure cooker no more than three-quarters full of grains and water.

Double Recovery

Another believer is Sam Axelrod of Lauderhill, Florida, who says he cured himself of cancer—not once but twice.

The first time he had prostate cancer. His doctor was in the process of setting up a series of 35 radiation treatments when a cousin told Axelrod about macrobiotics. After a lifetime of "pigging out," he says he never felt better than he did on the macrobiotic regimen. "I lost 50 pounds. I had so much confidence that this diet could cure me, I refused the radiation treatments." Within a year, he was cancer-free.

After several years of slipping from macrobiotics and following his sweet tooth, he had another cancer episode. "My urologist found a 3½-centimeter mass on my left kidney," says Axelrod. "All the signs were cancerous, so they wanted to take samples of the kidney. I wanted to wait." Six months later—with Axelrod still indulging his sweet tooth—the mass had grown to 5½ centimeters. "The doctor said, 'You have to have that kidney taken out right away.'"

Instead, Axelrod consulted Kushi, who recommended a strict macrobiotic diet—no deviations, no indulgences. "In two years, I had the best blood test I ever had," Axelrod recalls. "My cholesterol was 117. The 5½-centimeter growth completely disappeared."

How does this happen?

"We're still trying to find out," says Dr. Castelli, who has met people in remission due to macrobiotics. "Clearly, the diet helps regulate the immune system, but you have to remember that diets high in cholesterol and saturated fat are associated with increased cancer. Tumors don't do well without cholesterol. There are studies at the National Cancer Institute using tremendous doses of cholesterol-lowering drugs to treat cancer. Macrobiotics lowers cholesterol naturally."

Potential Healing

In addition to fighting cancer, advocates say, macrobiotics may offer an alternative way to help recover from other kinds of disease. In fact, many advocates of macrobiotics swear by its broadly curative powers.

According to Kushi, practitioners of macrobiotics see a connection between eating chicken and various forms of arthritis, so the macrobiotic diet, which excludes chicken, has benefits for arthritis sufferers.

Kushi claims it can help with diabetes, too. He points out that the dietary guidelines set by the American Diabetes Association (ADA) are similar to those for the macrobiotic diet. The ADA guidelines emphasize eating 50 to 60 percent of your daily diet as carbohydrates and cutting out fat. They also warn against sugar, especially glucose and glucose-containing natural sugars like sucrose and lactose, which are both found in milk.

"Macrobiotics does a great job of keeping blood sugar in control," says Dr. Castelli. "Like atherosclerosis and high cholesterol, diabetes is not a problem for vegetarian societies in central China that basically follow a macrobiotic diet."

Not surprisingly, macrobotics can also be effective if you're overweight—a factor that raises your risk of diabetes, heart disease and many other conditions. "Eating macrobiotically is good for weight loss because it focuses on whole foods, which have a higher mass-to-calorie ratio than processed foods, so you need to eat less to feel full," says Dr. Shintani, who uses a macrobiotic diet to help his patients lose weight. "Too many people now are focusing on low-fat foods, which are often loaded with sugar and white flour. By giving people whole, natural foods instead, people become healthy and the weight just comes off."

Other advocates claim that macrobiotics can help control Crohn's disease, a deterioration of the intestinal wall that impairs digestion and nutrient absorption.

It's also said that macrobiotics can lift depression and put a lid on aggression. "All the animal protein and sugar in the American diet can lead to pretty aggressive behavior," observes Gale Jack.

"We see mood changes all the time when people start macrobiotics," adds Kushi. "They become more peaceful and happy. Even their tastes change—instead of listening to rock music, they prefer jazz."

Discharging Your Disease

Those who promote macrobiotics for treating disease note that macrobiotic healing is not like taking medication, where you often feel better shortly after the pill hits your stomach. In fact, macrobiotics counselors teach that, depending on the severity of your condition, you may end up feeling worse before you feel better.

"When you start doing macrobiotics, you eliminate the accumulated excess, like mucus, from poor eating," explains Kushi. The process is called discharging.

The macrobiotic theory is that your body is filled with accumulated toxins from years of eating bad foods, and you've grown accustomed to the stimulating effects of those foods. When you stop eating them, your body goes through an adjustment period. Common discharge symptoms can include fatigue, mild aches and pains, fever, chills, coughing, perspiration, frequent urination, skin discharges or rashes, unusual body odor, diarrhea or constipation, decrease in sexual appetite, temporary cessation of menstruation and irritability.

But advocates insist these symptoms—if they occur—are temporary, and you'll feel better once the toxins have been discharged from your body.

The Macrobiotic Makeover

So you're ready for a macrobiotic makeover, but you're not sure where to begin. Before you put coals in your cookstove and start simmering brown rice, your best plan is to find an easy-to-follow macrobiotics cookbook and enroll in some cooking classes, advises Wendy Esko, macrobiotics cooking teacher at the Kushi Institute and co-author of *Aveline Kushi's Introducing Macrobiotic Cooking*.

"Macrobiotics isn't easy, because the food is unfamiliar to most people," says Esko. "You need hands-on training, so you know how the finished product is supposed to taste. It takes a while before you get comfortable enough to be creative."

But even before you start cooking, you have to restock your kitchen. You'll need to purge your pantry of all the "improvements" of modern cookery—including any food containing sugar, food that is artificially colored or flavored, processed food and food containing animal products (except fish). You'll also have to expunge all dairy products and eggs. Then bring in the new.

Pucker Up for Pickles

While most Americans think of pickles as something to toss on burgers, macrobiotic eaters believe that they aid digestion and stimulate appetite, so they should be eaten daily.

Unlike the typical conventional pickles most of us know, macrobiotic pickles are generally not made from cucumbers and are almost never dill. Instead they're made from a wide variety of vegetables, from turnips to cabbage. And instead of being aged in vinegar, they're pickled in sea salt, soy sauce or miso, a paste made from fermented soybeans and grains. In macrobiotics, the strength of the pickles is based on how long the pickles are fermented. Short-time, or quick pickles, are made in a few hours, while long-time pickles can take months.

You can make your own pickles—a popular practice in macrobiotic cooking—with a small pickle press that can be ordered from Asian food supply companies. It's a clear glass or plastic container with a screw-down plate attached to the inside of the lid. Put in the sliced vegetables, add salt, miso or another fermenting agent, tighten the plate on top of the food and let it sit in a cool dark place. Leave it just a few hours if you want short-time pickles, or months, if you want to try the flavor of long-time pickles.

Unfortunately, many of the foods that make up the "bread and butter" of the macrobiotic diet haven't yet found their way into mainstream grocery stores, so you'll probably have to bypass your usual supermarket and find a natural foods store. If there are none in your area, you can order macrobiotic foods from a variety of mail-order companies, including those that are listed in "Resources for Healing" on pages 56 and 68.

Cooking Power

Just as a fine Italian chef needs a pasta maker and a garlic press, a macrobiotic cook needs the proper tools to make the best meals.

The basics include pots and frying pans, but none of this cookware should be aluminum, since aluminum is considered toxic in macrobiotics. Apart from the basics, though, the one item that you'll certainly want most in your macrobiotic kitchen is a pressure cooker. With its heavy-walled construction and gasketed lid, this handy item works by cooking foods at higher temperatures than you could ever reach with a conventional cooker. You'll save hours when you're cooking dried grains and beans.

Many macrobiotic meals include pickles. But since you're not supposed to eat the chemicals, preservatives and extreme spices often used in commercial pickles, another helpful appliance is a pickle press. This utensil, which you can order from macrobiotics product distributors like the Kushi Institute store (see "Resources for Healing" on page 56), allows you to turn almost any vegetable into a pickle in a matter of hours.

And finally, since the slicing and dicing of vegetables is almost as important in macrobiotic cooking as the vegetables themselves, you may want to invest in a fine-bladed Japanese vegetable knife.

"How you slice a vegetable yields different tastes and energies," says Esko. "Grated or finely sliced carrots, for instance, are lighter in taste and energy than thick, round slices." Following the theme of yin and yang, macrobiotic cooks suggest that you use a wide array of shapes and sizes in each meal. If you already have fat florets of broccoli in your soup, for instance, add thin carrot slivers for balance.

Getting Set for a Macro Meal

As you might imagine, with all of this slow cooking and attention to detail, macrobiotic meals take longer to cook than your average instant microwave dinner. In fact, they generally take more than an hour, although macrobiotics proponents swear that every minute you devote to this cookery is eminently worth it.

"People have to set priorities, and health should be on top of that list," says Gale Jack.

The hardest part is the withdrawal that some people experience when giving up foods they're used to, especially those that contain sugar and caffeine. After that, you have to get used to new foods. It's easy to enjoy brown rice and vegetables, but your first sample of seaweed may taste like a sip from the ocean. When you add soy sauce, sea salt, miso soup and pickles, don't be surprised if your mouth begins to pucker.

Macrobiotics counselors aren't kidding when they say that macrobiotics is more than a diet: It's a way of life.

To Supplement or Not to Supplement

Although macrobiotics counselors often advise against vitamin and mineral supplements because they aren't natural, nutritionists say that if you're on macrobiotics, you'd better supplement your diet with vitamin B_{12}. Stored in the tissues of animals, vitamin B_{12} does not exist in the plant kingdom. Although it can be produced during fermentation, and some macrobiotics experts say you can get enough B_{12} from fermented soybean foods like miso, doctors say it's best not to take chances. Because vitamin B_{12} deficiency can cause permanent nerve and cell damage, you should get at least 3 micrograms per day, according to Elson M. Haas, M.D., medical director of the Preventive Medical Center of Marin in San Rafael, California, and author of *Staying Healthy with Nutrition*. Just to make sure you're getting enough, Dr. Haas says you can take supplements every two or three days to get a total of about 100 micrograms per week.

These supplements are especially important for children who are eating macrobiotic diets, say researchers. In one population-based study conducted in the Netherlands, researchers found that babies between 4 and 18 months of age who were fed macrobiotic diets were deficient in vitamin B_{12}, protein, vitamin D, calcium and riboflavin, which resulted in retarded growth, fat and muscle wasting and slower psychomotor development. Although macrobiotics practitioners say that such deficiencies are the result of children not eating a wide enough variety of foods, Dr. Castelli recommends giving multivitamins to any children who are on a macrobiotic diet.

As for adults, "you won't make it as an interior lineman on this diet," says Dr. Castelli, "but if you eat the right amount of greens, the right variety of beans and vegetables and some fish, you can get everything you need. I would still recommend that children, pregnant women and people just starting macrobiotics supplement the B vitamins, especially B_{12} and folic acid, because they can be difficult to get."

The bottom line, says Dr. Haas, is that while the macrobiotic diet is clearly healthier than the average American diet, it's still possible to miss some important nutrients.

"As long as people feel well, they can continue following the diet without worrying about supplementation," he says. "If they start to notice symptoms of deficiency, such as fatigue, coldness and hair loss, they need to make adaptations. It's not uncommon for people following a macrobiotic diet to take a multivitamin/mineral supplement as well as some extra vitamin C, vitamin E, calcium and magnesium."

If you want to switch to a macrobiotic diet to help alleviate the symptoms of a specific disease, that's fine, too, says Dr. Haas. Just make sure you clear it with your doctor and don't forgo any regular treatments that may have been prescribed for you.

Resources for Healing

Organizations

The International Macrobiotic Directory
c/o Bob Mattson
1050 40th Street
Oakland, CA 94609

The Kushi Institute
P.O. Box 7
Becket, MA 01223

One Perfect World
P.O. Box 10
Becket, MA 01223
(Operator of Macrobiotics Online—
www.macrobiotics.org)

Mail-Order Food Source

Kushi Foundation Store
P.O. Box 38
Becket, MA 01223

Books

Aveline Kushi's Complete Guide to Macrobiotic Cooking
Aveline Kushi with Alex Jack
Warner Books

Aveline Kushi's Introducing Macrobiotic Cooking
Aveline Kushi with Wendy Esko
Japan Publications

The Cancer Prevention Diet
Michio Kushi with Alex Jack
St. Martin's Press

Holistic Health through Macrobiotics
Michio Kushi with Edward Esko
Japan Publications

4 Chinese Nutrition

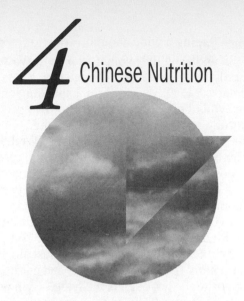

Three Thousand Years of Healing with Food

After 17 years of living with Crohn's disease, Gabriel decided he'd had enough.

The disease is far more than an uncomfortable annoyance. Crohn's causes progressive deterioration of the intestine. People who have it are plagued with constant episodes of diarrhea, bloating, pain and fatigue. Doctors often prescribe steroids, but when Gabriel took the medication, it only made him feel worse. As a last resort, this Los Angeles resident went to see a doctor of Chinese medicine in L.A.

Gabriel says the doctor diagnosed him as a "yang" person. "He put me on a strict cooling (yin) diet to counteract the Crohn's, which is considered a heat, or yang, condition," says Gabriel. "I ate lots of vegetables and grains—no meat, dairy, spices, salt or refined sugar. Within two months I was off the steroids, and though I'm still not off all of my medications, I hardly have any symptoms."

Welcome to the world of Chinese nutrition, where your body, your food and your health all hang in delicate balance. Tilting this balance toward better—or worse—health are the two opposite yet complementary forces of yin and yang. According to Chinese philosophy, these two forces are present in everything in the universe, and in Chinese medicine, all health treatment boils down to keeping yin and yang in balance.

Like Night and Day

Although yin and yang may sound strange to Western ears, you can remember them easily by thinking of night and day. Yin is like night—cool, contracting and dark. Yang is day—warm, expanding and light. In the well-known yin-yang symbol that looks like two polliwogs chasing each other's tails, the dark portion is yin, while the light is yang.

How do these qualities express themselves? Well, imagine a tanned, pumped Sylvester Stallone standing next to a milky, cerebral Meryl Streep, and you can see how the qualities are reflected in people. Sly would be considered a yang—a hard-driving, take-no-prisoners, Type-A personality. Yang folks are dominating, outgoing and aggressive.

According to Chinese medicine experts, those traits make the yangs susceptible to all kinds of hyper-energy problems. You can expect a yang person to suffer from tension and congestion, musculoskeletal pains, headaches, constipation, high blood pressure and cardiovascular disease.

Directly opposite the hot oven is the fridge—yin people, who are considered cool, collected types. They're the ones you'll find sitting on mountaintops reflecting about life. And because they'd rather toss around ideas than lift dumbbells, they tend to have small, softer builds. If they become too yin, however, they can have problems with lethargy, overweight, intestinal problems like diarrhea and headaches.

Somewhere in the Spectrum

Even though the yin-yang differences are clear-cut, people are not. Streep, for instance, is unlikely to have much of a problem with overweight, and if you saw her in *The River Wild*, you know she and Sly have a lot in common when it comes to toughing it out. So we're really talking about a tendency rather than a formula.

"Although most people fall somewhere in the middle of the yin-yang spectrum, they clearly lean one way or the other," says Roger Jahnke, O.M.D., a doctor of Oriental medicine who practices Chinese medicine in Santa Barbara, California. He compares these traits to a marriage in which each person provides a temperamental balance to the other. "One's always cold and trying to warm themselves against the other, who's always warm," he observes.

Your goal for optimum health is to be like the swirling black and white of the yin-yang itself—perfectly balanced. And one of the best ways to do that, say Chinese medicine experts, is by choosing carefully what you eat every day.

"Food is *so* important in Chinese health and healing," observes Martha Howard, M.D., a physician in private practice and co-director of Wellness Associates in Chicago, who has studied and practices both Chinese and Western medicine. "In fact, there are whole restaurants in China dedicated to making dishes according to people's diagnoses."

In the Balance

Although you've probably never said "Gosh, I'm yin today," if you've ever felt sluggish and cold, you've been yin. Likewise, if you've ever felt hot and hyperactive, you've been yang. And even though we all have a mixture of these qualities that are recognized by Chinese medicine experts, those doctors say that we're generally dominant in one or the other.

To determine which is dominant for you, put a checkmark beside the traits listed below that most describe you.

Yin	Yang
_____Low-energy, lethargic	_____High-energy, hyperactive
_____Intuitive	_____Intellectual
_____Introverted	_____Outgoing
_____Weak voice	_____Loud voice
_____Low appetite	_____Ferocious appetite
_____Pale complexion	_____Ruddy, flushed complexion
_____Gain weight easily	_____Lose weight easily
_____Small, flaccid body	_____Large, firm body
_____Delicate features	_____Coarse features
_____Exercise-avoidant	_____Exercise-oriented
_____Prone to lethargy, diarrhea oversleeping	_____Prone to tension, constipation or or insomnia
_____Tends to feel cold and/or damp	_____Tends to feel warm and/or dry

If you lean one way or the other, look at these lists of warming and cooling foods for food recommendations. If you're not generally at either of the extremes but somewhere in the middle, you're balanced, so you may choose a balance of foods from both groups.

Warming Foods (Yin)	Cooling Foods (Yang)
Chicken	Wheat
Lamb	Mung beans
Garlic	Watermelon
Ginger	Fresh fruit juices
Onions	Most vegetables
Black beans	

NOTE: Yin should not eat cold, raw foods, and yang should not eat hot, spicy foods.

Some restaurants in San Francisco now do the same, according to Elson Haas, M.D., medical director of the Preventive Medical Center of Marin in San Rafael, California, and author of *Staying Healthy with Nutrition*.

From Soy to Shining Seaweed

Surely it comes as no surprise that a Chinese nutrition diet requires one special ingredient—Chinese food. There's always takeout, of course. But to do this right, you really need to get in the habit of shopping and cooking Chinese-style.

Here's a short guide to some of the new foods that await you in the world of Chinese nutrition. If you don't have a bona fide Chinese market nearby, look for these foods in natural food stores or check the mail-order sources listed in "Resources for Healing" on page 68.

Beans and Beyond

Legumes such as beans and peas are nutritious, and they're high in protein. Beans and bean products like tofu are an especially important component of the mostly vegetarian Chinese diet.

Mung beans. Favored in Asian cooking, these green beans are small and slightly sweet. They go well in soups and with grains.

Soy milk. Soybeans are mashed, boiled and filtered to make this milk substitute, which doesn't really taste like milk. It's sweet and slightly thick.

Tempeh. Tempeh is a product made of processed soybeans that have been fermented. It's chewy and light, with a sweet, mushroom-like aroma. Like tofu, tempeh makes a good filler, but it should always be cooked.

Tofu. Developed thousands of years ago in China, tofu is made of processed soybeans that are shaped into a white, rectangular cake. Almost tasteless on its own, tofu absorbs other flavors like a sponge and makes a great filler. You can cut it into chunks and use it raw in salads or add it to lasagna instead of cheese. (An added benefit is that tofu contains genistein, a compound that some researchers believe may be a powerful cancer preventive.)

Great Grains

Whole grains are considered to be the heart and soul of a balanced Chinese diet. Chinese nutritionists prefer unprocessed grains, although they take much

Minding Your Yins and Yangs

A principle of Chinese medicine is that food keeps you healthy or makes you ill by generating either yin or yang energy in the body—that is, either cooling you down or warming you up. "This is much more important to understand than how many vitamins or minerals a food has, because it's these properties that affect balance," says Maoshing Ni, Ph.D., co-founder and vice-president of Yo San University of Traditional Chinese Medicine in Santa Monica, California, and co-author of *The Tao of Nutrition*.

Cooling and warming do not refer to the immediate state of food, like whether it's refrigerated or hot off the stove, says Dr. Ni. What you really have to consider are its long-term effects on your body. Black tea, for instance, produces cool energy even if you drink it hot. A chili pepper is

longer to cook than instant grains. They are generally soaked and boiled or pressure-cooked.

Barley. Commonly sold as hulled barley, this grain is light brown and a little fatter than rice. You'll find it soft, chewy and bland, but it adds a nice texture to soups and vegetable dishes.

Couscous. A fine, round grain that comes from the heart of duram wheat, couscous tastes sweet and goes well with fruits and vegetables.

Millet. Like couscous, millet is small and compact. It fluffs up when cooked, has a nutty flavor and goes well with beans or other grains.

Wheat. Wheat is used in many forms in Chinese cooking, from wheat noodles to "wheat meat," or wheat gluten, which is a salty, tender meat substitute made from wheat, seaweed and soy.

Deep-Sea Vegetables

Seaweeds are a daily staple in Chinese cooking because they are rich sources of minerals, especially iron, calcium and iodine. They can be boiled or sautéed with other foods or toasted and crushed as a condiment for soups, salads and grains. They have a delicate texture, but you may have to get used to their salty, fishy taste.

Arame. This is one of the milder sea vegetables. Resembling wiry black threads, it makes a good side dish, especially when cooked with vegetables.

Kombu. A popular accompaniment to grains, beans and root vegetables, kombu comes in dried sheets that are cut for cooking. Chinese cooks believe that adding kombu to beans increases their digestibility.

Nori. Mild-flavored nori comes in dried sheets in which you can roll up grains, vegetables and fish. You can also toast it and crush the pieces to sprinkle on salads, soups and grain dishes.

Wakame. This seaweed is similar to kombu except that it is thinner and cooks more quickly.

warming even if you pop it into your mouth straight from the fridge.

And it's not an either/or proposition. Foods fall somewhere in a spectrum ranging from hot to cold. Chinese nutrition actually recognizes five different, distinct degrees of food "temperature"—hot (yang), warm, neutral, cool and cold (yin).

For balance, it's helpful to determine your constitution—whether you're more yin or more yang—and eat accordingly, say Chinese nutrition experts. "Very basically, if you're hot and dry, you need to emphasize raw, cooling, juicy foods. If you're cool and feeling sluggish, you need to stress cooked, warming foods," says Harriet Beinfield, L.Ac., a licensed acupuncturist and Chinese medicine specialist at Chinese Medicine Works in San Francisco and co-author of *Between Heaven and Earth: A Guide to Chinese Medicine.*

Try It for a Week

A typical Chinese nutrition menu varies with the seasons. If you try the menu shown here, keep in mind that it's for spring and summer. For fall and winter eating, replace the cooling tropical fruits and green salads with hearty soups and cooked autumn vegetables like yams and black beans. You can find foods like seaweed and soy milk in natural food stores. The following dietary recommendations are from *The Tao of Nutrition* by Maoshing Ni, Ph.D., and Cathy McNease.

Monday Breakfast—Cream of rice or wheat with raisins and cinnamon; steamed apple slices
Lunch—Tofu and Spinach Soup; rice cake with nut butter
Dinner—Stir-fried vegetables with tofu and wheat gluten, served over brown rice

Tuesday Breakfast—Scrambled tofu with tomato and zucchini; brown rice with pecans
Lunch—Mushroom soup with whole-wheat noodles; couscous with steamed peanuts; papaya slices
Dinner—Baked yam; tofu with seaweed on rice

Wednesday Breakfast—Cornbread with banana, apple, pineapple and soy milk
Lunch—Fruit salad with soy yogurt and almonds; rice milk
Dinner—Tomato-mushroom sauce over whole-wheat noodles and tempeh cubes; steamed broccoli

Thursday Breakfast—Couscous with grated apples and raisins; soy milk
Lunch—Nori wrapped around rice and steamed carrots with cilantro
Dinner—Vegetable and tofu stir-fry on rice

Friday Breakfast—Steamed pineapple cornbread; almond pudding
Lunch—Pita with sprouts, lentils and carrots; green salad with tofu
Dinner—Tofu sautéed with mushrooms and bell peppers; brown rice; steamed eggplant

Have a Taste

How are you supposed to know if you're eating the right foods to cool you off or warm you up? Taste them, says Henry C. Lu, Ph.D., director of the Academy of Oriental Heritage in British Columbia and author of several books on Chinese medicine, including *The Chinese System of Food Cures*.

It sounds simple, but think about it. While eating a Western diet, we're likely to say "It tastes good" or "I don't like it"—and our judgment stops right there. In fact, we're so used to thinking that nutritious foods are unappetizing that people sling around phrases like "If it tastes good, it can't be good for you!"

In Chinese culture, however, judging which foods to eat and which not to eat goes way beyond basic likes and dislikes. Taste is an indicator of a food's quality, particularly its yin and yang energy. And yes, according to

Saturday Breakfast—Cereal with dates, raisins and sunflower seeds

Lunch—Summer vegetable soup; whole-wheat pita bread with avocado and bean sprouts

Dinner—Couscous with millet and assorted vegetables; green salad with sesame seeds

Sunday Breakfast—Scrambled tofu with egg; couscous and vegetables; soy milk

Lunch—Pureed chick-peas spread on whole-wheat bread; apple slices

Dinner—Vegetable stir-fry; brown rice with soybeans, peanuts and pecans

....

Tofu and Spinach Soup

Yield: 4 servings

This soup nourishes the brain as well as soothing the heart, fighting cholesterol and cleaning the blood vessels. It is rich in protein and other nutrients.

- 3 cups water
- $\frac{1}{2}$ cup vegetable broth
- 1 package tofu, rinsed and cubed
- $\frac{1}{2}$ bunch spinach, cleaned and chopped
- 1 tomato, peeled, seeded and sliced
- 1 teaspoon salt, or to taste
- $\frac{1}{4}$ teaspoon hot-pressed sesame oil
-    Pepper to taste

In a 2-quart saucepan, bring the water and broth to a boil. Reduce the heat and add the tofu, spinach, tomatoes and salt. Add the sesame oil and pepper and simmer.

....

this system of belief, sweet foods can be good for you.

Chinese nutrition experts say that food is divided into five flavors—*pungent*, such as green onions, chives and parsley; *sweet*, such as sugar, chestnuts and bananas; *sour*, such as lemons, pears and plums; *bitter*, such as hops, lettuce and vinegar; and *salty*, such as table salt and seaweed. As a rule of thumb, foods that are sweet and pungent have yang, or warming energy, and those that are sour, salty and bitter have yin, or cooling energy.

A Rainbow of Flavors

You can also tell whether most foods are yin or yang simply by looking at them, notes Paul Pitchford, director of the Oriental Healing Arts Program at the Heartwood Institute in Garberville, California, and author of *Healing with Whole Foods*.

If the foods are cool in color—such as blue, green or purple—they are generally yin. If they are red, orange or yellow—warm colors—they're most likely yang. Also, foods that grow quickly (are less dense) like lettuce are more yin, as are raw foods, says Pitchford. Those that take longer to grow (are more dense) or are slow-cooked are more yang. In general, the higher the caloric content, the more yang the food probably is.

But what about a food like chicken? Experts admit that it's hard to tell. "You just have to study and learn them," says Dr. Lu. "Chinese doctors learn by studying books that are thousands of years old. This is ancient wisdom." Here are some examples.

- Cold foods include clams, bamboo shoots, lettuce and watermelon.
- Cool foods include spinach, strawberries, cucumbers, eggplant and wheat.
- Neutral foods include milk, mushrooms and corn.
- Warm foods include onions, garlic, walnuts and chicken.
- Hot foods include ginger and red and green peppers.

As for scientific evidence that this "balance" produces better health, the usual range of Western-style research just doesn't exist. Those who follow the diet advice of Chinese medicine practitioners take it on faith that their advice works. The real track record here is history, they claim.

"Everything doesn't have to be analyzed at the molecular level," adds Pitchford. "Western science would be able to explain these properties if they chose to. It's just the science of observation." Pitchford and other experts in Chinese nutrition believe that if we would all become more in tune with our bodies, we'd be able to feel these warming and cooling reactions for ourselves.

A Balanced Diet

Recognizing that most people aren't accustomed to thinking of foods in terms of yin and yang and may need some help in negotiating the narrow path between the two, Dr. Ni has developed a meal plan that includes a number of uncommon foods. (If you need to hunt down foods like seaweed, look in natural food stores or order from one of the sources listed in "Resources for Healing" on page 68.) For optimum yin and yang balance, Dr. Ni recommends eating the following foods daily.

- Whole grains—including rice, millet, wheat, barley, corn and rye—should comprise 40 percent of the diet.
- Freshly prepared vegetables—especially dark, leafy greens, broccoli, cabbage and root vegetables—should make up another 40 percent of the diet.
- Fresh fruits in season should make up no more than 10 percent of the diet.
- Legumes, seeds and nuts—including peas, beans, peanuts, lentils, almonds and sunflower seeds—should comprise 10 to 20 percent of the diet, with meat-eaters eating less and vegetarians eating more.

What It's Like

Want to try a Chinese diet for a week? Here's how it might go.

Let's suppose, just as an example, that you're generally a yang person by Chinese medicine standards—high-energy and warm, with dry skin and a large appetite. And let's further suppose that your cravings tend to be for equally yang foods. That could certainly be a problem if you're striving for balance.

The first thing you'll have to do, if you're giving Chinese nutrition a try, is toss out the red-pepper sauce and other hot stuff. Fill your fridge with cooling foods like watermelon, seaweeds, grapefruit juice, cucumbers, whole-wheat pitas and other breads.

You can help yourself to lots of salads, stir-fries, beans and rice dishes. But you might need to make some strategic substitutions, using sweet peas instead of hot peppers and cucumbers instead of onions.

Preparing dinner can be a lengthy chore if you follow Chinese nutrition recommendations and use dried beans instead of canned. Soaking beans overnight and boiling them for an hour and a half the next day is tedious, but you can prepare them more quickly if you have a pressure cooker.

If you haven't had seaweed before, be patient until you get used to the flavor and find out how much to use. Nori, the seaweed that comes in big green sheets, is fun and easy to cut up and cook. You can wrap it around cooked carrots, crush it up and sprinkle it on salads or even boil it with beans and rice.

But before you do any of that, be sure to taste it. At first, eating nori is a bit like eating the ocean. It's salty and fishy to the untested palate. While it's okay in small doses, it's not what you'd want in everything.

If you can stick with the diet long enough to feel the difference, you may find that these yin foods accomplish their mission. If you have the kind of hot yang stomach that often feels the afterburn of a five-alarm Mexican meal, you may discover that you're much more calm on this new diet.

- Animal products, including dairy foods, poultry and eggs, should count for no more than 10 percent of the diet.
- Seaweeds like nori, wakame, kombu and arame are good in small amounts.

Dr. Ni also advises avoiding chemical additives, fried and greasy foods, excessive sugar, ice cream and coffee.

Other Parts of the Picture

When it comes to healing disease, doctors of Chinese medicine unanimously agree that you cannot divorce Chinese nutrition from other healing practices that make up the total system of Chinese medicine. An accepted part of this tradition is acupuncture, where doctors use needles to stimulate the body's healing energy. That goes along with acupressure, applying pressure with the fingertips to specific points on the body to provide relief or promote healing. Herbal treatments also come with the territory: A Chinese doctor or practitioner will help restore the proper balance of yin and yang by preparing decoctions (adding herbs to water and then boiling them until a concentrated liquid is left) with large amounts of potent herbs.

Ideally, all of the other healing treatments and procedures in Chinese medicine tie in with dietary recommendations. You can't rely on diet alone, according to practitioners, but also they say that diet does play a major role in the cause, prevention and treatment of disease.

"Over 50 percent of disease conditions are directly caused by diet," says Dr. Ni. "And frequently, diet by itself can be a treatment."

"As a rule, the earlier you start to treat a disease, or the closer the person is to health, the easier the illness is to treat with diet alone," adds Dr. Jahnke. "As they get further away, you need more therapies like acupuncture."

What a Diet Can Do

For many specific health problems, Chinese medicine has a tradition of prescribing certain remedies. To be certain that you're getting the right treatment—which may include other therapies as well as diet—you would have to consult a doctor of Chinese medicine. But expert practitioners say diet can go a long way toward remedying some specific conditions. Here are some guidelines.

Acne. According to Dr. Ni, acne is a condition associated with heat. To treat it, he recommends eating yin foods that will help cool your skin, such as cucumbers, watermelon, brown rice and lettuce.

Arthritis. According to Chinese medicine, there are four different types. The cold kind is characterized by jabbing pain. Damp pain is dull, aching and lingering. Wind pain is transient, strikes suddenly and quickly passes. Hot joint pain is characterized by redness and swelling. In Chinese medicine, a doctor will first try to identify the specific type of arthritis before prescribing a therapy.

For the cold, damp and wind types of arthritis, experts recommend turning up your internal thermostat with warm to hot foods like peppers, garlic, scallions, beans and grains. They suggest avoiding cold, raw foods and staying away from dairy products.

For hot arthritis, practitioners recommend the opposite: Cool your joints with plenty of yin-style fruits and vegetables, especially cabbage.

Asthma. Asthma is generally broken down into either a hot or cold type, says Dr. Ni. Both kinds can benefit from similar treatments. Dr. Ni and Dr. Lu both recommend apricots, pumpkins, mustard greens and honey as superior food cures for asthma.

Chronic bladder infections. According to Dr. Ni, these infections are a condition of damp heat and are best treated by serving yourself cooling foods such as watermelon, celery and cantaloupe. Avoid heat-producing foods such as meat, onions, scallions, ginger and black pepper.

The common cold. This is an example of a transient disease, says Dr. Lu. "It begins as a cold condition and usually becomes a hot disease as the patient moves from the shivering to the feverish stage."

Treatments of choice are pungent foods, like green onions and ginger, which can be sliced and sautéed and added to soups, warming the body and inducing perspiration. If a fever hits, however, you should switch to cooling foods to help bring your temperature down, says Dr. Lu.

Constipation. According to Chinese medicine experts, this is most frequently a condition of heat and dryness. Both Dr. Ni and Dr. Lu recommend sweet, cooling foods as a remedy. To cure chronic constipation, they suggest eating bananas on an empty stomach. Then make sure you include figs, Chinese cabbage and potatoes in your diet.

Coronary heart disease. This is often a problem for yang people who have a tendency toward high blood pressure. Many factors can contribute, including a high-fat diet and lack of exercise, says Dr. Haas. The fast-paced lifestyle often leads to clogged arteries and, along with the high blood pressure, a susceptibility to heart disease, says Dr. Ni. "Their condition is likely to get worse if they also eat a very yang diet that is heavy on fats, meats and proteins," he says.

To reverse heart disease, "they must reverse their diet to a more yin diet, which emphasizes vegetables and grains," says Dr. Ni. He emphasizes that yang people also need to participate in more passive or yin activities like tai chi (a Chinese exercise characterized by slow, fluid movement) to complement the diet. Other doctors, like Dr. Haas, emphasize that any complete program for reversing heart disease should also include exercise and stress relief.

Crohn's disease. As with most inflammations, Crohn's disease is deemed a heat disorder in Chinese medicine. Although it's generally considered incurable, some doctors of Chinese medicine claim to have made major advances using acupuncture along with a restrictive cooling diet, including lots of vegetables, pasta and grains. In Chinese practice the person who has Crohn's disease is allowed no meat, dairy, spices, salt or refined sugar.

Diabetes. Diabetes generally stems from a depletion of yin, according to Dr. Ni. "They call it exhaustion syndrome in Chinese medicine. It comes from eating foods that are too yang—lots of sugar, spicy foods, dairy products, fried foods, fats and meats, which tend to deplete the body of yin."

For people who have diabetes, Dr. Ni sees diet as a way to correct the exhaustion syndrome. "They need to eat a bland, yin-nourishing diet that emphasizes vegetables, beans and greens, and no sugar, although fruits are

Resources for Healing

Organization

American Association of Oriental
Medicine
433 Front Street
Catasauqua, PA 18032

Mail-Order Food Sources

Gold Mine Natural Foods
3419 Hancock Street
San Diego, CA 92110
1-800-475-3663

Mountain Ark Trading Company
799 Old Leicester Highway
Asheville, NC 28806
1-800-643-8909

Books

*Between Heaven and Earth: A Guide
to Chinese Medicine*
Harriet Beinfield, L.Ac., and Efrem Korn-
    gold, L.Ac., O.M.D.
Ballantine Books

The Chinese System of Food Cures
Henry C. Lu, Ph.D.
Sterling Publishing

Healing with Whole Foods
Paul Pitchford
North Atlantic Books

The Tao of Nutrition
Maoshing Ni, Ph.D., and Cathy McNease
Seven Star Communications

okay in moderation."

Hemorrhoids. These pain-ful, swollen varicose veins in the rectum are generally related to constipation and are caused by dryness and heat, say Chinese medicine experts. The best treatments, therefore, are cooling, yin foods such as bananas, figs, cucumbers and bamboo shoots, says Dr. Ni.

High blood pressure. This tends to be a heat disorder, says Dr. Jahnke. To put your blood on ice, doctors of Chinese medicine recommend cool and cold foods like bananas, watermelon, lemons and tomatoes. But for best results you'll probably want to combine these dietary measures with exercise, weight loss and stress relief, according to Dr. Haas.

Impotence. In Chinese medicine, impotence is viewed as a common symptom of yang deficiency of the kidney. To reignite that yang fire, experts recommend warm foods such as chicken, scallions, soybeans, lentils, wine, ginger and walnuts.

Overweight. People who have cool, inactive natures are especially likely to have problems with their weight. Yin people are more likely to pack on some extra pounds than yang people, say Chinese medicine experts. To avoid weight gain or shed unwanted inches, doctors of Chinese medicine advise people with yin qualities to warm up their bodies with heat-producing, yang foods such as beans, spices, grains and fish.

Premenstrual syndrome (PMS). According to Dr. Ni, PMS is due to our love affair with cold beverages. He notes that there's a very high incidence of women in the United States who suffer from the bloating, cramping and irritability that are all symptoms of PMS. According to Chinese medicine, cold beverages cause our blood to stagnate, and that's what leads to PMS. Dr. Ni recommends canning the cool drinks and filling up on pungent foods such as green onions, ginger and black pepper to restore heat.

Ulcers. Ulcers are a condition of excess heat, according to Chinese medicine. To heal ulcers caused by inflammation, practitioners recommend cooling foods such as bananas, lettuce, cucumbers, soy milk and avocados. They advise patients to give the cold shoulder to heat-producing foods such as red meat, coffee, hot spices, alcohol and vinegar.

Getting Off to a Good Start

As you've probably noticed, eating the right diet by Chinese nutrition standards is a bit more complicated than ordering takeout from your favorite Hunan House. It means becoming familiar with foreign concepts and uncommon foods as well as developing a whole new understanding of who you are.

To make the transition between a typical American diet and a Chinese one, experts say that you should make like a tortoise and take it slowly. "People are more likely to be successful if they take it easy and don't change everything in their diet at one time," says Pitchford. "Start by using more vegetables and less meat. Then keep reducing the amount of meat, especially red meat, that you eat, as well as dairy products and eggs, and replacing them with foods like tofu."

Although a good text on Chinese medicine can give you a better understanding of how to eat for your specific body type, Beinfield suggests that to more fully understand your own profile, you might want to see a Chinese medicine practitioner for a thorough diagnosis. "It's like we are all different kinds of locks, and our diets are our keys," she concludes. To find a practitioner, Beinfield recommends contacting the American Association of Oriental Medicine for referrals and more information (see "Resources for Healing").

5 Religion-Based Diets

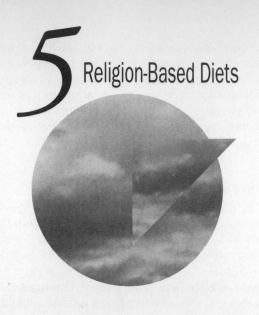

Food for the Spirit and Health

Now, what in heaven does religion have to do with food?

A lot, apparently—at least if you look at the prescriptions and proscriptions on diet advocated by the various religions of the world.

Of course, religious differences are more than spiritual, dialectical and inspirational. They're also intestinal. What you eat is part of what you are, tradition seems to say. And when it comes to the dietary laws of different faiths, contradictions abound.

Eating a pork chop can mean lasting punishment for a devout Muslim, but burgers are okay anytime. A Jew who follows the letter of kosher law can eat burgers, but never with milk. Hindus can have milk whenever they want but can't touch beef. And Jains—followers of a branch of Hinduism—are so vigilant about not eating meat that they've been known to carefully strain their drinking water to avoid swallowing tiny insects!

From Xanadu to Timbuktu

Food rules help to define religions and build community, say religious scholars.

"Historically, there were a lot of practical facets to dietary laws and restrictions, especially with regard to meat," says Philip Jenkins, Ph.D., head of the Department of Religious Studies at Pennsylvania State University in University Park. "One school of thought maintains that in hot climates, many foods like pork were unsafe to eat, so Islam and Hebrew dietary laws forbade pork consumption. These laws became ritualized over time, and they served to define a religion and build community."

Today, studies show that people who are active in their religions benefit from a lower incidence of major diseases like heart disease and cancer. Researchers say that these benefits are probably due to the community support, spiritual tranquillity and healthful lifestyle that often accompany a religious life, but, they say, dietary practices can be a positive contribution.

One of the shining examples of the benefits of faith—often cited by health researchers—is the very diet-conscious group of Christians known as Seventh-Day Adventists. This sect is largely vegetarian, and its community members have a much lower incidence of many kinds of serious health problems than the general population. Is it their faith—or their eating practices? Scientists tend to believe it's the latter, but on the other hand, the Adventists wouldn't be such strict vegetarians unless it was a fundamental part of their religion.

In other religions the health benefits may not be as prominent—or may even be nonexistent. But differences abound and are linked to a rich, distinctive diversity of religious life.

Here are just some of those religions and the diets followed by some of their sects and their strongest believers, along with some of the health benefits that researchers have noted.

Christianity

"Behold, I have given you every herb bearing seed, which is upon the face of all the earth, and every tree, in which is the fruit of a tree yielding seed; to you it shall be for meat."
—Genesis 1:29

Despite some biblical phrases alluding to vegetarianism, one glance at the hot dogs, sausage links and ice cream sandwiches served up at most church picnics and it's clear that Christians today generally see food and faith as separate issues.

"Christian theology says we are justified by faith, not by law or how we eat," explains the Reverend Glenn Asquith, Jr., Ph.D., professor of pastoral theology at Moravian Theological Seminary in Bethlehem, Pennsylvania. "The dietary laws in the Old Testament reflect the customs of the time, but then Jesus Christ came and moved his followers away from the law."

Although modern Christians like Dr. Asquith don't follow the old detary laws, a few Christian groups have delved deeply into the Good Book and have taken to heart what they believe to be the key to proper Christian eating.

When Pigging Out Was Risky

The terms *clean* and *unclean* crop up more than 30 times in chapter 11 of Leviticus in the Old Testament, the critical passages from which Seventh-Day Adventist and Jewish leaders derived dietary laws.

Are there underlying health reasons for those ancient laws?

"The dietary rules in the Old Testament reflected customs of the times," explains the Reverend Glenn Asquith, Jr., Ph.D., professor of pastoral theology at Moravian Theological Seminary in Bethlehem, Pennsylvania. "Since food preparation and preservation weren't as sophisticated as they are today, people had to be careful. Eating pork was dangerous, so the dietary laws against it helped people avoid the spread of illness."

Today, of course, religious law rather than health concerns dictate the dietary laws of Seventh-Day Adventists and Orthodox Jews. But the categories of clean and unclean are still the same as defined in Leviticus.

Healthy Adventists

The Seventh-Day Adventists, as already noted, have reaped a host of benefits from using their sacred text as a daily meal planner. Originating in the 1860s, the sect was co-founded by Adventist authority Ellen G. White, who was considered a messenger with a special light from God.

Extracting nutritional guidance from the Old Testament books of Genesis, Ecclesiastes, Deuteronomy and Proverbs (to name just a few), White advocated vegetarianism about 100 years before the appearance of the first veggie burger. She championed a diet that was based on fruits, whole grains, vegetables, nuts and seeds.

In the Bible, White noted, a number of foods, primarily shellfish and pork, were deemed unclean and were strictly forbidden. Some other meats were permitted but not encouraged. The Adventist diet adds to these restrictions, making coffee, tobacco and alcohol strictly off-limits.

Today about 45 percent of Adventists living in the United States are ovo-lacto-vegetarians—that is, they'll eat eggs and dairy products but no meat. Some Adventists adhere strictly to the laws, while others are less observant.

But whatever their commitment, Adventists in general still have a cleaner bill of health than the rest of the country's population. For one thing, they have less artery-clogging cholesterol chugging through their veins than non-Adventists. In a study of 222 Adventists, the cholesterol levels of both strict and not-so-strict Adventist men and women were 15 and 10 percent lower, respectively, than those of the general population.

Cancer rates are also lower among all Adventists. A study of 34,000 Adventists showed that both men and women are less likely to die from cancer than members of the general population. Adventist men seem to be particularly safeguarded, showing an overall cancer incidence that's one-quarter less than that of men in the general population.

Among Adventists who follow a strictly vegetarian diet, the health benefits are even more pronounced, according to epidemiologist William Castelli, M.D., former director of the Framingham Heart Study and currently medical director of the Framingham Cardiovascular Institute in Framingham, Massachusetts.

"The vegetarian Adventists have only 10 to 15 percent of our heart attack rate and 40 percent of our cancer rate," he says. "They outlive us by about seven years. And their elderly can run circles around the majority of people in their fifties and sixties in the rest of America."

The Advent of New Foods

In the second half of the nineteenth century, Sylvester Graham and John Harvey Kellogg were two spiritual-minded Americans who were particularly inventive in creating new foods, leaving a legacy that's now in every supermarket.

Experimenting with food as a way to get people's nutritional and sexual lives in order, Graham created the cracker that bears his name. And Kellogg came up with cornflakes, the crisp, crunchy foundation of a dry-cereal empire. Both believed that their new foods were so nutritious that they could keep the body pure and minimize sexual urges.

Are there any spiritual benefits to following the dietary laws? "I wouldn't go so far as to say that it's a sin to eat the wrong foods," says Patricia Johnston, R.D., Dr.P.H., associate dean of the School of Public Health at Loma Linda University in California. "But Paul said that our body is a temple, and there is definitely a connection between good health and spirituality."

Essenes: In the Fasting Lane

Although the original Essene order died out at the end of the first century A.D., there may still be a few people carrying the torch for this very rigid, celibate vegetarian community.

Some modern-day Essenes, deriving inspiration from teachings in the Dead Sea scrolls—which were unearthed in 1947—believe that fasting has a special place in their spiritual lives. In fact, if you want to be a modern-day Essene, you should eat no more than two meals a day, according to Edmond B. Szekely, author of *The Essene Science of Fasting and the Art of Sobriety*. And you should follow a strict vegetarian diet. Overeating, according to Szekely, drives angels out of your body and lets Satan in. Since Satan is the root of disease, according to Szekely's interpretation of Essene beliefs, you're curing yourself of satanic influence when you fast.

For optimal health, Szekely recommends fasting as often as one day a week to "detoxify" the body. But if you've never fasted, don't dive in head-first, because you may have an excessive buildup of waste products, he warns. In his book, Szekely says you need to follow a well-balanced, detoxifying diet for a couple of months before you begin. After that, short fasts of a day or even a half-day can be undertaken to benefit both the body and the spirit, in Szekely's view.

Not surprisingly, these lifestyle recommendations are questioned by modern theologians. While it is known that Jesus fasted for extended periods, even his lifestyle wasn't as rigid as that of the Essenes, says Dr. Jenkins.

"We know that the Essenes had absolutely strict, unbending adherence to the law," says Dr. Jenkins. "And one of the things we know for sure about Jesus is that he did not. Put the two together, and they don't mesh."

As for the health benefits of fasting, some doctors believe that it may indeed be the key not only to conquering common diseases like arthritis, heart disease and diabetes but also to significantly lengthening our lives. (For more on fasting, see chapter 11.)

Fasting is the only scientifically well-documented approach for extending the life span of laboratory animals, according to Joel Fuhrman, M.D., a nutritional medicine specialist, director of the Amwell Health Center in Belle Mead, New Jersey, and author of *Fasting—and Eating—for Health*. He also stresses that anyone who fasts should be supervised by a doctor.

Judaism

"No soul of you shall eat blood, neither shall any stranger that sojourneth among you eat blood."
—Leviticus 17:12

Back in the days when Moses was reading the riot act to the troubled people of Israel, food sanitation practices weren't what they are today. Eating meat was a dangerous proposition. Plus, it meant animal suffering, which God denounces in the Old Testament books of Deuteronomy and Exodus—two of the five books of Moses that comprise the Torah and form the foundation of the Jewish faith.

Though it isn't clearly spelled out in the Torah, many biblical scholars believe that God answered the Israelites' food dilemma by giving them the *kashrut*—the kosher dietary laws detailed in the book of Leviticus in the Torah. "These laws were given to the Israelites in order to establish a spiritual relationship with food," says Rabbi Reuven Flamer, founder of the Chai Center in White Plains, New York, where he combines instruction on Jewish practices with lessons on healthful living.

Going Kosher

The kosher laws described in the Torah focus primarily on which meats are clean, meaning fit for consumption, or unclean, meaning off-limits in Judaic law. In addition, clean meats must be slaughtered and prepared for eating under strict guidelines in accord with God's word. According to the kashrut laws, explains Rabbi Flamer, meats that are identified as kosher are literally "fit to be used."

The Old Testament says that these sanctioned meats can come only from animals that have cloven hooves and chew their cud, all fish with fins and scales and fowl that aren't considered birds of prey. Prohibited meats include pork, all shellfish and all predator birds. Also, the Old Testament says that using blood for food is strictly forbidden, so every drop must be drained from meat before it earns the kosher seal of approval.

The herculean task of enforcing kosher law begins at the slaughterhouse, according to Rabbi Flamer. That task falls under the guidance of a *shochet*, a religious person trained in slaughtering directives. The shochet wields a razor-sharp knife to kill the animal quickly. The blood is drained at once, and the animal is inspected for blemishes by a kosher inspector called a *bodek*. If it passes inspection, says Rabbi Flamer, the meat is deveined, soaked, washed, salted and washed again three more times before it is awarded the kosher seal.

Kosher law also forbids mixing meat and dairy products, which means you can't cook them together, eat them together, put them on the same plate or even eat them with the same utensils. You can eat them on the same day, but by kosher law, you should wait six hours after eating one before eating the other. That means no cheeseburgers and no baked goods made with both animal shortening and dairy products.

Kosher food producers make life easier for consumers by labeling kosher products with a kosher stamp. The most common seals are a bold *K* with a star or a circle around it and a bold *U* with a circle around it. Food is also labeled as meat or dairy. Another label, *pareve*, means it's neither meat nor dairy, or neutral.

Is Kosher Healthier?

Interestingly, only a fraction of the people who scan their foods for kosher seals are actually Jewish. Some are Muslims and Seventh-Day Adventists—two other religious sects whose members don't eat "unclean" animals. But others eat kosher in the belief that kosher food, especially meat, goes through such rigorous inspection that it must be better.

This may or may not be true, say the experts. Kosher animals must get a nod of approval from two sets of critical eyes—federal inspectors and bodeks. But the bodek isn't really a backup. He's checking meat to see that it passes spiritual criteria, not necessarily health criteria.

"Bodeks essentially check the flesh and the lungs for blemishes," explains Rabbi Flamer. He says that bodeks don't normally check places like the glands, where diseases may begin, as federal inspectors are required to do.

Produce that's labeled kosher also benefits from inspection, according to Judith Eaton, R.D., a food therapist and nutritional consultant to companies seeking kosher certification. "The Torah forbids the consumption of insects, so every single leaf, berry and legume is inspected," says Eaton, "And those 'natural' dyes that are derived from insects aren't allowed in kosher food, either."

Still, says Eaton, food is not automatically healthier just because it bears a kosher label. Typically, kosher cuts of meat, like beef brisket and veal shank, are notoriously fatty. Kosher hot dogs can be just as fat-filled and cholesterol-laden as regular franks, and junk foods like kosher soda pop are just as nutritionally barren as every other soft drink. Eaton warns that people on salt-restricted diets actually need to be extra careful to check the sodium content of kosher meats. Since these meats are salted, they're often higher in sodium, she says, and should be soaked in water before cooking to remove as much salt as possible.

Islam

"O believers, eat what is good of the food We have given you,
and be grateful to God, if indeed you are obedient to him."
—Koran 2:172–73

When it comes to dietary laws, Islamic disciples don't mince words.

"God says I allow *this* for you and I disallow *that* for you, so we have to obey," says Abdel Rahman Osman, Ph.D., director of the Islamic Center of New York in New York City. "Pork is forbidden. Those who disobey will be punished."

Founded in the seventh century A.D. by the prophet Muhammad, the Islamic faith is a relatively young world religion. Its followers, called Muslims, believe that God, or Allah, revealed His wisdom to Muhammad, and it is documented in the sacred text of the Koran. They believe that the Christian and Jewish people before them were given imperfect information.

Swine and Punishment

Essentially, Islamic dietary laws are like the kosher laws, only with higher stakes. If Muslims knowingly indulge in forbidden foods, there is literally hell to pay. Fortunately, if they unknowingly eat pork, they will not be punished. Or if a Muslim happens to be stranded on an island with nothing but wild pigs and poisonous plants, he can opt for the porker. But in normal circumstances, any Muslim who eats pork is risking the anger of Allah.

In Islamic as in Jewish tradition, pork, birds of prey, fanged beasts of prey and meat that contains even a drop of blood are forbidden. But Muslims are allowed to mix meat and dairy foods, and there are no rules regarding the preparation of food. Because there are no Islamic seals of approval in this country, most Muslims buy kosher meats, explains Dr. Osman.

Also like followers of the Jewish faith, Muslims have no assurances from Allah that if they eat according to the dietary laws, they will enjoy better health while they are here on Earth, although there may be some other rewards, according to Dr. Osman. "The benefits are the rewards that Allah bestows upon you for following the law," he says.

Although you don't have to be a vegetarian to follow the teachings of Islam, Muslims do support nonviolence to animals. "That's why the Muslims are advised not to slaughter animals in front of other animals and to slaughter in the name of God for the soul they are taking," according to Dr. Osman.

Don't Prey on the Predator

Like the children of Israel in the Old Testament, early Muslims got word from a prophet, Muhammad, that certain animals were okay to eat but others were best left to roam. According to the Koran—Muslim sacred scripture—the following foods are forbidden.

• The blood and flesh of swine.
• Any meat from animals that were killed by other animals or died of natural causes.
• Any food that was not slaughtered while alive and healthy.
• Any bird of prey or fanged beast of prey.
• Food killed in the name of a god other than Allah.

Hungriness Is Next to Godliness

Like the Essenes, Muslims also believe that a little rumbling in the tummy is a virtuous thing.

Not only do the Muslims have obligatory fasts from sunrise to sundown during Ramadan—a holy month in Islam—but they also believe that people should fast often and keep their "fuel tanks" just over the halfway mark.

"Food is only to live," explains Dr. Osman. "When you feed yourself until you are full, you are burdened with digesting food and your spirituality is diminished. Being a little hungry makes you appreciate the sufferings of the poor and be charitable."

Hinduism

"Let him eat vegetables that grow on dry land or in water, flowers, roots, and fruits, the productions of pure trees, and oils extracted from forest fruits . . . Let him avoid honey, flesh, and mushrooms growing on the ground."
—Laws of Manu 6.12–13, from the Vedas

Hinduism is the granddaddy of religions: It is —so old that no one can even figure out where it came from. And since the religion began, as far as anyone can tell, Hindus have been vegetarians. Started around 500 B.C. in India, Hinduism is grounded in the Vedas—ancient sacred texts written by Indian sages about 5,000 years ago. The Vedas hold universal truths that everyone is expected to recognize. And according to the Rules set forth in the Vedas, eating meat is akin to murder.

No Meat Is Good Meat

Unlike other religions that give humans dominion over animals and often rank the animals as clean or unclean, Hindus put us all on the same playing field. To them God is every bit as present in the dog next door as he is in you.

Although only one entity, God takes many divine forms—some of which resemble animals or actually are animals. The Lord Ganesha, lord of plenty, for instance, is part elephant and part man. And the cow is considered so sacred that the Supreme Lord Krishna's holy paradise is called *Goloka*—literally, "cow place."

Goodwill toward animals also helps improve your karma—the force that determines your standing in the next incarnation, say Hindu scholars. Since Hindus believe that existence is nothing but a continuous cycle of births and rebirths until you get everything right and become one with the divine being, every bit of good karma helps.

Eating meat results in bad karma, explains Virender Sodhi, M.D. (Ayurvedic), N.D., a naturo-

---

Reverence for Cows

"Mother cow is in many ways better than the mother who gave us birth," said Mahatma Gandhi, a venerated leader of the Hindu people. Your mother may nurture you for a few years, said Gandhi, but then she tosses you from the nest. In the Hindu view, the cow never stops giving, even after she dies.

Cow worship has been central to Hindu religion for thousands of years, as is evidenced by the 200 million cattle now roaming the Indian countryside. The Supreme Lord Krishna celebrated his love for the cow and proclaimed it in the sacred texts, the Vedas. According to scripture, everything that comes out of a cow—from milk to dung—is sacred as well. So while a cow may not be used for porterhouse steak, her urine, called *go-mutra*, is actually still drunk by pious Hindus in many parts of India.

---

pathic physician and director of the American School of Ayurvedic Sciences in Belle-vue, Washington. "You get inherent weaknesses from a previous life's transgressions. Eating meat disturbs your peace and carries on in your karma."

The Ayurvedic Contradiction

To those familiar with Ayurveda—the ancient Indian healthcare system that is also based on the Vedas—the Ayurvedic prescriptions

of eating meat for certain illnesses may seem to contradict the sacredness of animals. But the apparent contradiction is easily explained, accord- ing to Vasant Lad, B.A.M.S., M.A.Sc., director of the Ayurvedic Institute in Albuquerque, New Mexico.

"Vegetarianism is the ideal, but there is a difference between using meat for food and using it for medicine," he explains. "Certain meats, aside from that of the cow, can be strengthening, and according to the Vedas, they have a place in curing diseases such as anemia."

Buddhism

"I undertake to observe the rule: to abstain from taking life; to abstain from taking what is not given; to abstain from sensuous misconduct; to abstain from false speech; to abstain from intoxicants as tending to cloud the mind."
—The Five Precepts

An early offshoot of Hinduism, Buddhism has a similar view of life as an endless cycle of misery, decay, births and rebirths. To Buddhists, the ultimate goal is to reach enlightenment and the state of Buddhahood, or Nirvana, which is achievable only through the right deeds and meditation.

Performing the right deeds largely means following the Five Precepts, or the fundamental rules of Buddhist ethics. The first and foremost of these precepts is not to take life. To many Buddhists and Buddhist scholars, this means that they must be vegetarians, period. Yet many Buddhists interpret this ethical code differently, and various factions continue to eat meat.

"Many Buddhists, like those in Thailand, believe that as long as they didn't do the killing or the meat wasn't killed specifically for them, it's okay," explains Sensei Sonja Kjolhede, a teacher at the Zen Center in Rochester, New York. "But eating meat is taking life. We're inextricably connected."

6 Ayurveda

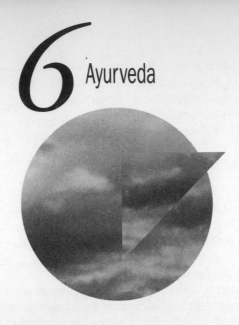

Customized Nutritional Healing

When it comes to food, most of us have heard the health news. We know we're supposed to order our fish poached, with no butter, and avoid fried food like the bubonic plague. And—oh, yeah—shovel five servings of fruits and vegetables onto our plates each day. At least that's what researchers, doctors and nutritionists are saying is good for us. But if you turn to a far more ancient and less scientific source, you'll hear a much different story. According to the nutritional wisdom of Ayurveda—"the science of life"—even if you follow this recommended diet to the letter, you still might be eating the wrong foods.

The followers of this ancient tradition are skeptical about the healing power of many foods that today's scientists deem terrific. "It's not that these things aren't important," says Hari Sharma, M.D., professor emeritus and former director of the Division of Cancer Prevention and Natural Products Research at Ohio State University College of Medicine in Columbus and author of *Freedom from Disease*. "It's that breaking down our diets in this way is terribly oversimplified."

Take everything you've read about nutrition and put it on a shelf, say the advocates of Ayurveda. This health system from India was first recorded in spiritual texts called the Vedas 5,000 years ago, but here's how the age-old plan looks under modern scrutiny.

You Eat What You Are

By Ayurvedic standards, the idea that everybody should eat the same diet for optimal health is nonsensical. That's because Ayurveda—even though it comes from a culture very different from our own—has a central tenet that is very American: You are an individual, and you have unique needs that must be satisfied in order for you to feel good.

Most of us probably think about our uniqueness in terms of our personalities. But Ayurveda says that your body also has a personality, and therefore it requires a highly personalized diet.

"That's why one person can drink a glass of milk and be fine, while another takes a couple of sips and gets diarrhea," says Virender Sodhi, M.D. (Ayurvedic), N.D., a naturopathic physician and director of the American School of Ayurvedic Sciences in Bellevue, Washington. It's also why some people can down three-alarm chili with glee while others end up running for a fire extinguisher, according to Dr. Sodhi. "The way we process food depends upon our biological makeup."

"Food can be medicine, or food can be poison," observes Vasant Lad, B.A.M.S., M.A.Sc., director of the Ayurvedic Institute in Albuquerque, New Mexico. "But it comes down to constitution, not nutrition." The constitution he's talking about isn't the one penned by our Founding Fathers. It's "the physical makeup of the individual comprising inherited qualities modified by the environment." That definition is straight out of the dictionary, and it describes quite well what Ayurvedic doctors mean by the word. Ayurveda says that you have two constitutions, the one you're born with—*pakruti*—and the one that reflects your body's condition from day to day—*vikriti*.

Your prakruti is a combination of what ancient Ayurvedic gurus called *doshas*, which are three primary forces. Each of the doshas, they believe, is made up of some combination of the five basic elements that comprise everything in the universe—ether (space), air, fire, water and earth. The vata dosha (ether and air), pitta dosha (fire and water) and kapha dosha (water and earth) are present in all living things.

The Combo You're Born With

At conception, you receive a vata-pitta-kapha combination from your parents. Ayurvedic experts say that combination forms the blueprint for who you are—the color of your eyes, how much sleep you need at night, your reaction to stress and a lot of other characteristics. Generally, people have two doshas that are primary, and one of those two is dominant. But everyone has some of all three, they say. And the combination that forms your prakruti remains constant from cradle to grave. Your vikriti—the day-to-day set of characteristics—is more fluid and changeable. Although it is supposed to remain relatively constant, forming a mirror image of your prakruti, it's affected by everything, including the weather, the seasons and especially your diet.

Your vikriti determines your current state of health. When you're feeling not quite right or downright ill, it's because your vikriti is out of whack, say Ayurvedic doctors. Keeping your vikriti in balance with your prakruti, they say, is the key to good health. While maintaining that balance ultimately requires many things, including positive attitude, internal cleansing, meditation and a healthy lifestyle, "the first step is nutrition," says Dr. Sodhi.

Building Better Balance

The easiest way to eat for balance, says Dr. Sodhi, is to determine the dominant dosha in your prakruti—which combination of elements in your system does the most to determine your basic characteristics. Then you should choose the foods that decrease or counteract the elements of that dosha, because it is those elements that are most likely to go out of balance.

Here's an example. If your prakruti is predominantly pitta, your essential characteristics are those associated with fire and water. Your diet, therefore, should be cooling, especially during the heat of summer. If you defy your prakruti and exist on pitta-increasing foods like hot chili and jalapeño peppers, it will essentially overload your vikriti, your day-to-day functioning system. Adding too much fire to fire, you'll pay the consequences with heartburn, ulcers and other "fire-related" ailments.

Conversely, you can eat foods that balance your pitta. By living in balance, you can achieve perfect health and longevity, say advocates of Ayurveda. You'll also attain mental clarity, compassion, love and happiness, says Dr. Lad.

To determine what your dominant dosha is, see "What's Your Dominant Dosha?" on page 84. But take note: Even though you're likely to have an excess of your dominant dosha, any of the three can become unbalanced.

Vata: Light on Its Feet

Being air and space, vata is the mover and shaker of the doshas. As the only traveling dosha, it can go anywhere in the body, but it's most prevalent in the colon, bladder, skin, bone marrow, nervous system and lumbar region.

Vata shepherds food through the digestive process and nutrients in and out of cells. It's the force that controls your breathing, balances your tissues and creates energy. Typical vata traits are anxiety, enthusiasm, impulsiveness and changeability.

It's easy to spot vata-dominant people. They have light, thin builds and are usually very short or very tall, with prominent features, joints and veins. Vivacious and moody, they tend to worry, overexert and sleep and eat at different times each day. Michael Jordan is tall, energetic, exuberant and so light that they named a sneaker (Air Jordan) after him. That's vata.

When you have too much vata, that light wind rustling through your body becomes a gale force, drying you out and causing vata conditions like rough skin, chapped lips, intestinal gas, lower back pain, arthritic joints, insomnia and fatigue.

"Unfortunately, vata is the first to go out of balance and the hardest to get back in," says Dr. Sodhi. Because they're so changeable, "vata-dominant people stick to the vata-balancing diet for about two weeks," Dr. Sodhi observes, and it's difficult for them to stay on one diet any longer than that.

Pitta: Hot Stuff

Fire and water combine in pitta to form one scorching dosha. Pitta is responsible for digestion, body heat, appetite, anger, perception and understanding. It's seated in the small intestine and dominates the sweat glands, heart, eyes, metabolic system, liver and blood. Pitta traits are like those of a good entrepreneur—concentration, perfectionism and orderliness.

In a word, pitta-dominant people are intense. With a sharp intellect, precise speech and a love of challenge, they are generally enterprising and successful. Physically, they have muscular builds, fair, ruddy skin and light eyes, and they are perpetually hungry.

To see a pitta in action, just tune in to *Nightline*. Anchorman Ted Koppel is a classic pitta, right down to the probing intellect and freckled complexion.

Although a pitta is usually warm and engaging, head for cover when this person boils over. Hell hath no fury like a pitta unbalanced. Besides fostering irritability, Dr. Sodhi says excess pitta can cause ulcers, acne, rashes, stress-related heart attacks and the intestinal inflammation of colitis.

"Pitta people tend to take their dietary advice way too seriously, and eating becomes a goal to achieve rather than a pleasure," explains Page Latham, R.N., of the Maharishi Ayur-Veda Medical Center in Lancaster, Massachusetts.

Kapha: Comforting

Pour cool water into soft earth and you have kapha—stable, moist and heavy. It's seated in the chest and dominant in the head, stomach, heart, joints, limbs and extremities.

Generating lubrication, such as mucus, and providing unity among the cells, kapha is what keeps us running like a well-oiled machine. Its qualities are those of the hardy—endurance, strength and courage.

We all know and love at least one kapha-dominant person. They're the ones with the ample frame and large, liquid eyes, who are relaxed, easygoing and empathic. Think of a tearful Oprah Winfrey embracing an anguished guest, and you have the epitome of kapha.

When kapha people become unbalanced, however, those positive attributes of stability and passivity become extreme, and kaphas can become impossibly lazy, stubborn, greedy and overattached. According to Dr. Sodhi, the usual manifestations of kapha imbalance include problems with overweight, allergies, high cholesterol levels, procrastination, cysts and stupor.

(continued on page 86)

What's Your Dominant Dosha?

If you're following the teachings of Ayurveda, practically every food choice you make is based on your dosha. But how do you determine your dominant dosha? The only sure way is to consult an Ayurvedic doctor (or two or three) to get a personal profile. But the following quiz is another good starting point, and it will help you find out how the advice and menus in this chapter may apply to you personally.

Be aware, however, that such quizzes can indicate an imbalance in your doshas rather than giving a total view of your constitution. Try to answer according to general patterns over your lifetime, not just how you've been feeling lately. Use the following rating system and respond to each statement with a number.

Characteristics	Vata
My hair texture tends to be	____Dry, curly, full of body
My hair color is	____Medium or light brown
My skin tends to be	____On the dry side
My complexion (when compared to others of my race) is	____Darker
Compared with others of my height, I have	____Smaller bones
My weight is	____Thin, I don't gain easily
My energy level	____Tends to fluctuate, to come in waves
Regarding temperature, I	____Dislike cold, am comfortable in the heat
My typical hunger level	____Can vary from excessive to no interest in food
I prefer my food/drink	____Warm, moist, oily
I generally eat	____Quickly
My sleep is most often	____Interrupted, light
My dreams often include	____Flying, looking down at the ground, mountains, chase scenes
My resting pulse rate (in beats per minute) is	____80–100 (women)
	____70–90 (men)
My sexual interest is	____Strong when romantically involved, low to moderate otherwise
I am most sensitive to	____Noise
My emotional moods	____Change easily, I'm very responsive
My general reaction to stress is	____Anxious, fearful
With regard to money, I	____Am easy and impulsive
My way of learning is	____To learn quickly, enjoy more than one thing at a time, I can lose focus
I learn new material best by	____Listening to a speaker
My memory is	____Best in short term
My way of speaking is	____Quick, often imaginative or excessive
If there was one trait to best describe me, it would be	____Vivacious
Regarding my relationships, I	____Easily adapt to different kinds of people
My family and friends might prefer me to be more	____Settled
This evaluation made me feel	____Indecisive
Totals:	____**Vata**

0 = Doesn't describe me at all   2 = Describes me quite well

1 = Describes me a little   3 = Describes me almost perfectly

Assessing Your Score

If one column total is 15 or more points higher than the others, this is clearly your dominant constitutional type—vata, pitta or kapha. If two of the column totals are 0 to 15 points apart, you are a dual-dosha constitutional type: vata-pitta (or pitta-vata), pitta-kapha (or kapha-pitta) or vata-kapha (or kapha-vata). And if all three column totals are within 0 to 10 points of each other, you are a tridosha type.

Pitta	Kapha
____Straight, fine	____Thick, wavy, shiny
____Blond or reddish tone, early gray	____Dark brown, black
____Delicate, sensitive	____Oily, smooth
____More reddish, freckled	____Lighter
____Average-size bones	____Larger bones
____Average	____Heavy, I gain easily
____Is moderate or high, I can push myself too hard	____Is steady
____Dislike heat, perspire easily, thrive in winter	____Dislike damp cold, tolerate extremes well
____Is Intense, I need regular meals	____Is usually low but can be emotionally driven
____Cold	____Warm, dry
____Moderately fast	____Slowly
____Sound, moderate	____Deep, long, I am slow to awaken
____Fire, waterfalls, battles, fights	____Oceans, clouds, romance
____70–80 (women)	____60–70 (women)
____60–70 (men)	____50–60 (men)
____Moderate to strong	____Slow to awaken but sustained, generally strong
____Bright light	____Strong odors
____Are intense, I'm quick-tempered	____Are even, I'm slow to anger
____Irritated	____Mostly calm
____Am careful, but I spend	____Tend to save, accumulate
____To focus sharply, discriminate, finish what I start	____To take my time, tend to be methodical
____Reading or using visual aids	____Associating it with another memory
____Good overall	____Best in long term
____Clear, precise, detailed, well-organized	____Soothing, rich with moments of silence
____Determined	____Easygoing
____Often choose friends on the basis of their values	____Am slow to make new friends, but am loyal forever
____Tolerant	____Enthusiastic
____Annoyed	____Sleepy
____ Pitta	____ Kapha

"The challenge with kapha people is getting them motivated enough to stick to a diet," says Dr. Sodhi.

It's a Matter of Taste

So what is the secret to a "balanced diet," according to Ayurveda? You won't find it by reading nutrition labels, that's for sure. In fact, you don't have to use your eyes at all. Just open your mouth and say "yum," because the key to Ayurvedic nutrition lies not in the way food breaks down into vitamins and minerals but in the way it tastes.

Before you drop this book and make a beeline for your local sundae shop, however, you should understand that the concept of taste in Ayurveda is much more complex than what you think tastes good and what you think tastes bad. In Ayurveda, the "taste" of the food depends on the elements in the food, so understanding taste is an absolute must if you want to choose the foods that don't unbalance the elements of your dominant dosha.

Like the doshas, tastes are considered to be derived from the five elements—ether, air, fire, water and earth—so they have the power to change the body's composition. If you're a kapha person, for instance, you already have water and earth as your predominant elements. Eat too many foods with tastes that are also derived from water and earth, and you're going to be a bloated kapha, say Ayurvedic doctors. Continue eating those foods indefinitely without correcting your kapha imbalance, and they say you'll get diabetes—a condition of prolonged, excess kapha.

There are six tastes that can lead you back to (or away from) Ayurvedic balance.
- Sweet: The taste of foods like milk or dates.
- Sour: Foods like citrus fruits or fermented food.
- Salty: Foods like anchovies.
- Bitter: Foods like rhubarb or coffee.
- Pungent: Foods like chili peppers.
- Astringent: The taste of foods like apples or cabbage.

Food also has six "qualities" that play a role in keeping your doshas balanced, but they're secondary to taste. They are: heavy, oily, hot (temperature), light, dry and cold.

Generally, Ayurvedic experts recommend that you favor foods that have qualities opposite those of your primary dosha. Rice cakes, for example, are light, cool and dry, so they would be a good choice for heavy, moist, kapha people.

"For optimum health, it's important to try to include all six tastes and qualities in every meal, although you obviously need more of some tastes than others," says Latham. "While this may sound difficult, it's quite easy when you include spices and tea with your meals."

"But artificial flavors don't count," adds David Frawley, O.M.D., doctor of Oriental medicine and director of the American Institute of Vedic

Studies in Santa Fe, New Mexico. "Artificial foods don't have any vital energy. They can't do anything good for you."

"Do's and Don'ts to Balance Dosha" on page 90 can help you choose the tastes and qualities that you need to regain balance. This table of food guidelines for basic constitutional types comes from *Ayurveda: The Science of Self-Healing* by Dr. Lad.

The guidelines in this table are general, according to Dr. Lad. You'll need to make specific adjustments, depending on your own health requirements. Some of the variables are food allergies that you might have, the strength of your digestion and the season of the year. In any Ayurvedic diet, you also need to give prime consideration to the degree of your dosha predominance or aggravation.

From this table you can begin to make up an Ayurvedic diet that will allow you to avoid aggravating foods and eat more balancing foods—which is the key to good health, according to advocates. (Note: Sometimes you will need to look for a specific kind of fruit or vegetable—such as sweet oranges instead of sour oranges or a sweet lettuce like iceberg as opposed to more bitter, leafy greens.)

Remember, you want to choose foods that decrease, not increase, your dominant dosha. Or use the simplified guidelines in the following list to help achieve balance.

• To decrease vata, eat sweet, sour, salty, heavy, oily and hot.
• To increase vata, eat pungent, bitter, astringent, light, dry and cold.
• To decrease pitta, eat sweet, bitter, astringent, cold, heavy and dry.
• To increase pitta, eat pungent, sour, salty, hot, light and oily.
• To decrease kapha, eat pungent, bitter, astringent, light, dry and hot.
• To increase kapha, eat sweet, sour, salty, heavy, oily and cold.

A Food for All Seasons

Once you have the gist of the foods that aggravate and pacify, you need to consider other factors that alter your vikriti, particularly the seasons, which have powerful dosha-shifting force.

"Seasonal eating is basically common sense," says Amadea Morningstar, a Western-trained nutritionist and author of *Ayurvedic Cooking for Westerners*. "If it's cold and wintry outside, you don't want to eat chilled pasta salad. You want warm, spiced soup." It's especially important to follow the seasonal diet that corresponds to your dominant dosha. These guidelines from Morningstar can help.

Winter. This is kapha season. You need heavy, warm foods to battle the cold, but don't neglect to eat some lighter, kapha-pacifying fare to avoid slipping into a hibernation-like stupor.

Spring. Kapha changes into pitta during this season. Now is the time to shake off kapha for the year with lighter, bitter foods, like the first leafy greens of spring.

Summer. This is pitta season, period. Give your body cool, soothing foods, especially if you're a pitta.

Fall. As summer turns to winter, vata turns into kapha. You need warm, moist, well-lubricated foods to balance biting winds and cold November rains.

The Healing Power of Ayurveda

Ayurveda is uniquely effective at preventing disease, say Ayurvedic physicians. "Ayurvedic physicians in India used to get paid only while their patients were healthy," says Jay Glaser, M.D., director of the Maharishi Ayur-Veda Medical Center. "When patients got sick, they stopped paying."

Ayurvedic doctors give their patients a detailed examination. They take your pulse and inspect your tongue, fingernails, eyes, skin and some key internal organs. To check the liver, for instance, the doctor asks you to lie flat on your back, then checks by feel, pressing with his fingers in the area of the organ. With this type of examination, Ayurvedic doctors say they can pick up imbalances that Western medicine would never see—imbalances that, left unchecked, would progress into disease.

"Health is not all or nothing," explains Richard Averbach, M.D., whose practice is affiliated with the College of Maharishi Ayur-Veda Health Center in Fairfield, Iowa. "There are six stages along the continuum between health and disease. During the first four, you often don't even know you're sick."

Top Treatments

"Ayurveda is also a wonderful complement to Western medicine as disease treatment," says Dr. Glaser, who has developed a program for treating 36 common chronic conditions. According to Dr. Glaser, Ayurvedic doctors are especially good at addressing chronic and degenerative diseases and common problems like allergies. While Western medicine is less effective in these areas—in Dr. Glaser's view—Western doctors are especially good at surgery, and they excel at treating trauma and acute disease.

Unfortunately for those who like their proof in print, there are scientific studies on the effects of meditation and Ayurvedic herbs on health but almost none on the effect of diet. "Diet studies are very complicated and require a lot of time and funding," says Dr. Averbach. "We've just reached the point of credibility where we are able to get the money to conduct them."

From proponents of Ayurvedic medicine, however, there are many clinical reports and personal anecdotes documenting Ayurveda's healing powers. Ayurvedic doctors believe that Ayurveda can heal practically anything. To treat disease, they say, you should first see an Ayurvedic doctor to identify which dosha imbalance is responsible for the condition. The doctor will describe the pacifying diet for that dosha, which you are supposed to follow at least until the condition clears up, and sometimes longer, integrating the new diet into your lifestyle. Other treatment regimens often include therapies like yoga or herbs in addition to diet.

While the following conditions might be helped by an Ayurvedic diet, experts emphasize that the best approach is to be under the care of an Ayurvedic practitioner. The goal of Ayurvedic medicine is to prevent these conditions in the first place, according to Elson Haas, M.D., medical director of the Preventive Medical Center of Marin in San Rafael, California, and author of *Staying Healthy with Nutrition*. But here's an overview of the Ayurvedic approach to a number of common health problems.

Circulatory System Disorders

Ayurveda's teachings about heart disease are similar to those of Western medicine. Stress, bad diet and heredity are all key culprits, according to Ayurvedic doctors. The prominent dosha problem is pitta, which fires the driving temperament that leads to heart attack and stroke.

Too much kapha also can contribute by creating blockages. And high vata can add to artery constriction. Here are some of the specifics.

Atherosclerosis. This condition tends to develop from a lifetime of building up too much kapha, says Dr. Frawley. "Generally, you follow the same treatment as you would for coronary heart disease."

Coronary heart disease. This is "a kapha problem," says Dr. Glaser. "The Pritikin and Ornish diets are very similar to what Ayurveda recommends—a kapha-pacifying diet that emphasizes very low fat foods. It works very, very well."

High blood pressure (hypertension). High blood pressure is common to all three doshas, says Dr. Lad. "Transient hypertension (it comes and goes) is vata, while malignant hypertension (which is dangerously high) is pitta. And chronic high blood pressure is kapha. Kapha is the easiest to treat with diet alone," according to Dr. Lad. For constant, kapha high blood pressure, Ayurveda recommends an anti-kapha diet that restricts dairy products, butter, eggs and high-fat foods, says Dr. Frawley.

"After my husband died, I put on ten pounds. I had high blood pressure and high cholesterol—the works," recalls Carol, a pitta-kapha from Seattle. Dr. Sodhi prescribed a kapha- and pitta-pacifying diet, which eliminated dairy products, wheat, caffeine and alcohol. "I lost ten pounds in a month, and now, several months later, I'm off both of my blood pressure medications," she says.

Digestive System Disorders

"Digestive diseases are the result of toxins," explains Dr. Frawley. "When the digestive fires are not working, toxins build up and back up into the system, manifesting themselves as disease. When you change your diet properly, your body is able to let the toxins drain out, so the disease clears."

Constipation. This common problem can be due to an imbalance of any dosha, but it's usually a vata condition, particularly when it's frequent or occurs in the elderly, says Dr. Sodhi. Vata constipation is the most severe and is often accompanied by gas. Kapha is medium, accompanied by lethargy and bloating. And pitta is the mildest, often following fever and accom-

(continued on page 92)

Do's and Don'ts to Balance Dosha

To use this table, look under the column that corresponds to your dominant dosha to find the foods that are recommended or are not recommended. In the "Yes" column are foods that are recommended because they help balance your dosha. In the "No" column you'll find foods that are not recommended because they aggravate that particular dosha.

	Vata		Pitta		Kapha	
	Yes	No	Yes	No	Yes	No
Grains	Oats (cooked) Rice Wheat	Barley Buckwheat Corn Millet Oats (dry) Rye	Barley Oats (cooked) Rice (basmati) Rice (white) Wheat	Buckwheat Corn Millet Oats (dry) Rice (brown) Rye	Barley Corn Millet Oats (dry) Rice (basmati, small amount) Rye	Oats (cooked) Rice (brown) Rice (white) Wheat
Animal Foods	Beef Chicken or turkey (white meat) Eggs (fried or scrambled)	Lamb Pork Rabbit Venison	Chicken or turkey (white meat) Eggs (white) Rabbit Shrimp (small amount) Venison	Beef Eggs (yolk) Lamb Pork Seafood	Chicken or turkey (dark meat) Eggs (not fried or scrambled) Rabbit Shrimp Venison	Beef Lamb Pork Seafood
Fruits	All sweet fruits Apricots Avocados Bananas Berries Cherries Coconut Figs (fresh) Grapefruit Grapes Lemons Mangos Melons (sweet) Oranges Papayas Peaches Pineapple Plums	All dried fruits Apples Cranberries Pears Persimmons Pomegranates Watermelon	All sweet fruits Apples Avocados Coconut Figs Grapes (dark) Mangos Melons Oranges (sweet) Pears Pineapple (sweet) Plums (sweet) Pomegranates Prunes Raisins	All sour fruits Apricots Berries Bananas Cherries Cranberries Grapefruit Grapes (green) Lemons Oranges (sour) Papayas Peaches Pineapple (sour) Persimmons Plums (sour)	Apples Apricots Berries Cherries Cranberries Figs (dried) Mangos Peaches Pears Persimmons Pomegranates Prunes Raisins	All sweet and sour fruits Avocados Bananas Coconut Figs (fresh) Grapefruit Grapes Lemons Melons Oranges Papayas Pineapple Plums
Oils	All oils		Coconut Olive Soy Sunflower	Almond Corn Safflower Sesame		No oils except almond, corn or sunflower (in small amounts)

	Vata		Pitta		Kapha	
	Yes	No	Yes	No	Yes	No
Vegetables						
	All cooked vegetables Asparagus Beets Carrots Cucumbers Garlic Green beans Okra (cooked) Onions (cooked) Potatoes (sweet) Radishes Zucchini	All raw vegetables Broccoli Brussels sprouts Cabbage Cauliflower Celery Eggplant Leafy greens* Lettuce* Mushrooms Onions (raw) Parsley* Peas Peppers Potatoes (white) Spinach* Sprouts* Tomatoes *These vegetables are okay in moderation with oil dressing.	All sweet and bitter vegetables Asparagus Broccoli Brussels sprouts Cabbage Cauliflower Celery Cucumbers Green beans Leafy greens Lettuce Mushrooms Okra Peas Parsley Peppers (green) Potatoes Sprouts Zucchini	All pungent vegetables Beets Carrots Eggplant Garlic Onions Peppers (hot) Radishes Spinach Tomatoes	All pungent and bitter vegetables Asparagus Beets Broccoli Brussels sprouts Cabbage Carrots Cauliflower Celery Eggplant Garlic Leafy greens Lettuce Mushrooms Okra Onions Parsley Peas Peppers Potatoes (white) Radishes Spinach Sprouts	All sweet and juicy vegetables Cucumbers Potatoes (sweet) Tomatoes Zucchini
Dairy						
	All dairy products (in moderation)		Butter (unsalted) Cottage cheese Ghee Milk	Buttermilk Cheese Sour cream Yogurt		No dairy except ghee and goat's milk
Legumes						
		No legumes except mung beans, tofu and black and red lentils	All legumes except lentils		All legumes except kidney beans, soybeans, black lentils and mung beans	
Nuts						
	All nuts (in small amounts)			No nuts except coconut		No nuts at all
Seeds						
	All seeds are okay (in moderation)			No seeds except sunflower and pumpkin		No seeds except sunflower and pumpkin
Sweeteners						
	All sweeteners except white sugar		All sweeteners except molasses and honey			No sweeteners except raw honey

Spice Up Your Digestion

If you follow the teachings of Ayurveda, there are many spices and herbs that are essential in preparing foods for health. Here are the ones that Ayurvedic doctors recommend for optimal digestion and food absorption.

If you're vata, all spices are good, and if you're kapha, you can eat any spice except salt. For pitta, you should avoid all spices except coriander, cinnamon, cardamom, fennel, turmeric and a small amount of black pepper.

Some of the following spices are available in any supermarket, but there are others that you may have to search for. Try Asian, Middle Eastern or Indian grocery stores if there are any in your area, or check out the nearest natural food stores. If there are none around, check "Resources for Healing" on page 99 to find suppliers.

Black mustard seed. Pungent. Pittas should use it sparingly.

Coriander. Sweet, astringent and cooling.

Cumin. Aromatic and medicinal.

Fennel. Sweet, pungent and cooling.

Ginger. Sweet and pungent.

Hing. A substitute for onion and garlic; use in very small quantities.

Trifala. A combination of three fruits—amla, haritaki and bahera—with an initially bitter taste. Also an antioxidant.

panied by burning and irritability. "All are easily treated with the appropriate dosha-balancing diet," says Dr. Sodhi.

Diarrhea. Typically a pitta condition, says Dr. Frawley, this type of diarrhea burns the rectum, is yellow and smells foul. Treatment includes an anti-pitta diet, which means avoiding hot spices, alcohol and oily, greasy or fried foods. Cooking with ginger and nutmeg is also recommended.

There can also be vata and kapha diarrhea. With vata diarrhea, you'll have alternating constipation and diarrhea. If it's kapha diarrhea, you'll detect mucus in the stool. Both improve with diets for their respective constitutions, says Dr. Frawley.

In Sue Grenager's case, a tridosha diet was necessary. Grenager, a vata-pitta from Pennsylvania, experienced diarrhea for two and a half years during a stressful time at her job. After trying other alternative medicine treatments, she found Ayurveda. Her treatment included a diet to pacify all her doshas, which she was told were "terribly out of whack."

Grenager now follows a vata- and pitta-pacifying regimen. "I eat very little meat, lots of lentils and rice, no corn, potatoes, peanuts or pizza, little wheat and warm food. I'm reasonable but not rigid about it. My stools are much more normal now."

Food allergies. Allergic reactions to foods are "weaknesses of digestive fires and often reflect constitution," says Dr. Frawley. "Vata people tend to have allergies to vata-aggravating foods like beans, soy and corn. Pitta people have allergies to tomatoes and sour fruit like strawberries. Kapha people are sensitive to dairy and wheat products." To treat food allergies, Dr. Frawley recommends strict adherence to the constitutional diet, then a slow introduction of restricted foods until the offending food is discovered.

Hemorrhoids. These painful, bulging veins in the anus are usually a vata or pitta condition, says Dr. Sodhi. Vata hemorrhoids are dry, rough and irregular, with little bleeding. They are caused by constipation and dry stool from too much cold, raw, dry and/or astringent food and are remedied by a vata-pacifying diet, he says. Pitta hemorrhoids swell, bleed and burn, and they require an anti-pitta diet.

Hepatitis. This infectious, damaging liver disease isn't caused by too much pitta, but too much pitta can increase the tendency for hepatitis, says Dr. Frawley. Ayurveda doesn't deal with acute hepatitis, but it can alleviate the after-effects, such as liver damage and potential recurrence, through herbs and a pitta-pacifying diet and lifestyle. On an Ayurvedic treatment plan, you would eliminate oily, greasy food, red meat, alcohol and too many sweets.

Intestinal gas. Gas is usually the result of excessive light, dry, vata-aggravating foods like beans, cabbage or peanuts, says Dr. Sodhi. It's easily remedied with a vata-pacifying diet, including almost any cooking spices, which expel gas.

Nausea. An imbalance in any of the doshas can cause nausea, says Dr. Frawley. Vata nausea is associated with dry vomiting, pain in the chest and palpitations, pitta nausea with the bilious, burning kind of vomiting, and kapha with a watery and mucusy type.

Overweight. Overweight is "often a cultural standard, not a disease," says Dr. Frawley, warning that Ayurveda is not meant to be a weight-loss diet for artificial thinness. It can remedy real overweight, however, which is generally a kapha condition. For people who have this condition, the Ayurvedic doctor recommends a light, kapha-pacifying diet with emphasis on digestion-improving spices such as ginger.

Ulcers. Ulcers, particularly peptic ulcer disease, are characteristically a pitta disorder, says Dr. Lad. Like most diseases involving acidity and burning, it is remedied with an anti-pitta diet.

Underweight. As you might expect, this is usually a vata condition, says Dr. Sodhi, and is easily remedied with a vata-pacifying diet.

Nervous System Disorders

According to vedic literature, nervous system disorders are typically attributable to vata, as nerve impulses are thought to be like a wind traveling through the body. When those communications are blocked, mental and physical faculties break down, often resulting in tremors, headache and even paralysis.

Anxiety. According to Dr. Lad, anxiety is characteristically a vata disorder. "As you would expect, the treatment relies on a vata-pacifying, grounding diet."

Depression. Depression can be either vata, pitta or kapha, says Dr. Lad. "Vata depression is associated with extreme grief, fear and anxiety. Pitta depression is generally that of highly successful people when they fail, causing them to be immobilized and often suicidal. Kapha depression is guilt and attachment. It leads to obesity and monotonous living. The required diet depends on the type of depression."

Headache. This common complaint can be attributed to all three doshas, says Dr. Lad. "Vata headaches are generally associated with constipation, dizziness and ringing in the ears, pitta with hyperacidity and pain in the temples and kapha with sinus congestion. Each is treatable with the proper dosha-pacifying diet."

Insomnia. This is a classic symptom of high vata, says Dr. Sodhi. It's often brought on by anxiety and ungroundedness and therefore requires heavy, grounding foods, like whole grains and dairy products, he says. "Stimulants, like coffee and tea, should be avoided, and warm milk is very helpful."

Reproductive System Disorders

Ayurvedic doctors agree that the health of the reproductive system is of great importance, not just for procreation but also for overall well-being. As with all health problems, any dosha imbalance can be the culprit, but hormonal problems are generally pitta problems, says Dr. Sodhi. Here are some common reproductive ailments that Ayurvedic diet can treat.

Amenorrhea. Cessation of menstruation is basically a high vata condition, says Dr. Frawley, who recommends an anti-vata diet, which includes meat, dairy, nuts, oils and whole grains.

Endometriosis. This condition occurs when the tissue that lines the uterus is implanted on other pelvic organs, causing excessive pain and bleeding. According to Dr. Sodhi, this is mostly a pitta imbalance. "I see a lot of women with endometriosis—women who are very successful, drink a lot of coffee, have a lot of stress and so on. This lifestyle taxes the liver until it can't cleanse the hormones properly. I've had a lot of success with herbs and a pitta-pacifying diet," he says.

Enlarged prostate. Prostate enlargement is a pitta-vata condition, says Dr. Sodhi. "It's pitta because it involves hormones and infection, and vata because it generally happens later in life, which is a vata time." Treatment involves dietary measures to pacify both pitta and vata and is best done under a physician's supervision, says Dr. Sodhi.

Fibrocystic breasts. This problem is most common in kapha women, says Dr. Sodhi, although it can appear as the result of any dosha imbalance. "You have to be diagnosed to know for sure."

Jean, a vata-pitta from Washington, used an Ayurvedic diet to treat large fibrocystic lumps in her breasts as well as a cyst on one ovary. Dr. Sodhi prescribed a diet to balance all three doshas and improve her liver function. His plan emphasized reducing kapha by eliminating wheat, dairy and red meat and allowing very little oil. "My lumps are all but gone," says Jean.

Genital herpes. Like other infectious diseases, herpes is primarily pitta, according to Dr. Sodhi. "I have seen a lot of people with herpes.

I haven't cured anybody, but they have fewer outbreaks—some have had no outbreaks for two or three years." The best dietary strategy is anti-pitta, especially avoiding alcohol and hot, spicy foods, he says.

Impotence. This is generally a vata condition, because it involves anxiety, stress and insufficient energy, says Dr. Frawley. Treatment includes temporary abstinence from sexual activity and a vata-pacifying diet supplemented with foods that increase semen production, such as ghee (clarified butter), nuts and shellfish.

Infertility. Difficulty conceiving is associated with vata, generally considered the least fertile of the three dosha types, says Dr. Frawley. "Ayurveda recommends using an anti-vata, kapha-building diet, with a special emphasis on dairy, especially milk."

Miscarriage. This "is most commonly a high pitta condition occurring in pitta-dominant women, because pregnancy increases their already high body temperature," says Dr. Frawley. Ayurvedic treatment includes avoiding spicy, oily and other pitta-aggravating foods while increasing dairy intake, especially milk.

Respiratory System Disorders

Diseases of the respiratory system tend to be kapha conditions, since they involve congestion and fluids such as mucus and phlegm. Because such congestion squelches digestive fires, digestive spices like ginger are often recommended along with a kapha-pacifying diet.

Allergies and hay fever. These are tridosha problems, says Dr. Lad. "Hay fever is due to kapha excess. An excess of pitta, on the other hand, can cause rashes. And vata allergies involve bloating, constipation and palpitations," Dr. Lad says. "These can all be treated by the appropriate diets."

Bronchial asthma. Constriction of the bronchial tubes that causes wheezing is the result of excessive vata, says Dr. Lad. Ayurvedic treatment includes a vata-pacifying diet along with herbal preparations.

Colds. These are primarily kapha disorders, says Dr. Frawley. "The treatment diet should be kapha-pacifying, with an emphasis on light, warm and simple foods, like steamed vegetables and grains."

Cough. Coughing is typically a kapha condition, characterized by mucus and heaviness in the chest. It can also be pitta, which is marked by yellow phlegm and a burning sensation in the chest, or vata, which is dry with little or no expectoration, says Dr. Frawley. For kapha and vata coughs, dosha-pacifying diets are helpful. An anti-pitta diet will prevent a pitta cough from becoming worse, but usually herbal treatment is also needed, he says.

Laryngitis. This can result from an excess of any of the three doshas, says Dr. Frawley. Kapha is indicated by white mucus, pitta by yellow mucus, sore throat and fever, and vata by a dry throat and low voice. It's treated similarly to cough, with vata and kapha types responding to dosha-pacifying diets. Pitta requires stronger treatment, Dr. Frawley says.

Sinusitis. Sinusitis is a kapha condition, says Dr. Glaser. "We have incredible success treating sinusitis through a kapha-pacifying diet." Along with this, however, Dr. Glaser recommends herbal drops in the nose, a treatment called nasya.

Bob Wartinger, a corporate manager who lives in Seattle, used a kapha-pacifying diet to clear up his congestion. A kapha-pitta, Wartinger was prone to sinus problems and colds and was seeing Dr. Sodhi for advice on boosting his energy for peak performance. Dr. Sodhi put him on a kapha-pacifying diet—no dairy products, wheat or sugar, including a ban on fructose in fruit juice. "It was hard, because I loved lasagna and orange juice," Wartinger says. "But I made the changes and felt better almost immediately. No more sinusitis. No more congestion."

Skin Conditions

"Skin diseases are more common in pitta people, but they can be attributable to any of the three doshas," says Dr. Frawley. Here are some skin problems that Ayurvedic doctors say are often caused by diet, and that they think diet can treat.

Acne. This is a pitta condition, says Dr. Lad. "It's very common among pitta people, especially in the summer." Ayurvedic treatment for acne is pitta-pacifying with an emphasis on avoiding sour foods, he says.

Boils. These skin eruptions are pitta conditions, says Dr. Frawley. "They can be triggered by eating too many pitta-causing foods—things that are overly spicy, greasy or oily." Treatment emphasizes a strongly anti-pitta diet, with many light, cool foods like salads and vegetable juices.

Eczema. According to Dr. Lad, eczema is mostly a pitta condition. He says it's best treated with a pitta-pacifying diet, and especially avoiding sour foods like citrus fruits, vinegar, cheese and fermented foods.

Psoriasis. Psoriasis "can be vata, pitta or kapha," says Dr. Lad. "Vata is dry, rough and scaly, pitta has a lot of inflammation, and kapha has silvery, crusty scabs." He suggests following the appropriate dosha-pacifying diet.

Urinary Tract Disorders

All three doshas can potentially be blamed in diseases of the urinary tract, but urinary infections are primarily pitta, says Dr. Sodhi. Here are the conditions that diet can help.

Kidney stones. These are usually a result of a pitta imbalance, says Dr. Sodhi. "Pitta causes calcium stones, but you can also have phosphorus stones, which are the result of high kapha." For pitta-caused stones, Dr. Sodhi recommends an anti-pitta diet, eliminating spinach, meat and dairy products. He also adds some herbal preparations. For kapha-caused stones, he suggests an anti-kapha diet and the herbs.

John, from New Zealand, had a history of kidney stones. When he came to Dr. Sodhi, John had several tiny calcium stones in one kidney and an inch-long stone in the other. "I wanted to try natural treatment, something that would get rid of the stones and keep them from coming back," he remembers.

Dr. Sodhi gave him herbs and prescribed a kapha-pacifying diet that

First Steps

If you decide to try an Ayurvedic diet, you'll first need to see an Ayurvedic doctor to determine your balance and the foods you require. Depending on your body type and temperament, the doctor might say something like, "You're extremely pitta, with some kapha and a small vata imbalance." If that's the situation, you'll probably be told to follow a pitta-pacifying diet in summer and a light, vata-pacifying diet after that—eliminating caffeine and alcohol and tempering your penchant for eating hot, spicy foods.

After two weeks of waking up without your mornng java and smacking your forgetful right hand every time it reaches for some off-limit delicacy, you arc likely to discover that Ayurvedic eating is not easy. But those who have tried it say that it can make a significant difference in the way you feel.

Many people experience more vitality. You may feel more alert and more awake even though you can't have caffeine. And there may be immediate side benefits. One of our editors said she'd always had cramps and bloating during her period. While she was on the diet, she discovered that her period came and went without the usual symptoms.

One thing you'll notice immediately on an Ayurvedic diet is that nothing compares to the taste of fresh food. Having all six tastes in every meal is like a food symphony—sweet, sour and satisfying. If you're in the habit of rummaging through your fridge an hour after a meal for that elusive "something else," you may find a big difference. "I felt light, healthy and energetic," noted our editor after just two weeks on the diet.

included no dairy and no meat. "After four months, all the stones in my right kidney were gone, and the one in the left was one-third of the size," John recalls.

Urinary tract infections. "Like most infections, these are generally caused by high pitta," says Dr. Frawley, "although it's possible to have a vata or kapha urinary tract infection, too." Pitta infections, which are acute and are characterized by difficult, frequent, burning urination, require a strong pitta-pacifying diet, says Dr. Frawley. He stresses the need to shun alcohol, spices and tomatoes.

Water retention. Also called edema, this condition is typically kapha, says Dr. Frawley, "because it's caused by excess water in the body, which is common in kapha-dominant people." For kapha-type edema, marked by significant swelling and moist, pale skin, he recommends a kapha-pacifying diet, which eliminates dairy products, oils, fats and cold drinks.

Chronic Diseases

"Ayurvedic physcians see a tremendous number of people with chronic diseases," says Dr. Sodhi, "because they are the diseases that Western medicine doesn't treat effectively." These are some chronic conditions commonly treated by Ayurvedic nutrition.

AIDS. This is generally a condition of low ojas, says Dr. Frawley, "which are vital energies that keep the immune system strong. They are also associated with strong kapha." Treatment, therefore, includes a pitta- and vata-pacifying diet, which stresses milk, yogurt and ghee and restricts spicy, sour, bitter and astringent tastes, he says.

"No one is saying that we can cure people of AIDS, but we have been able to make their lives better," stresses Dr. Sodhi. "One man I treated who had full-blown AIDS, with Karposi's sarcoma, was able to gain about 15 pounds and avoid some of the common complications, like blindness."

Alzheimer's disease. According to Dr. Glaser, Alzheimer's disease "is one that Ayurveda doesn't discuss directly, but we use treatments based on ancient recommendations for dementia, memory loss and senility," says Dr. Glaser. "Like other neurological problems, it's a condition of excess vata and requires vata-pacifying treatments. Ghee is also very important."

Diabetes. Diabetes "starts out as a kapha imbalance but becomes a vata imbalance if left untreated," says Dr. Sodhi. "With dietary treatment alone, we can get the best results with early Type II (non-insulin-dependent), kapha-type diabetes." At this stage, Ayurvedic doctors recommend a long-term, anti-kapha diet, which emphasizes the bitter taste.

Even in later stages of severe diabetes, where kidney failure can lead to long-term dialysis, Ayurveda sometimes helps, say Ayurvedic doctors.

Inflammatory bowel disease. This is primarily a problem of too much pitta, says Dr. Lad. "The treatment diet needs to be strongly pitta-pacifying."

Marcia Goldberg of Sumneytown, Pennsylvania, battled Crohn's disease, a type of inflammatory bowel disease, for 30 years. After some success with hospitalization and experimental drugs, she tried yoga and meditation and eventually found relief. She now follows a vata- and pitta-pacifying diet to keep her symptoms in check.

Low energy. Lack of energy, which translates into steady fatigue, is a problem that brings many people to Ayurvedic physicians. "There's not much that Western physicians can do for people with chronic fatigue. We put them on their feet again," says Dr. Glaser.

"It's the result of too much pitta, which leads to low digestive fire and low energy," adds Dr. Lad. "Treatment includes digestive herbs and a pitta-pacifying diet."

Multiple sclerosis. Multiple sclerosis is a condition of both pitta and vata, says Dr. Lad. "I recommend following a pitta-pacifying diet in pitta season and a vata-pacifying diet in vata season."

"I generally emphasize a vata-pacifying diet," says Dr. Glaser. "By using diet and a complete treatment program, including daily massage, yoga and transcendental meditation, we've had some great success."

Parkinson's disease. A progressive condition that attacks the brain, causing muscle tremors and rigidity, Parkinson's disease is typically a vata imbalance. The diet for it should focus on lowering high vata, says Dr. Lad, noting that vata-pacifying herbs would also be in order.

Rheumatoid arthritis. This type of arthritis, which disrupts the normal functioning of the joints and the tissues surrounding them, is a vata condition, says Dr. Lad. Its name in Ayurveda is amavata, because it is believed to result from a buildup of toxins (ama.) Complete therapy involves detoxification and massage, but an anti-vata diet combined with good digestive spices can help, he says.

A Taste of Ayurveda

So you're ready to join the nutrition fraternity of vata, pitta, kapha, but you don't know where to start. " The first step is to relax," advises Morningstar. "Ayurveda is simply about developing a better, more intimate relationship with food." The primary rules are eat fresh, eat for optimum digestion and eat constitutionally. "But go slowly," she adds. "If you eat nothing but canned and frozen foods, make gradual substitutions. Start by eating fresh vegetables once a week. Then aim for buying fresh organic foods whenever possible."

On the following pages, you'll find sample menus for an Ayurvedic diet, along with some recipes. They are not season-specific, which is of primary importance in Ayurveda. To plan season-specific meals, you need an Ayurvedic cookbook.

Resources for Healing

Organizations

American School of Ayurvedic Sciences, Ayurvedic and Naturopathic Medical Clinic
2115 112th Avenue NE
Bellevue, WA 98004

Ayurvedic Institute
11311 Menaul NE, Suite A
Albuquerque, NM 87112

The College of Maharishi Ayur-Veda Health Center
P.O. Box 282
Fairfield, IA 52556

The Maharishi Ayur-Veda Health Center
679 George Hill Road, P.O. Box 344
Lancaster, MA 01523

Ayurvedic Physician Referrals

Alternative Yellow Pages
Future Medicine Publishing
21½ Main Street
Tiburon, CA 94920

Mail-Order Sources

Ayush Herbs, Inc.
2115 112th Avenue
Bellevue, WA 98004
1-800-925-1371

Maharishi Ayur-Ved Products International
P.O. Box 49667
Colorado Springs, CO 80949-9667
1-800-255-8332

Books

Ayurveda: A Life of Balance
Maya Tiwari
Inner Traditions

Ayurvedic Cooking for Self-Healing
Usha Lad and Vasant Lad, B.A.M.S., M.A.Sc.
Ayurvedic Press

Ayurvedic Cooking for Westerners
Amadea Morningstar
Lotus Press

Try It for a Week

Here are sample menus for each of the three doshas. You can also make dishes that suit all three constitutional types, which is known as tridoshic.

All meal plans and recipes are excerpted and/or adapted from *The Ayurvedic Cookbook* by Amadea Morningstar with Urmila Desai and *Ayurvedic Cooking for Westerners* by Amadea Morningstar.

Vata Menus

In general, focus on warm, cooked foods and foods with oily properties and sweet, sour and salty tastes.

Sunday   Brunch—Whole-wheat crepes
Snack—Fresh fruit
Dinner—Nice Burger (page 107), tossed salad and basmati rice and steamed vegetables with ghee* and Indian spices

Monday   Breakfast—Oatmeal or Cream of Wheat cereal
Lunch—Hot vegetable soup and bread
Snack—Fresh fruit or fruit juices
Dinner—Pasta with cream sauce and hot tea

Tuesday   Breakfast—Poached, soft-boiled or scrambled eggs and whole-wheat toast
Lunch—Cream of broccoli soup
Snack—Nuts and seeds and a warm drink
Dinner—Egg noodles with Light Basil Sauce (page 103)

Wednesday   Breakfast—Cinnamon rolls and hot milk
Lunch—Cottage cheese, pasta salad and a small lettuce salad
Snack—Yogurt and/or a warm drink
Dinner—Pasta Primavera (page 105)

Thursday   Breakfast—Shredded wheat cereal and whole-wheat toast
Lunch—Hot Korean Vegetables and Noodles (page 104)
Snack—Sunflower seeds or nuts
Dinner—Vegetarian Stroganoff (page 103)

Friday   Breakfast—French toast
Lunch—Cheese sandwich with Avocado Spread (page 107) and/or vegetable soup
Snack—Fresh fruit or fruit juice
Dinner—Vegetarian burritos or cheese enchiladas with whole-grain breads and/or muffins

Saturday   Brunch—Pancakes with blueberries
Snack—Whole-wheat crackers and guacamole
Dinner—Pasta with Pesto Sauce (page 105), zucchini salad and tea

Desserts are optional, but common vata-calming desserts include tapioca pudding, rice pudding and pumpkin pie. Beverage choices include hot herbal tea, hot chocolate, hot milk and fruit juices.

*Ghee, which is used often in Ayurvedic cooking, is simply clarified butter.

Pitta Menus

In general, pitta people should seek cool foods and drinks. Favor those foods with predominantly sweet, bitter and astringent tastes.

Sunday Brunch—Scrambled Tofu (page 106) with cinnamon rolls
Snack—Fresh melon, apple or pear
Dinner—Vegetarian Stroganoff (page 103)

Monday Breakfast—Waffles with maple syrup
Lunch—Broccoli-stuffed baked potato
Snack—Fresh vegetables: celery, jícama, peas
Dinner—Pasta Primavera (page 105)

Tuesday: Breakfast—Oatmeal or Cream of Wheat or Cream of Rice cereal
Lunch—Salad with vegetables, beans and cottage cheese
Snack—Dried fruit, figs or raisins
Dinner—Bean burrito and salad or pasta

Wednesday Breakfast—Oat bran muffins and Mint Tulip (page 104)
Lunch—Sweet chick-peas and whole-wheat tortillas
Snack—Toasted sunflower seeds
Dinner—Chinese tofu stir-fry with rice and Chinese vegetables

Thursday Breakfast—Shredded wheat cereal
Lunch—Cream of broccoli soup and hot whole-wheat tortillas
Snack—Cut-up raw vegetables
Dinner—Pasta with Light Basil Sauce (page 103), zucchini salad and tea

Friday Breakfast—French toast and tea
Lunch—Salad with kidney beans and cottage cheese
Snack—Sunflower or pumpkin seeds
Dinner—Red beans and rice with vegetables

Saturday Brunch—Pancakes with maple syrup and hot milk
Snack—Hummus (very easy on the garlic) and whole-wheat or rice crackers
Supper—Nice Burger (page 107), tossed salad and basmati rice with ghee and Indian spices

Desserts are optional, but common pitta-calming desserts include tapioca pudding, rice pudding and fresh fruits. Beverage choices include grape juice, apple juice, water, herbal tea and milk. If you're pitta, you should have no caffeine and only moderate alcohol—a maximum of two drinks per week.

(continued)

Try It for a Week—Continued

Kapha Menus

Whenever possible, kaphas should seek food and drink that are light, dry and warm. Always try to find foods that are pungent, bitter and astringent in taste.

Sunday   Brunch—Corn cakes with applesauce
        Snack—Dry-roasted chick-peas
        Supper—Buckwheat egg noodles with Light Basil Sauce (page 103)

Monday   Breakfast—Scrambled Tofu (page 106)
        Lunch—Chinese stir-fry with black bean sauce and Chinese vegetables
        Snack—Fresh fruit in season
        Dinner—Hummus and rye crackers

Tuesday   Breakfast—Poached eggs and rye toast
        Lunch—Hot vegetable soup and/or cornbread
        Snack—Popcorn
        Dinner—Spicy Chinese stir-fry

Wednesday   Breakfast—Cornflakes with goat or soy milk
        Lunch—Bean nachos with chili (no cheese)
        Snack—Fresh fruit in season
        Dinner—Salad with chick-peas, beets and plenty of vegetables

Thursday   Breakfast—Puffed-oat cereal with goat or soy milk
        Lunch—Cream of broccoli soup and salad
        Snack—Toasted corn chips
        Dinner—Broccoli-stuffed baked potato

Friday   Breakfast—Granola cereal with goat or soy milk
        Lunch—Fresh Dilled Eggplant (page 106)
        Snack—Popcorn
        Dinner—Beans, corn tortillas and salad

Saturday   Brunch—Buckwheat pancakes with blueberries, honey and ghee
        Snack—Fresh fruit: apple, pear, apricot
        Supper—Hot Korean Vegetables and Noodles (page 104) and a large salad with sprouts

Desserts are optional, but common kapha-calming desserts include any fresh fruit in season, eaten a few hours after the meal. Beverage choices include spring water, herbal teas and hot ginger tea.

Light Basil Sauce

Preparation time: 20 minutes   **Yield:** 2–3 servings

> 2 cup fresh raw cow's milk or soy milk
> 1 clove garlic, unpeeled
> 6 black peppercorns
> ½ cup raw walnuts
> 1 cup finely chopped fresh basil leaves

In a medium saucepan, combine the milk, garlic and peppercorns. Bring to a boil over medium-high heat. Remove from the heat. As desired, discard the garlic or peel and return to the milk mixture.

Place the walnuts in a blender and grind finely. Add the milk mixture and basil. Blend until pureed.

Vegetarian Stroganoff

Preparation time: 15 minutes plus soaking time   **Yield:** 2–4 servings

> 1½ ounces dried shiitake mushrooms
> ⅓ cup blanched raw almonds
> 2 cups boiling water
> ⅛ teaspoon freshly ground nutmeg
> ⅛ teaspoon freshly ground black pepper
> 1 pound firm tofu
> 1–2 tablespoons ghee
> 1 tablespoon finely chopped onions
> ½–1 teaspoon paprika
> Salt (to taste)

In a medium heatproof bowl, combine the mushrooms and almonds. Add the water. Cover with a lid or plate and let stand for 2 hours, or until the mushrooms are very plump.

Pick out the mushrooms and slice thinly.

Pour the almonds and liquid into a blender and blend until the almonds are pureed. Pour back into the bowl and stir in the mushrooms, nutmeg and pepper.

Rinse and drain the tofu. Pat dry and cut into ¾" cubes.

Warm the ghee in a large no-stick frying pan over medium heat. Add the onions and sauté for 2 minutes, or until soft. Add the tofu and the mushroom mixture. Cover and cook for 5 minutes, or until hot. Stir in the paprika and salt.

(continued)

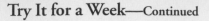

Hot Korean Vegetables and Noodles

Preparation time: 45 minutes   **Yield:** 3– 4 servings

   2 ounces cellophane noodles (mung bean noodles)
4–8 dried shiitake mushrooms
   1 tablespoon plus 1 teaspoon sunflower oil
   1 leek (white part only), thinly sliced, or ¹/₂ small onion, thinly sliced
   1 clove garlic, unpeeled
   1 cup thinly sliced carrots or ¹/₂ cup snow peas
   1 cup finely chopped spinach or broccoli
   1 cup thinly sliced yellow crookneck summer squash
   1 cup bean sprouts
   1 tablespoon tamari
   2 teaspoons ground coriander
   1 teaspoon Sucanat
   3 small cloves garlic, minced
¹/₂ teaspoon ground red pepper or 1 dried hot Chinese pepper, crumbled

Combine the noodles and mushrooms in a medium bowl. Add hot water to cover and let soak for 30 minutes. Drain. Slice the mushrooms thinly. Set aside with the noodles.

Warm 1 tablespoon of the oil in a large no-stick frying pan over medium heat. Add the leeks or onions and the unpeeled garlic. Sauté for 5 minutes. Remove and discard the garlic.

Add the carrots (if using), spinach or broccoli, squash and the reserved mushrooms. Sauté for 3 to 5 minutes, or until the vegetables are tender and bright in color. Add the snow peas (if using) and sauté for 1 minute. Stir in the bean sprouts and cook for 30 seconds. Add the tamari, coriander, Sucanat and the reserved noodles. Toss well to combine. Cover and set aside.

Warm the remaining 1 teaspoon oil in a small no-stick frying pan over medium heat. Add the minced garlic and cook for 1 minute, or until tender. Stir in the ground pepper or crumbled pepper. Serve as a garnish for the noodles.

Note: Sucanat is a natural sugar substitute, available in the baking section at health food stores.

Mint Tulip

Preparation time: 10 minutes   **Yield:** 4 servings

   3 cups water
   1 cup fresh or frozen pineapple juice
      Juice of ¹/₂ lemon
   1 tablespoon frozen orange juice concentrate
 10 fresh mint leaves or 1 tablespoon dried mint
 10 dates, pitted and chopped
1–8 tablespoons flaked or grated coconut

In a blender, combine the water, pineapple juice, lemon juice, orange juice concentrate, mint, dates and coconut. Blend until pureed. Serve cool.

Pasta Primavera

Preparation time: 15–20 minutes **Yield:** 2–4 servings

    4–8 ounces pasta
    ⅓   cup extra-virgin olive oil
      1 clove garlic
      2 small yellow crookneck squash, thinly sliced
      1 small zucchini, thinly sliced
    1½   cup fresh peas
      2 tablespoons chopped red onions
      1 tablespoon dried sage
         Salt and pepper (to taste)
         Freshly grated Parmesan or gomasio (ground toasted sesame seeds),
         optional

Cook the pasta in a large pot of boiling water until just tender. Drain and return to the pot.

While the pasta is cooking, combine the olive oil and garlic in a blender and process until the garlic is pureed. Transfer to a large no-stick frying pan. Place over medium heat for 1 minute. Add the squash, zucchini, peas and onions. Cook, stirring occasionally, for 5 to 10 minutes, or until the vegetables are tender but not limp. Add the sage, salt and pepper.

Pour the vegetables over the pasta and toss to mix well. Serve sprinkled with the Parmesan or gomasio (if using).

Pesto Sauce

Preparation time: 10 minutes **Yield:** 2 cups

      1 large clove garlic, unpeeled
    ½   cup pine nuts or walnuts
      2 cups loosely packed fresh basil leaves, chopped
      1 cup loosely packed fresh Italian parsley leaves, chopped
    ½   cup water
      3 tablespoons raw sesame tahini
      2 tablespoons extra-virgin olive oil
      2 teaspoons miso

Place the garlic in a steamer basket and steam, tightly covered, over boiling water for 5 minutes.

Meanwhile, grind the pine nuts or walnuts in a blender until finely powdered. Add the basil, parsley, water, tahini, oil and miso. Blend until creamy (if needed, add more water to facilitate blending).

Peel and mince the garlic. Add to the sauce. Blend briefly to incorporate.

(continued)

Scrambled Tofu

Preparation time: 5–10 minutes   **Yield:** 2 servings

1 tablespoon ghee or sweet unsalted butter
¼ teaspoon mustard seeds
8 ounces tofu
¼ teaspoon turmeric
¼ teaspoon salt
¼ teaspoon freshly ground black pepper
⅛ teaspoon hing
⅛ teaspoon ground cumin

In a large no-stick frying pan over medium heat, warm the ghee or melt the butter. Add the mustard seeds and cook for 30 seconds, or until they begin to pop. Add the tofu and mash with a fork into small pieces.

Stir in the turmeric, salt, pepper, hing and cumin. Cook, stirring, for 3 to 5 minutes, or until heated through.

Fresh Dilled Eggplant

Preparation time: 25–30 minutes   **Yield:** 5–6 servings

3 tablespoons sunflower oil
1 medium eggplant, peeled and cut into 1" cubes
1 bunch fresh dill, finely chopped
½ teaspoon turmeric
⅛ teaspoon hing
1 cup water
¼ green pepper, chopped , optional
2 tablespoons honey or barley malt
2 tablespoons lemon juice
1 teaspoon curry powder
1 teaspoon ground coriander
¾ teaspoon salt

Warm the oil in a large no-stick frying pan over medium heat. Stir in the eggplant, dill, turmeric and hing; cook for 1 minute. Add the water. Cover and simmer for 10 minutes.

Add the peppers, honey or barley malt, lemon juice, curry powder, coriander and salt. Cover and cook for 5 minutes.

Avocado Spread

Preparation time: 10 minutes   **Yield:** 2 servings

  1 **ripe avocado**
  1 **tablespoon lime juice or lemon juice**
  1 **tablespoon chopped fresh coriander leaves**
$1/8$ **teaspoon freshly ground black pepper**
$1/8$ **teaspoon garlic powder, optional**

Mash the avocado in a small bowl. Add the lime juice or lemon juice, coriander, pepper and garlic (if using). Mix well.

Nice Burgers

Preparation time: 1½ hours   **Yield:** 16 burgers

  3 **cups water**
$1^1/3$ **cups brown basmati rice**
$1/4$ **cup whole-grain teff, optional**
  1 **cup sprouted mung beans**
  2 **stalks celery, finely chopped**
$1/2$ **cup grated carrots**
$1/3$ **cup finely chopped tender leek greens**
$2/3$ **cup finely ground pumpkin seeds**
$2/3$ **cup finely ground almonds**
  1 **clove garlic, minced**
  4 **teaspoons dried basil**
  2 **teaspoons dried oregano**
2–4 **tablespoons finely chopped fresh parsley**
  1 **teaspoon chopped fresh sage**
  1 **teaspoon salt**

In a medium saucepan, combine the water, rice and teff (if using). Bring to a boil over high heat. Reduce the heat to medium-low, cover and cook for 40 minutes, or until the rice is nearly tender. Stir in the mung beans and cook for 5 minutes, or until the liquid is absorbed. Remove from the heat.

Preheat the oven to 350°. Lightly oil 2 baking sheets.

In a large bowl, combine the celery, carrots, leek greens, pumpkin seeds, almonds, garlic, basil, oregano, parsley, sage and salt. Mix well. Add the rice mixture and stir well to combine.

Form the mixture into 16 patties. Place on the prepared baking sheets and bake for 30 to 35 minutes, or until golden and heated through.

Note: Teff is a tiny, sweet-flavored Ethiopian grain, available at health food stores.

7 The Ornish Program

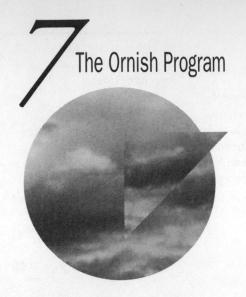

Eating to Open Your Heart

It takes a lifetime to clog an artery.

It takes truckloads of greasy meals and fatty snacks, countless hours of inactivity and years of emotional stress and strain. And once that artery is blocked, only major surgery can open it up again.

Tell that to Werner Hebenstreit.

After surviving two heart attacks, Hebenstreit expected to be incapacitated for the rest of his life. At 71, his coronary arteries were so blocked that even crossing the street brought on excruciating chest pain. He swallowed as many as 14 different pills a day to control his elevated blood pressure, sky-high cholesterol and other cardiac symptoms.

And yet, by age 80, he had the energy of a man decades younger. In the intervening years, he'd also taken up a new, favorite pastime—hiking with his wife, Eva, sometimes for as long as six hours. '

Such a change in the span of just nine years would seem impossible. Yet Hebenstreit never had open-heart surgery. He took no drugs, except a baby aspirin every other day.

Werner Hebenstreit owes his return to health, he says, to Dean Ornish, M.D., a Harvard-trained heart specialist who's changing the way medicine views heart disease.

The Total Program

While the Reversal Diet is crucial for anyone fighting heart disease, there are three other components to Dr. Ornish's program. While each of the four parts is valuable by itself, it's the combination that's been proven to reverse heart disease, according to Helen Roe, R.D., nutritionist at Dr. Ornish's Preventive Medicine Research Center in Sausalito, California, and the chief nutritional consultant for his research studies.

"Based on our research, all the people who actually reversed their signs of heart disease did the whole program, not just the diet," says Roe. "And the more closely they adhered to all four parts of the program, the more dramatic their reversals were."

Stress management. Stress affects the heart in a number of ways. Besides increasing blood pressure and cholesterol levels, it stimulates the production of hormones that constrict blood vessels and make blood more likely to clot, upping your risk of heart attack.

People on Dr. Ornish's program spend a minimum of one hour a day practicing stress-management techniques—30 minutes in the morning and 30 minutes later in the day. The techniques include deep breathing, stretching, visualization and meditation.

Exercise. Regular exercise helps the heart work more efficiently, increases endurance and can help you cope with emotional stress. It also helps control blood sugar and keeps blood pressure and cholesterol levels in the healthy range, says Lee Lipsenthal, M.D., medical director of the Preventive Medicine Research Institute.

The program includes at least 30 minutes a day of aerobic exercise like walking, biking, jogging or swimming. Walking is the preferred form of exercise for most people, since it's convenient and causes fewer injuries than other types. But before they begin any kind of exercise program, participants in the Ornish program get a physical exam.

Group support. People in the program also take part in support groups. They share their feelings about the program and also discuss how they're coping with other challenges in their lives. The groups are designed to provide a sense of community and connectedness that many people with heart disease are sorely lacking, according to Dr. Ornish.

Dr. Ornish believes that feelings of isolation play a key role in heart disease, both by creating chronic stress and by leading to destructive behavior like smoking and dangerous, unhealthy eating habits.

"The heart is more than just a physical pump," he says. "There is also an emotional and spiritual side to heart disease. The heart needs to be nurtured and to be connected with other people."

A Way with Foods

Instead of touting wonder drugs and using high-tech surgical techniques, Dr. Ornish teaches people to heal themselves with some of the oldest healing techniques under the sun.

A Week at Camp Ornish

While thousands of people adopt Dr. Ornish's program just by following the advice in his books, there's no better way to get started than by attending one of Dr. Ornish's week-long Open Your Heart retreats. Held four times a year at the Claremont Resort in Oakland, California, the retreats teach people everything they need to know to make the program a permanent part of their lives.

Participants include people of all ages, some with extensive medical histories, others apparently fit and well. Here are some of the people our editor met on one retreat.

• Jack Kirsch. Sick of dealing with heart problems, Kirsch was prepared to make dramatic lifestyle changes in order to regain his health. After two bypass surgeries, he started following the program a few months before coming to the retreat, after reading one of Dr. Ornish's books.

• A fit, athletic man in his forties, who looked as if he should have been out running a marathon instead of waiting in line to have his blood pressure taken (he asked that his name not be used.) He inherited a tendency toward sky-high cholesterol that puts him at high risk for a heart attack. By age 40, he'd already been through one angioplasty, a procedure that allows for increased blood flow through a partially blocked artery.

• Los Angeles real estate developer Harry Topping, a young, healthy self-confessed workaholic who admits he rarely makes time for exercise. "Healthwise, I've been lucky so far, but I know I need to get in better shape and pay more attention to what I eat," says Topping. "I live on take-out food."

Major Meal Revisions

Three times a day, participants are treated to delicious, satisfying meals that are cooked according to Dr. Ornish's stringent dietary guidelines. "This is really important, because you learn how good the food can taste," says Roe. "It gives you confidence that you can continue to eat this way for the rest of your life, without losing the enjoyment of food."

Roe and her staff make every effort to give their guests the tools they need to continue the diet once the retreat is over. Participants take a tour of a local grocery store and learn how to choose healthy, low-fat foods that fit into the diet.

Cooking demonstrations by Jean-Marc Fullsack—the French chef who devel-

As part of his program. Dr. Ornish insists that participants get regular, gentle exercise and attend support groups, where they are urged to talk about their fears and frustrations. While helping people learn to manage stress with yoga and meditation, he also promotes a simple, healthful and tasty vegetarian diet.

"We don't have to wait for a new drug," says Dr. Ornish. "We simply

oped the recipes for Dr. Ornish's books—reveal some of the techniques he uses to make low-fat vegetarian fare taste good. While Fullsack's techniques seem over-ambitious to many participants, everyone enjoys tasting his creations afterward.

Even though the Ornish diet is far from what most participants are used to eating, there's very little grumbling about the food. The hardest part for many participants is starting the day without coffee.

For the first couple of days, there is a pot each of regular coffee and decaf at breakfast, and participants are encouraged to mix the high-test with the unleaded to get weaned from caffeine. Around the middle of the week, the caffeinated coffee is taken away, and participants have two choices—either do without or sneak a cup from the coffee shop down the hill.

Beyond the Food

But the Ornish program is much more than a diet—and the retreats let people road-test every part of the program, with expert guidance from Dr. Ornish and his staff. Every morning and evening, trained instructors guide the program's guests through half-hour stress-management sessions that include a combination of slow stretching, yoga postures and meditation. Participants also attend daily support groups led by experienced counselors.

The expert guidance is particularly helpful when it comes to exercise, especially for those with heart disease, who are very cautious about physical exertion—and sometimes afraid of it. But before the retreat, all participants are required to have a full medical workup so that Dr. Ornish's staff knows their medical history and can help them find a level of exercise they can handle. And many are surprised to learn that they can exercise safely within their physical limitations.

Some participants try a new activity each day. Along with exercise like walking, jogging and aerobics classes, the program also offers weight-lifting, swimming and water exercise.

All of this individual attention comes at a price: The week-long program will cost you well over $3,000. But most of the participants seem to feel that their money was well-spent. "The way I look at it, I could have spent that much on a vacation, on a cruise or whatever," says Jack Kirsch. "But this is more than a vacation. It's an investment in the rest of my life."

---

have to put into practice what we already know about diet and exercise and lifestyle." If we all did that, Dr. Ornish claims, heart disease would be as rare as malaria.

One key to Dr. Ornish's program is his Reversal Diet—a very low fat vegetarian eating plan. This approach to eating has been shown to lower cholesterol and blood pressure and bring about safe, steady, lasting weight loss in numerous people. And it gets these results, says Dr. Ornish, whether or not you have heart disease.

What's more, when you combine the Reversal Diet with the rest of Dr. Ornish's program, you have an approach that can actually reduce the buildup of plaque—a mixture of cholesterol and other fats that accumulates in our arteries like rust on the inside of a pipe, says Elson Haas, M.D., medical director of the Preventive Medical Center of Marin in San Rafael, California, and author of *Staying Healthy with Nutrition*.

Counteracting a Killer

Dr. Ornish's simple, natural approach to treating heart disease has generated considerable interest in recent years, and with good reason: Heart disease is America's number one killer, claiming more lives than all other causes of death combined. Forty million Americans have heart disease and don't even know it. Many won't find out until they have a heart attack.

Conventional treatments for heart disease can be risky, painful and expensive. According to the American Heart Association (AHA), Americans spend over $13 billion a year on bypass surgery—a procedure that means "splicing in" new blood vessels to bypass a clogged-up site. That amount is more than we spend on any other operation, says Dr. Ornish.

Many people turn to surgery in hopes of beating heart disease once and for all. But about half of all bypasses clog up again within ten years. Angioplasty—the process of opening a clogged artery by inserting a small balloon—has been little more than a stopgap measure for many people. About a third of all arteries opened with angioplasty clog again within four to six months.

Heartening Discoveries

Dr. Ornish was still a medical student when he first put his theories about lifestyle and heart disease to the test. He recruited ten people with heart disease and chest pain who, for one reason or another, had decided against bypass surgery. Based on his conclusions about effective treatment, Dr. Ornish put all ten on a "test-flight" version of his stress-reducing, exercise-enhancing, very low fat eating program.

After a month of following Dr. Ornish's regimen, all of the recruits reported having more energy and stamina and much less chest pain. Their cholesterol and blood pressure readings dropped. By the end of the study, tests showed, they were actually getting better blood flow to their hearts.

Encouraged, Dr. Ornish began a second study. He divided 48 people with heart disease into two groups. One group followed their doctors' advice, while the second group followed Dr. Ornish's program of diet, exercise and stress management.

After 24 days, Dr. Ornish's group had 91 percent fewer episodes of chest pain than they'd reported only a few weeks earlier. Their cholesterol levels dropped an amazing 21 percent.

New Test on the Block

While these results were very encouraging, they only showed that lifestyle changes could reduce the symptoms of heart disease. Dr. Ornish was convinced that there was more to it than that. He believed that his program not only prevented further clogging of the arteries but could also actually begin to undo the damage that had already been done.

"When you get your fat and cholesterol intake down low enough, instead of just trying to get rid of the fat and cholesterol you ate at breakfast, your body can start to get rid of what's been building up in your arteries all these years," he explains.

He believed that a very low fat vegetarian diet would give the body an opportunity to start healing itself—that it could actually begin to reverse heart disease in people who already had it.

This was a radical theory. At the time, heart specialists believed that people with heart disease never got better. Surgery and drugs could ensure that their condition deteriorated a little more slowly, but doctors thought that there was no turning back.

Dr. Ornish's new "reversal" theory was also tough to prove. It wouldn't be enough to show improvements in blood pressure and cholesterol. He would need to show that the people who made lifestyle changes actually reduced the amount of blockage in their arteries and improved blood flow to their heart muscles.

Fortunately, by the 1980s a sophisticated new test was available. Re-

The Reversal Diet Pyramid

Most of us are familiar with the Food Guid Pyramid that's been publicized to help promote healthy eating. The pyramid for Dr. Ornish's Reversal Diet has some similarities to the official U.S. Department of Health version, but the proportions of foods are different. Here's what you should get in your daily diet according to the Reversal Diet pyramid.

• Six or more servings each day of grains. For breads, one slice of whole-grain bread is considered a serving, and for cereals, rice or pasta, a serving is ½ cup.

• Five or more servings of fruits and vegetables. One piece of fruit is considered one fruit serving, and a vegetable serving is ½ cup. Try to eat dark green, leafy vegetables, dark yellow fruits and vegetables and cruciferous vegetables like broccoli and cauliflower.

• One to two cups of nonfat milk products—skim milk, nonfat cheese or nonfat yogurt.

• Four to eight egg whites or one to two cups of beans or peas.

• If you eat sweets, have no more than two ounces of packaged sweets a day. If you drink alcohol, you should drink no more than one serving of an alcoholic beverage—either 4 ounces of wine, 12 ounces of beer or 1½ ounces of "hard" liquor.

searchers had developed positron emission tomography—the PET scan. This scanning device actually produces an image of your heart and its blood flow. It gives doctors a highly accurate picture of how far heart disease has progressed.

Proving a PET Theory

To test his reversal hypothesis, Dr. Ornish assembled a group of people who had serious heart disease and took readings with the PET scan and with angiograms (x-rays that show the blood vessels). He then divided the participants into two groups: One followed standard dietary advice, while the other went on the newly formulated Reversal Diet. In a study that came to be called the Lifestyle Heart Trial, those on the standard diet trimmed their fat intake somewhat, eating fewer eggs, less red meat and more chicken and fish. The other group ate a very low fat vegetarian diet that was based on fruits, vegetables and whole grains. They also followed Dr. Ornish's program of exercise and stress management, and they participated in group support sessions.

A year later, Dr. Ornish had findings to support his theory. The PET scan showed that those in the first group had more serious arterial blockages than they'd had at the beginning of the study. And that happened even though they followed the diet recommended by most doctors.

The people in the second group—the ones who'd followed Dr. Ornish's program—showed clear improvement. In fact, 82 percent actually had less arterial blockage than they had when Dr. Ornish started the study. Not every blockage in every artery improved—some got better, some got worse—but the overall effect of the new program was positive. At the beginning, the average blockage for the whole group was a little more than 61 percent. A year later, that number was down to nearly 56 percent.

That may not sound like much of a difference, but even a small decrease in blockage translates into much better blood flow to the heart, says Dr. Ornish.

The Heart of the Matter

In Dr. Ornish's view, when you're healing heart disease, you're improving your outlook on life as well as your chances of living longer. "People start the program because they want to unclog their arteries or lose weight, but the reason they stay on it is that it really makes them feel better," he says.

It's these other, less tangible benefits that motivate people to stay on the diet for the rest of their lives, Dr. Ornish believes. Whether or not people have heart disease to begin with, when they follow the program, they notice a big difference in their sense of well-being.

"It's hard to define," says Dr. Ornish, "because it's not something that shows up on an angiogram or a PET scan. People have more energy, think more clearly and just feel better."

Why So Many Diets Don't Work

Many people who lose weight on Dr. Ornish's Reversal Diet have tried to diet before, often without success.

In fact, Americans in general seem to be addicted to diet fads. To mention just a few, there was the grapefruit diet, the Beverly Hills diet, the "I Love New York" diet, the amino acid super-diet and—just to pare off all the pounds that we gained in between the hundreds, if not thousands, of diets we've tried—even a "yo-yo syndrome" diet.

And yet, Americans are heavier than ever. Why?

"You cannot weigh less by eating less," says Ken Goodrick, Ph.D., assistant professor of medicine and director of the Behavioral Medicine Research Center at Baylor College of Medicine in Houston. "The most you can do is eat healthy, low-fat meals and exercise, so your weight falls to a naturally healthy level."

What's wrong with weight-loss diets?

• Restricting food makes us crave it even more. "In one study, men who dieted down to 80 percent of their ideal body weight were obsessed with food for the rest of their lives, even after they regained the lost weight," Dr. Goodrick says. "Food became even more interesting than sex and football. When you restrict food, it becomes a powerful negative force instead of something nutritious and enjoyable."

• Prohibiting favorite foods is a recipe for disastrous bingeing. Any eating plan that eliminates your favorite food—even chocolate or bacon—is a setup for failure. "If you know it's okay to eat a small piece of cheesecake, you'll probably enjoy that small piece and not overeat," says Patricia Giblin Wolman, R.D., Ed.D., professor of human nutrition and chairman of the Department of Human Nutrition at Winthrop University in Rock Hill, South Carolina. "But if you fear the foods you really like, eating even a small amount could make you feel you've blown it and lead to a binge."

• Eating less prompts your body to guard its fat cells. "Traditional dieting actually lowers metabolism and leads to increased absorption of calories from the food," says Dr. Goodrick. "Your body defends its fat reserves that way."

• Cutting calories can drain energy. "Dieter's fatigue" is sign that your metabolism has slowed down to conserve calories and body fat, he says.

• Setting a low goal weight may be unrealistic because it's more than your body can accomplish. "You can't set a goal weight ahead of time," Dr. Goodrick says. "Depending on your body and your heredity, you may never weigh 120 or 130, even if the weight charts say that's your ideal weight. All you can do is eat wisely, exercise regularly, and see where your weight naturally falls."

Another benefit? Well, the people enrolled in Dr. Ornish's Lifestyle Heart Trial also lost a significant amount of weight—an average of 25 pounds. "It was a surprise, since we weren't even trying to get people to

Fat-Free Shopping

Following a very low fat diet has never been easier: As more and more people try to trim the fat, manufacturers are coming up with a huge variety of healthy options. The following list is just a sampling of the very low fat foods available at your supermarket, gourmet shop or health food store. New products are being introduced all the time, so keep reading labels to find new foods to add to your menu.

Soups
- Fantastic Foods Soup Cups
- Health Valley Fat-Free Soups
- Nile Spice Soup Cups
- Swanson Clear Vegetable Broth
- VegeX Vegetable Bouillon

Cereals (no added fat)
- Cheerios
- Corn Chex, Rice Chex and Wheat Chex
- Cornflakes
- Grape-Nuts
- Kashi and Puffed Kashi
- Nabisco 100% Bran
- Quaker Multi-Grain Oatmeal
- Quaker Old-Fashioned or Quick Oats
- Rice Krispies
- Shredded Wheat
- Shredded Wheat 'n Bran
- Special K
- Total, Total Cornflakes and Total Raisin Bran
- Weetabix

Snacks
- Entenmann's Fat-Free Cookies
- Guiltless Gourmet Baked Not Fried Tortilla Chips
- Guiltless Gourmet Fat-Free Bean Dips
- Health Valley Fat-Free Cookies (except chocolate and chocolate chip varieties)
- Jell-O Fat-Free Pudding Snacks
- Keebler Reduced-Fat Pecan Sandies
- Louise's Fat-Free Potato Chips
- Mr. Phipps Fat-Free Pretzel Chips
- Quaker Rice Cakes (including white Cheddar, butter and Monterey Jack varieties)
- SnackWells Cinnamon Grahams
- Stella D'Oro Fat-Free Bread Sticks
- Swiss Miss Fat-Free Pudding Snacks

lose weight," Dr. Ornish observes. People were told to eat whenever they were hungry, and no one monitored the sizes of the portions, so they could eat as much as they wanted.

The weight-loss results were particularly remarkable since many of the participants had long histories of unsuccessful dieting. In the past, whenever they'd tried to lose weight, they'd failed. Now, when they weren't even trying to slim down, the pounds came off almost effortlessly.

These days, practically everyone who tries the program notices significant weight loss. Typical of an Ornish program participant is Barbara Sharp, a college professor from San Diego. Severely overweight when she began the program, after three months Sharp lost more than 27 pounds.

Dairy Products, Egg Products and Milk Alternatives

- Alpine Lace Fat-Free Cheese
- Borden Lite Line Cheese Slices
- Carnation Evaporated Skim Milk
- Coffeemate Fat-Free Liquid Creamer
- Dannon Fat-Free Yogurt
- Egg Beaters
- Frigo Fat-Free Ricotta
- Philadelphia Brand Fat-Free Cream Cheese
- Second Nature Egg Substitute
- Smart Beat Fat-Free Cheese

Meat Substitutes

- Arrowhead Mills Quick Seitan Mix
- Boca Burger
- Green Giant Harvest Burgers for Recipes
- Meat of Wheat
- Mori Nu Lite Silken Tofu
- Morningstar Farms Ground Meatless
- Smart Dogs

Pasta and Sauces

- DeCecco Penne Pasta
- Golden Grain Pasta
- Healthy Choice Pasta Sauces
- Millina's Finest Pasta Sauces
- Ragu Light Pasta Sauces
- Ronzoni Pasta

Condiments

- Good Seasons Fat-Free Dressing Mix
- Hidden Valley Ranch Fat-Free Salad Dressings
- Ken's Steakhouse Fat-Free Dressings
- Kraft Free Salad Dressings
- La Victoria Salsa
- Old El Paso Salsa
- Pace Picante Sauce
- Paula's No-Fat Dressings
- Polaner Spreadable Fruit
- Pritikin Salad Dressing
- Seven Seas Fat-Free Dressings
- Smart Beat Mayonnaise
- Sorrell Ridge Spreadable Fruit
- Weight Watchers' Italian Salad Dressing
- Weight Watchers' Light Mayonnaise

During those months, she said she never counted calories, nor did she ever feel hungry. "I've struggled with my weight for a long time, and it's hard to believe I'm losing weight without even trying to," she says.

Taking the Low-Fat Road

What makes the Reversal Diet such an effective method of weight loss?

Part of the answer, says Dr. Ornish, is simple mathematics. Fat is the greatest source of calories in most people's diets: A gram of fat has nine calories, versus only four calories from a gram of protein or carbohydrate. So when you take most of the fat out of your diet and replace it with carbo-

Low-Fat Cooking Techniques

To keep your meals as low in fat as required by the Reversal Diet, you need to be careful how you cook. No more sautéing in oil, for sure. But here are some alternative cooking techniques that work well.

Baking. This is a cooking method that uses dry heat. To bake without excess fat, use nonstick cookware or spray the pan very lightly with cooking spray. Always preheat the oven: This keeps food from drying out.

Blanching. This is a way of partially cooking vegetables before adding them to a stir-fry or other mixed dish. To blanch vegetables, cook them briefly in boiling water. Allow two minutes for julienned carrots or celery, a minute for green beans, peas, snow peas or summer squash and a mere ten seconds for fresh spinach.

Blanching is also a great way to cook dried beans without having to soak them overnight. Bring the water (use ten times as much water as beans) to a boil. Add the beans and boil for six minutes, then rinse under cold water. Another bonus: Beans cooked this way are less likely to cause flatulence.

Braising. Braising is a method of cooking vegetables in enough liquid to make a sauce. Chop vegetables into uniform-size pieces, put them in a pot and partially cover them with liquid (use wine or vegetable stock for extra flavor). Cover and cook over low to medium heat until they reach the desired tenderness.

Grilling. This is a great way to prepare vegetables without adding fat. For best results, use a very hot, clean, nonstick grill. It's also important that you cut the vegetables to a uniform thickness so that they'll cook evenly. If you use salt, save it until the vegetables are almost cooked; otherwise, it can dry them out.

Roasting. Roasting also cooks with dry heat. To roast vegetables such as squash, peppers, onions and garlic, use a rack or roasting pan and leave the vegetables in their skins—they stay sweeter that way. Just remember to peel before serving.

Steaming. Steaming uses moist heat to seal in flavors and helps vegetables retain their nutrients. Use a steamer rack or basket over a pot of water at full boil and don't let the food come into contact with the water. You can add more water as needed.

hydrates—as people on the Reversal Diet do—you're automatically getting a lot fewer calories even though you're still eating the same amount of food.

"If you change the type of food you're eating, you don't have to be so concerned about the amount of food," says Dr. Ornish. "That's why you will lose weight on a very low fat diet even without restricting portion sizes."

The Reversal Diet is also easy to follow. There's no need to keep track of calories and fat grams. All you have to do is stick to whole, unprocessed grains, fruits and vegetables—and eat plant protein foods that are in the legume family, such as peas and beans.

And because you're not starving yourself, the Reversal Diet is an eating plan that you can stick with for life.

"Most weight-loss diets don't work because they're based on deprivation, counting calories and restricting portion sizes," Dr. Ornish says. "That might work for a little while, but studies show that about 97 percent of the people who go on a diet and lose weight gain it all back within five years. That's because sooner or later people get tired of feeling hungry and deprived, and they go back to the eating patterns that caused them to be overweight in the first place."

On the Reversal Diet, Dr. Ornish contends, maintaining weight loss isn't a struggle because people never have to experience feelings of deprivation. "If you eat this way, you never have to feel hungry. If you stay within the guidelines, you can eat as much food as your body needs and still lose weight safely and easily."

Feeding Your Heart

When it comes to fighting heart disease, low-fat diets are nothing new: Both the AHA and many government health agencies recommend cutting back on fat and cholesterol.

What's different about the Ornish diet is just how low it goes. Whereas the AHA recommends a diet that gets no more than 30 percent of its calories from fat, the Ornish diet is a mere 10 percent fat.

If you've been eating like a typical American, getting your fat intake that low will require some major changes in your diet. For instance, it's not enough to replace lean beef (which gets over 30 percent of its calories from fat) with chicken breast (19 percent of calories from fat) or flounder (12 percent of calories from fat). On the Reversal Diet you'll have to give up meat, poultry and fish altogether. You'll also have to do without nuts and whole eggs (although egg whites are okay) and switch to nonfat dairy products. And you have to cook without any butter, margarine or oil whatsoever.

What you will be eating is lots of whole grains, fruits, vegetables and beans, with a little nonfat milk or yogurt and an occasional egg white. This will drastically cut down on the amount of fat and cholesterol in your diet. "There is no cholesterol in fruits and vegetables and grains and beans— none at all," notes Dr. Ornish.

Dishing It Out

If this diet seems a little extreme to you, you're not alone: Many people feel that way at first, says Dr. Ornish. "In the beginning everyone thought that the program would be impossible to follow. Doctors would tell me they couldn't even get their patients to eat chicken instead of beef, much less become vegetarians. They thought it was just too hard, and nobody could possibly do it."

But Dr. Ornish and his staff have found that for many people, these kinds of big dietary changes are actually easier to make than small ones.

"If you make small changes in your diet—like eating fish instead of beef and taking the skin off your chicken—you're probably not going to feel a difference," he says. "In a way you're getting the worst of both worlds: You feel the deprivation of not being able to eat whatever you want, but you're not making changes big enough to get much benefit."

A 30 percent fat diet is certainly better than what most Americans are eating, but it simply doesn't go far enough, in Dr. Ornish's view. If you're still getting 30 percent of calories from fat, you haven't made big enough changes to reverse blockage in your arteries, he says.

"Your cholesterol might come down 4 or 5 percent on this kind of diet, but if you have chest pain, it tends to stay there," Dr. Ornish says. "If you have high blood pressure, it probably won't get better. And worst of all, if you have heart disease, it gets worse. You may get worse a little more slowly, but you still get worse."

Dr. Ornish emphasizes that getting 10 percent of your calories from fat is only part of the life-changing program. "If you make these dramatic changes in your diet and do the exercise and meditation and group support, you'll feel so much better so quickly that you'll have a lot more incentive to stick with it."

A Meaty Question

If you're used to eating a typical American diet, the Reversal Diet introduces some major changes in your dining style. The biggest challenge for most of us is learning to do without meat.

As other advocates of vegetarian diets point out, meatless eating is actually the norm for millions of people around the world. Studies of these people show that their diets dramatically reduce their risk of developing heart disease. In China, for instance, millions of people follow a traditional plant-based diet. They also have low blood pressure and cholesterol levels and very low rates of heart disease.

In fact, it's been shown that a vegetarian diet protects the heart in a variety of different ways. First, by cutting out meat, poultry and seafood, you eliminate the principal sources of cholesterol that permeate the American diet. What's more, you also cut way back on saturated fat, which the body converts into cholesterol.

Besides dumping loads of cholesterol into your body, meat is also rich in iron, and too much iron in your diet can up your risk of heart disease. Iron and cholesterol are a dangerous combination, according to Dr. Ornish, because iron converts cholesterol into a form that's more easily absorbed

How to Try the Reversal Diet

To get a full-scale experience with the Reversal Diet, you'd have to spend several days at one of Dr. Ornish's Open Your Heart retreats. There you would probably be handsomely fed by Jean-Marc Fullsack, a classically trained French chef who develops recipes for the program. Many people are surprised at how delicious low-fat vegetarian food can be when it's prepared by a master.

Back at home, however, getting ready for a Reversal Diet meal can be a little more complicated. To do it right, you'll probably want to try some of the recipes in Dr. Ornish's book *Eat More, Weigh Less*. At first glance, some of these recipes may look complicated. It's hard to find much time for blanching asparagus, seeding tomatoes or soaking pounds of dried beans if you're rushing to get food on the table.

The other problem is that many of the recipes call for exotic ingredients like soba noodles and fat-free phyllo dough. While these products may be easy to come by in New York or San Francisco, it's a bit more difficult if you happen to live in, say, a small town in eastern Pennsylvania. Don't count on finding kombu seaweed at the local Buy n' Bag supermarket.

But it's still possible to go the route of the Reversal Diet without trying to duplicate Fullsack's fabulous cuisine. Stir-fried vegetables and pasta dishes are likely to become the core of your menu, as long as you leave out meat or cheese. Here are some "lessons" in practical Reversal Diet cookery, suggested by a *Prevention* editor who tried it for a week.

Lesson 1: When you take the fat out of a dish, you have to put something else in. If you browse through the Ornish recipes, you'll see that Fullsack cooks with a great variety of different flavors, from chili peppers to poppyseeds to fresh lime juice. Some other flavorings—like paprika, red-pepper flakes and red wine vinegar—may be right on your kitchen shelf. It's just a matter of using them more often.

Lesson 2: When you do it right, low-fat food can be delicious. In *Eat More, Weigh Less,* you'll find truly wonderful meals like Jean-Marc's Spinach and Roasted Pepper Tart with Pico de Gallo Salsa. But the first time you make these dishes, they may take the better part of an afternoon to do all the blanching, peeling and roasting. The result is a hearty, flavorful dish.

The verdict: You can eat really well on this diet—if you like to cook and are willing to spend some serious time in the kitchen. But for those who aren't that ambitious, there is hope: Dr. Ornish has a new book of recipes that can be prepared in a half-hour or less, *Everyday Cooking with Dr. Dean Ornish: 150 Simple Seasonal Recipes for Family and Friends*.

The book includes a section called "Jean-Marc's Top 17 Techniques for Cooking with No Added Fat," along with complete recipes for full meals and ten recipes for low-fat breakfasts. The meals are divided up seasonally, so you'll find recipes that are appropriate for spring, summer, fall and winter. Most of the ingredients are easy to find in a supermarket or natural food store.

into your arteries. So a meat-based diet delivers your arteries a one-two punch—a hefty dose of the stuff that blocks your arteries and also the iron that makes it more likely to stick there.

Bonus Benefits

The benefits of a vegetarian diet go a long way beyond preventing heart disease. Among people who eat vegetarian diets, "rates of osteo-porosis, diabetes, high blood pressure and obesity are a fraction of what they are in people who eat meat," Dr. Ornishexplains..

A vegetarian diet may also offer some protection from many types of cancer, studies suggest. In parts of China where the people eat a plant-based diet, colon, breast and prostate cancer are much less common than in regions where the traditional diet includes meat.

Meatless doesn't mean tasteless, however—and Dr. Ornish's nutri-tionists have gone the extra mile to put a multitude of tempting flavors into the Reversal Diet.

"For a lot of people, the idea of vegetarianism is a little scary," says Helen Roe, R.D., a nutritionist at Dr. Ornish's Preventive Medicine Re-search Center in Sausalito, California, and the chief nutritional consultant for his research studies. "They think of it as brown rice and bean sprouts and worry that we're going to make them eat some kind of weird food that they won't even recognize."

But many people who attend Dr. Ornish's Open Your Heart Retreat to learn more about his program are pleasantly surprised by the variety and abundance on a typical Ornish menu. From pasta dishes to vegetarian burgers and from oven-baked "fries" to pizza loaded with roasted vegetables (minus the cheese), the food is satisfying, well-seasoned and familiar.

Roe admits that for most people, adopting a vegetarian diet means changing the way they think about food. "At first, people can't imagine how they're going to plan their meals, since we're so used to thinking of meat as the main dish and grains and vegetables as the side dishes," she says. On the Ornish program, vegetables and grains are the main dishes, too.

Oil, No

To keep fat intake below 10 percent of calories as Dr. Ornish pre-scribes, you have to do more than trim meat from your diet. You also have to ferret out the other hidden fats, Dr. Ornish points out.

Unlike some experts who maintain that certain oils (like olive oil) are beneficial, Dr. Ornish discourages any type of oil on the Reversal Diet. All oils—whether they're corn, olive, peanut or safflower oil—contain 14 grams of fat per tablespoon, he points out. Use just a splash on your lunchtime salad and a spoonful to stir-fry your dinner, and you've used up your entire fat budget for the day. That doesn't leave much room for more nutritious foods like whole grains and vegetables, most of which contain tiny amounts of fat.

But what about reports that one type of oil—olive oil—might actually reduce your risk of heart disease?

Contrary to popular belief, cooking with olive oil won't lower your cholesterol levels, says Dr. Ornish. "Compared to lard or butter, olive oil isn't quite as bad because it contains less saturated fat," he observes. "It won't raise your cholesterol levels as much as lard or butter will, but it will raise them, because all oils contain at least some saturated fat."

This is why the Reversal Diet excludes all oils—even those touted as healthy, like olive and canola. "In fact, if you did nothing more on your diet than eliminate all oils, you would lose weight and your cholesterol levels would come down, because oils are pure fat," says Dr. Ornish.

For most people, omitting oil means learning new ways of cooking. Instead of frying or sautéing food, you'll begin to experiment with grilling, steaming, baking and poaching. You'll also have to check the ingredients of prepared foods. You'll find that mayonnaise, salad dressings, snacks like chips and crackers and even some types of bread contain oil.

The Reversal Diet also excludes other, less obvious sources of dietary fat like seeds, nuts, peanut butter and avocados. These foods contain mostly unsaturated fats. Altough these aren't as bad as the saturated kind, they can still cause problems for people concerned about heart disease, according to Roe.

"Unsaturated fats don't raise blood cholesterol, so they're less harmful than the saturated fats found in animal products," Roe explains. "Still, they're very high in calories and contribute to weight gain, which plays a very important role in heart disease."

No More Bad Yolks

Eggs and milk are rich in protein and other important nutrients, but they contribute a lot of fat to the average person's diet. What to do?

With a few modifications, it turns out that eggs and nonfat dairy products can be part of the Reversal Diet.

Most health-conscious people have heard that eggs are high in cholesterol, but many don't know that all of an egg's fat and cholesterol are found in the yolk. Egg whites, on their own, contain no cholesterol and no fat. So while you'll have to do without egg yolks—as well as pasta, bread and other baked goods made with whole eggs—egg whites are allowed.

Whites work just as well as whole eggs when you're making omelets and many other egg dishes, says Roe. In place of each whole egg, use two egg whites, she suggests.

When you're selecting dairy products for the Reversal Diet, just choose skim milk and nonfat cheese or yogurt. Low-fat milk that's labeled 2 percent may seem like a good choice, but it's not. "The 2 percent fat means 2 percent of the weight, not 2 percent of calories," says Roe. The fat is actually about 38 percent, which is way too much for people with heart disease, she notes.

(continued on page 126)

Five Days of Reversal Diet Menus

If you're wondering what it's like to go the Reversal route, here are sample menus for five days in a row—with a minimum of repetition—from Helen Roe, R.D., nutritionist at the Preventive Medicine Research Center.

Day 1

Breakfast 1 cup shredded wheat

½ banana

1 cup fortified soy milk

Lunch 1 cup barley-lentil soup (no added fat)

Veggie sandwich made with 2 slices whole-wheat bread, 1 slice nonfat cheese, leaf lettuce, sliced red bell pepper, sliced zucchini, sliced yellow squash, tomatoes, sprouts, mustard and nonfat mayonnaise

Apple

Dinner 1½ cups mixed field lettuces, shredded carrots, tomatoes and radishes with nonfat Italian dressing

1½ cups whole-wheat pasta topped with 1 cup nonfat marinara sauce with ½ cup chick-peas

½ cup steamed broccoli florets

2 slices crusty French bread

1 cup sliced nectarines and blackberries

Snack 10 baked corn tortilla chips

½ cup fat-free bean dip

Day 2

Breakfast 1 cup cooked rolled oats

½ cup fresh blueberries

½ cup fortified soy milk

Lunch Vegetarian burrito made with 1 whole-wheat flour tortilla (no added fat) spread with ½ cup nonfat refried beans, stuffed with ½ cup steamed diced red peppers, squash and onions and ½ cup steamed brown rice and topped with ¼ cup fat-free salsa

1 cup fresh watermelon

Dinner 1 cup arugula salad sprinkled with ½ cup corn and garnished with sliced red onions

2 slices bruschetta made with 1-inch slices of toasted French bread spread lightly with nonfat mayonnaise and topped with diced fresh tomatoes, onion, garlic and fresh basil and heated under the broiler

1 cup cooked risotto (Arborio rice) with mushrooms and red peppers

1 cup steamed kale

½ cup fresh peaches

Snack 1 cup plain nonfat yogurt

½ cup mixed fresh fruit

Day 3

Breakfast Soy milk "smoothie" made with 1 cup fortified soy milk, ½ banana and ½ cup strawberries

½ toasted whole-wheat bagel

Lunch 1 cup black bean soup (no added fat)

2 cups wild rice salad made with 1 cup cooked wild rice, 1 cup chopped onions, carrots, peas and broccoli and nonfat dressing

6 fat-free crackers

1 fresh pear

Dinner 1½ cups spinach salad made with sliced beets, cucumbers and red onions

Large baked potato

Corn on the cob

1 cup steamed asparagus

1 slice whole-grain bread (no added fat)

Snack Fat-free crumpet, toasted

3 tablespoons nonfat plain yogurt

¼ cup strawberries

Day 4

Breakfast Omelet made with 2 egg whites, ¼ cup diced asparagus and ¼ cup fresh mushrooms

1 slice whole-wheat toast

½ cup fresh peaches

Lunch 1 cup fat-free zucchini potato soup

Sandwich made with ¼ block firm tofu, sliced and seared in hot, non-stick pan, grilled or broiled, served on a whole-wheat bun with nonfat barbecue sauce and grilled or roasted onions

1 cup coleslaw made with green and red cabbage, apples and nonfat mayonnaise dressing

Dinner 1 cup white bean salad made with cooked white beans, diced raw zucchini, tomatoes and fresh basil with nonfat Italian dressing, served on a bed of 1 cup shredded fresh spinach

1½ cups pasta with fat-free marinara sauce

2 slices whole-grain bread

½ cup fresh apricot halves

Snack 1 cup shredded wheat

½ cup fresh berries

1 cup fortified soy milk

(continued)

Five Days of Reversal Diet Menus—Continued

Day 5

Breakfast   1 cup mixed whole-grain cereals (mix your own, such as kamut, spelt, All-Bran and Grape-Nuts)

½ cup mixed fresh fruit

1 cup fortified soy milk

Lunch   1 cup fat-free split-pea soup (instant soup cups or canned)

1 cup cooked whole-wheat couscous with diced fresh tomato and cucumber, chopped parsley and fresh mint

1 pita bread cut in triangles

1 apple

Dinner   2½ cups pasta primavera made with 1½ cups whole-wheat pasta and 1 cup turnips, carrots, shallots, mushrooms, green peas and sugar snap peas sautéed in vegetable broth

1 cup Swiss chard with roasted onions

2 slices French bread

½ cup fat-free strawberry sorbet

Snack   ½ cup vanilla nonfat frozen yogurt

But even though skim milk and nonfat dairy products contain almost no fat or cholesterol, you should be careful not to eat too much of them, says Roe. "We tell people to stick to one or two servings a day," she says. That amounts to an eight-ounce glass of skim milk, six ounces of nonfat yogurt or an ounce of nonfat cheese. "Also, some people choose not to eat them at all, and that's fine, too. You don't need dairy products to have a well-balanced diet," she says.

Even if you have trouble digesting dairy products or just don't like them, you don't have to eat your cereal dry. For a lean milk substitute, try soy milk, made from the liquid left over after soybeans are cooked. Fat-free varieties are available at most health food stores.

Protein? No Problem

When contemplating a no-meat, low-fat diet, some people worry about getting enough protein. But on the well-balanced Reversal Diet, getting adequate protein is never a problem, says Roe.

"Our protein requirements depend mostly on our body size: The recommended daily protein intake for a 140-pound woman, for example, is about 50 grams a day. If you eat a typical fast-food lunch—a cheeseburger, large fries and a chocolate shake—you've more than covered your protein needs for the day, and you've still got two more meals to think about," says Roe.

"If you're eating a typical American diet, with meat at least twice a day, you're getting two or three times as much protein as your body really needs," Roe observes. And eating this much protein isn't healthy: It's been linked to a higher risk of osteoporosis, the brittle-bone disease that strikes half of all American women after menopause. Studies show that a high-protein diet can also increase the risk of atherosclerosis, or hardening of the arteries—even if the diet is also low in fat.

Of course, you do need a certain amount of protein—or rather, you need amino acids, the usable particles that your body gets from protein. Amino acids are important for building new muscle, maintaining healthy skin and hair and producing hormones and digestive enzymes.

It's easy to follow the Reversal Diet and get all of the nutrients you need, including protein, according to Roe. A vegetarian diet like Dr. Ornish's plan offers a sufficient amount of protein through beans, peas and whole grains (including brown rice, cereals and pastas). All whole foods have healthy levels of amino acid without the negatives of a meat-based diet. As long as you consume enough calories from a wide variety of foods, there's no need for you to worry about your protein intake, says Roe.

Another easy way to get all of the essential amino acids is by eating nonfat dairy products: Like meat, they're complete proteins. For a combination that's rich in amino acids, try eating your grains or legumes with a little skim milk or nonfat yogurt. Have oatmeal or cold cereal with skim milk. Or enjoy a bean burrito topped with some nonfat yogurt. These are quick, easy,ways to add protein-rich meals to your menu.

Great Grains

There's a lot more to a grain-based diet than rye toast and cold cereal. The grains in the following list aren't just nutritional superstars; their appealing textures and hearty flavors will keep your diet interesting as well as healthful.

Barley. Its slightly sweet, oatlike flavor goes especially well with onions and garlic. It's most often used in soups and stuffings and can be as soft or as chewy as you like, depending on how long you cook it.

Buckwheat. Despite its name, buckwheat isn't actually wheat. In fact, it's not even a grain, although it looks, cooks and tastes like one. The best-known form of buckwheat is kasha, roasted buckwheat kernels with a nutty, toasted flavor. Buckwheat is also ground into flour, which is often used to make pancakes or pasta.

Bulgur. This is a wheat kernel minus its hard outer layer, known as the bran. It cooks quickly, has a nutty flavor and texture and is the main ingredient in Middle Eastern salads such as tabbouleh. It can also be used in salads, stews and stuffing or sautéed with herbs or vegetables for a nutritious side dish.

Quinoa. This grain is one of the best vegetarian sources of protein; in fact, it's the only grain that's a complete protein, providing as many essential amino acids as meat or fish. It's also a significant source of iron, fiber and B vitamins. Rinse quinoa in cold water before cooking; otherwise it can taste bitter.

Dipping into Amber Waves

Once you stop eating meat, fish and poultry and cut back on dairy products, you'll probably find that there's a whole lot of empty space left on your dinner plate.

On the Reversal Diet, you fill up much of that space with starchy foods like bread, rice, pasta and cereals. All of your favorite starches fit into the diet as long they don't contain egg yolks or added fats. (You have to read labels to find out whether they have these ingredients.) But some starches are better than others, Roe says, and these should show up on your plate more often.

The carbohydrates favored in the Reversal Diet are found in whole grains like oats, wheat, brown rice and barley and in foods made from them, like whole-wheat pasta and whole-grain breads and breakfast cereals. Foods made with whole grains not only have a heartier taste than more refined products like regular pasta, white bread and white rice, they're also richer in vitamins and minerals. And whole-grain foods are also higher in fiber than their more refined cousins.

Fiber Fill-Up

Grains contain two different types of fiber, soluble and insoluble. Both kinds offer important health benefits, so they're an integral part of the Reversal Diet.

Soluble fiber is the kind found in oats, rice bran, fruits and beans: It seems to lower cholesterol levels by increasing the amount of cholesterol you excrete. Insoluble fiber keeps your digestive system running smoothly, ending constipation and helping to prevent hemorrhoids, diverticular disease and irritable bowel syndrome. The best sources of insoluble fiber include wheat bran and many of the foods that contain it, such as whole-wheat bread and breakfast cereals.

But apart from these benefits, fiber is an important part of the Reversal Diet for another reason: It also helps control your appetite. "When the food is very bulky, it fills you up before you get too many calories," says Dr. Ornish.

If you switch to the Reversal Diet, you'll eat many more grains like oats, wheat and brown rice. But before long, you'll probably want to vary these grain servings with any of the lesser-known or little-served grains like barley, buckwheat and bulgur. Each has its own unique flavor and texture.

If the grain selection at your supermarket is limited, visit some health food stores. Many of them carry a wide variety of unprocessed whole grains that could include lesser-known varieties. Also, health food stores usually carry whole-grain flours, breads, cereals and pastas.

The Garden of Reversal

Already a fan of fruits and vegetables? Well, go wild. Just about any fresh food from the produce section is a shoo-in for the Reversal Diet. In fact, the only exceptions you're likely to see there are avocados, olives, coconuts,

nuts and seeds, all of which are high in fat. That leaves a nearly endless variety of greens, root vegetables, seasonal fruits and exotic tropicals to choose from.

And you're almost as well off in the frozen food section, according to Roe. Not only does the freezer keep you supplied with frozen veggies when fresh ones are out of season, it also saves time. With frozen vegetables, you don't have to worry about washing and chopping, which gives you a break when you're in a hurry.

Another bonus: Frozen vegetables often contain more nutrients than so-called fresh veggies, which may not arrive at stores until a week or more after they've been picked.

There is one warning from Roe, however: Be careful of frozen vegetables that come with sauces or seasonings, since they frequently contain added fat.

The Good in Canned Goods

When shopping in the canned foods section, look for fruits packaged in their own juice, without added sweeteners, suggests Roe. She adds that canned vegetables can also fit into the Reversal Diet, as long as they don't have added fat. But if you are sodium-sensitive, you should scan the labels for sodium content as well as fat, since many canned foods are heavily salted.

You'll also find flavorful extras among the canned goods. Capers, artichoke hearts, water chestnuts and bamboo shoots add flavor to salads and stir-fry dishes. True, some of these products are packed in oil, but most are not. Just read labels to make sure.

Exotic Tropical Fruits

The Reversal Diet is an invitation to explore the vast selection of fruits and vegetables in your supermarket, natural food stores and specialty markets. Here are two exotic tropical fruits that you might want to try as you're expanding your fresh-food diet.

Carambola. Also known as starfruit, carambola has an oval shape and four to six prominent ribs. Slice it crosswise and you'll have a handful of star-shaped pieces to spice up your next fruit or vegetable salad. Carambola has a sweet, complex flavor that some describe as a blend of grape, apple and grapefruit.

Carambola is delicious added to a stir-fry or whipped into a mousse or sorbet for dessert, but it's also tasty all by itself. You don't even have to peel it! When fully ripe, carambola has a deep, vibrant yellow color. It's rich in vitamin C and has only 42 calories per fruit.

Kumquats. You'll find these bite-size, orange-skinned treats in the produce section from November through March. Their flavor is part orange, part tangerine. Kumquats are high in vitamin C and have only ten calories a pop. Best of all, you don't even have to peel them: The skin isn't just edible, it's actually the sweetest part of the fruit.

And don't forget that farmers markets, pick-your-own farms, health food stores and ethnic groceries can all be great sources of fresh, healthful produce. The greater the variety of fruits and vegetables in your diet, says Roe, the more interesting and nutritious your meals will be.

Juices can also help you meet your daily requirement of fruits and vegetables on the Reversal Diet, but be careful not to overdo them. "It's always better to eat the whole fruit or vegetable instead of drinking the juice," says Roe. "The fiber makes them take longer to digest, so they're less likely to cause sharp jumps in your blood sugar. They're also more satisfying."

Fruit juices in particular can be high in calories and sugar—and even "natural" sugars, eaten in excess, can lead to weight gain. They can also raise your triglycerides, a type of fat found in the blood. (Elevated triglyceride levels are associated with an increased risk of heart disease.) In general, vegetable juices contain less sugar than fruity ones and are better choices for most people, says Roe. Just be careful of canned varieties if you're sensitive to sodium, since many are loaded with salt.

A Little Sweet Talk

Sure, sugar is a carbohydrate—but that doesn't make it an honored guest on the Reversal Diet list. "Sugar is empty calories," says Roe. "It provides a quick energy source, but it doesn't last, and it leaves you feeling more tired and less energetic than ever. Also, eating sugar has the side effect of raising your triglycerides."

Sugar can also sabotage your efforts at weight loss. "You can eat an unlimited number of calories in the form of sugar without feeling full," says Dr. Ornish.

And eating sugar makes your blood sugar rise very quickly, causing the pancreas to secrete insulin, a hormone essential for converting your food into energy. This sudden rush of insulin is necessary for your body to process the sugar, but it makes your body convert calories into fat more easily. It also raises cholesterol and blood pressure and accelerates the buildup of plaque in your arteries, according to Dr. Ornish.

The Reversal Diet doesn't forbid an occasional sweet treat. "It's certainly better to eat sugar than to eat fat," says Dr. Ornish. With this in mind, though, try to limit sweets to two moderate servings a day, he advises. And moderation is the key. "A serving is not an entire Entenmann's fat-free cake," says Roe. If your sweet treat is a packaged food, be sure to check for the serving size on the label and eat just one serving or less.

For those with a sweet tooth, limiting luscious desserts may be a little difficult at first, but most people learn to satisfy their cravings for sweetness with other foods, says Roe. "We encourage people to get in the habit of eating a piece of fruit when they have an urge for something sweet."

In the absence of high-protein foods, which can help reduce cravings for sweets, try to eat more complex carbohydrates, especially whole grains like oats, barley and brown rice, suggests Roe. "They give you longer-

A Salty Tale

Years ago, if you had high blood pressure, cutting back on salt was standard advice, and many doctors still recommend it. Why doesn't Dr. Ornish?

"We don't give a blanket recommendation to eliminate salt, since research indicates that only about 25 percent of people with high blood pressure are sodium-sensitive," he says.

What's more, even people whose blood pressure increases in response to salt seem to become less salt-sensitive on the Reversal Diet, says Lee Lipsenthal, M.D., medical director of Dr. Ornish's Preventive Medicine Research Institute. That's because all the complex carbohydrates in the diet actually make your body more efficient at getting rid of sodium, he says.

"When you increase the amount of complex carbohydrates in your diet— and that's mostly what you're eating on the Reversal Diet—your body breaks them down into water and carbon dioxide," he explains. "All that extra water means you that excrete more urine, and when you create more urine volume, you eliminate more sodium."

Dr. Lipsenthal has seen this happen to many of the 430 people with heart disease who have been enrolled in Dr. Ornish's studies.

"Many of them were taking diuretics to control their blood pressure when they started," he says. "Within a month on the Reversal Diet, they no longer needed them, because the diet has a natural diuretic effect."

Of course, you should never stop taking a prescription without your doctor's approval. If you take diuretics to control high blood pressure, the best advice is to schedule an appointment with your doctor after a few weeks on the Reversal Diet so he or she can decide whether you still need your medication.

---

lasting energy and help keep your blood sugar levels stable. That may take the edge off sugar cravings."

Shaking Up the Sodium Question

When it comes to heart disease, doctors and nutritionists have traditionally taken a hard line on sodium. Not Dr. Ornish.

For most people who are on the Reversal Diet, moderate salt won't raise blood pressure, according to Dr. Ornish. He says it's acceptable to use a small amount of salt when you're cooking dishes that could use a little lift. This can even help some people stick to a very low fat diet, Dr. Ornish notes, since a little salt can make a lean entrée a lot more palatable. That's why many of the recipes in Dr. Ornish's books call for a small amount of salt.

Of course, that doesn't mean you should go crazy with the saltshaker. "Essentially, this is a no-added-salt diet," says Lee Lipsenthal, M.D., medical director of the Preventive Medicine Research Institute. "You don't want to add salt to your food at the table or get in the habit of eating lots of salty processed foods, like fat-free potato chips. If you've got high blood pressure, that would probably get you into trouble."

If your doctor has told you to cut back on salt, however, you can certainly do this while following the Reversal Diet, says Roe. "If you're following the diet consistently, you'll only be getting about 2,000 to 4,000 milligrams of sodium per day," she says. That's because whole grains, beans and fresh fruits and vegetables are all naturally low in sodium. Eat more of these foods and fewer salty snacks, canned foods and other highly processed items, and your sodium intake will stay in the healthy range.

Say No to Stimulants

Besides swapping eggs for oatmeal, you'll have to make another notable change in your morning routine. The Reversal Diet prohibits tea and coffee, both regular and decaffeinated.

"It's not that caffeine plays a direct role in heart disease, but it affects the way we deal with stress. And stress management is an integral part of the program," says Dr. Ornish.

That means you'll have to wean yourself from coffee, black tea, cola drinks and chocolate, all of which contain significant amounts of caffeine. And decaffeinated coffee is off-limits because it also contains small amounts of caffeine. If you like having a hot drink in the morning, have some herbal tea or a roasted grain beverage like Postum, which has a coffeelike aroma but contains no caffeine.

Dr. Ornish's program also discourages the use of alcohol. Aside from the well-known health hazards caused by excessive drinking, some people also use alcohol to avoid dealing with stress, says Dr. Ornish.

But what about reports that light drinking—the equivalent of one or two glasses of beer or wine a day—might actually offer some protection from heart disease? All the evidence isn't in yet, but according to several studies, moderate drinkers seem to be less likely than teetotalers to die of heart disease. So does that mean that a daily cocktail is actually good for people concerned about heart disease?

"We don't encourage people to start drinking," says Dr. Ornish.

"There isn't enough evidence to recommend it. If you already drink, you're limited to one drink a day." If you drink more than that, in Dr. Ornish's view, the disadvantages will outweigh whatever benefit there might be.

Good Policy: Supplements for Insurance

With its emphasis on fruits, vegetables and whole grains, the Reversal Diet is far more nutritious than "standard" American fare. But that doesn't mean it's perfect. Taking the right vitamin and mineral supplements can be a sensible way to get a little extra nutritional insurance, says Roe.

"The ideal is to get the nutrients the way nature intended, through the food we eat," she says. "But some nutrients are so important, it may be worthwhile to take a supplement if you're not sure you're getting enough."

Among the vital nutrients are vitamins C and E and beta-carotene, called antioxidants. The antioxidants act as a kind of nutritional SWAT team, fighting to protect the body's cells from damage. They work by disarming harmful molecules called free radicals, which, if left unchecked, damage cells through a chemical reaction known as oxidation. Researchers think the cellular damage caused by oxidation plays a role in a number of different illnesses, from cataracts to cancer to heart disease.

If you choose to take antioxidants, Dr. Lipsenthal recommends staying within the following ranges: 100 to 400 international units of vitamin E and 1,000 to 3,000 milligrams of vitamin C. (Vitamin C in doses of more than 1,200 milligrams daily may cause diarrhea in some people.) He suggests, however, that you avoid beta-carotene supplements and get the antioxidant in food sources, such as yellow and orange vegetables.

The simplest way to get these nutrients is by taking a multivitamin. Just make sure it doesn't contain iron, cautions Roe. "Some studies have shown an increased risk of heart disease with high iron intake," she says.

Should you choose to take individual supplements instead of a multivitamin, be especially careful not to get too much of any one nutrient. "Those ranges are the total amount for the day, so you don't want to take 400 international units of vitamin E if you're also taking a multivitamin that has vitamin E," says Roe. Most multivitamins have 30 to 100 international units of vitamin E, but some have as much as 400 international units.

A calcium supplement may also be important, especially for women, who are more likely than men to have bone loss or osteoporosis in later years. "We don't recommend calcium for everybody," says Roe. "It really depends on what your diet is like and a number of other factors, including your sodium intake."

If you do take calcium, you also need to get adequate magnesium to make sure the calcium is assimilated, says Dr. Haas. Good food sources of magnesium include tofu, quinoa, toasted wheat germ and spinach, or you may take a supplement. Magnesium is especially important for anyone who's at risk for cardiovascular disease.

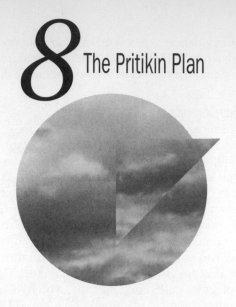

8 The Pritikin Plan

From the Folks Who Invented Low-Fat

Today, we think of it as commonsense, healthy eating: low in fat, high in fiber, heavy on the fruits and vegetables and easy on the salt and sugar. But a generation ago, there was a special name for eating this way—"eating Pritikin."

The Pritikin Eating Plan, now well-known as a therapeutic diet, first made headlines in 1977, when its colorful founder, Nathan Pritikin, was interviewed on TV's *60 Minutes*. He described a novel plan that jolted the medical community—a diet intended for people with heart disease. Soon after, the Pritikin diet was being "discovered" by people across the country as an effective way to lower cholesterol, banish high blood pressure and peel off excess weight.

Renewing Life's Lease—With Food

The keenest advocates of the Pritikin diet, if they know they need it and can also afford it, spend a few weeks at the one of the exclusive Pritikin Longevity Centers, located in Santa Monica, California, and Miami Beach. A respite at the center combines a healthy vacation with intensive counseling on nutrition and exercise.

But thousands more follow the Pritikin Eating Plan without ever making this pilgrimage, striving for the health benefits that are now within affordable reach of everyone. They have bought Pritikin's books and followed the diet themselves at home. And they keep to the prescribed diet, often with the aid of the Pritikin line of soups, sauces, cereals and pastas that are now found in many supermarkets.

It's not exaggerating to say that the Pritikin program has given thousands of people a new lease on life. Since 1976, some 60,000 people have passed through the center's doors, and countless others are doing the program on their own.

Many people who turn to the Pritikin diet have advanced coronary artery disease: Their hearts are so weakened and their arteries so clogged that they have recurring chest pain and get winded while climbing a flight of stairs. A number have survived heart attacks, while others have had extensive medical treatments such as angioplasties (in which clogged arteries are expanded by a surgically inserted "balloon") or bypass surgeries.

Other Pritikin advocates have diabetes that they're struggling to control, and many are dangerously obese. The staff at the Santa Monica Longevity Center notes that many of their visitors arrive at the center with enough medication to open a small pharmacy—insulin for their diabetes, nitroglycerin to head off angina attacks and pills to control blood pressure or high cholesterol.

But not everyone who comes to a Pritikin center is in danger: Some just want to feel more energetic and lose a little extra weight. Either way, they find in the Pritikin Eating Plan a safe, natural way to take control of their health.

The Pritikin Revolution

Today, it strikes us as an obvious, commonsense approach: fighting heart disease by addressing its root causes, like excess weight, a sedentary lifestyle and a high-fat, high-cholesterol diet. This was not the case when Nathan Pritikin first came on the scene.

In the 1970s, the days of eight-track tapes and microwave ovens as big as televisions, notions about the connections between diet and heart health were largely guesswork. Nathan Pritikin was definitely out of step with mainstream medicine when he insisted that a high-fat diet and a sedentary lifestyle were direct causes of heart disease. And he ran the risk of being called a crank or worse when he asserted that changing those habits could help even people with severe heart disease regain their health and lead more active lives. He even suggested that people could live longer by following his plan.

The medical establishment was shocked by both the message and the messenger. For one thing, Nathan Pritikin wasn't a doctor, just a layperson with a lifelong curiosity about health and nutrition. And he was far from unbiased or dispassionate. He became interested the way most people do—when he learned that his own health was in jeopardy. In his early forties,

Are You at Risk?

Some six million Americans have elevated risk of heart disease because of their habits, health conditions, family history or even age and gender. According to Elson Haas, M.D., medical director of the Preventive Medical Center of Marin in San Rafael, California, and author of *Staying Healthy with Nutrition,* here are some of the conditions and behaviors that may raise your risk of heart disease.

Smoking. If you're still smoking cigarettes, your risk is double that of a non-smoker. People in their thirties and forties who smoke are five times more likely to die of a heart attack than those who don't.

Diabetes. People with diabetes are another high-risk group. Men with diabetes are twice as likely to develop heart disease as other men. Women with diabetes have five times the risk.

Blood pressure. High blood pressure makes your heart work harder and can damage the lining of your arteries, making them more likely to become clogged. In fact, a person with high blood pressure is six times more likely to have heart failure than someone with normal blood pressure.

Cholesterol. A total cholesterol level of 200 mg/dl (milligrams per deciliter) is considered healthy. If your readings are higher than that, your heart disease risk increases.

Weight. If you're overweight, you're at higher risk than someone of normal weight.

Lifestyle. If you have a sedentary job and spend most of your leisure time reading or watching TV, your inactivity may be putting you at increased risk for heart disease. Studies have shown that sedentary people tend to have higher levels of LDL (low-density lipoprotein, the bad cholesterol) and lower levels of HDL (high-density lipoprotein, the good cholesterol) than those who get regular exercise.

Family history. Heart disease runs in families. Having several close relatives who've had heart disease increases your risk.

Gender. Men in their thirties and forties run a higher risk of heart disease than women of the same age, but once a woman hits menopause, her risk increases.

The Pill. Women over 35 who take oral contraceptives and smoke cigarettes have a significantly higher risk of heart disease than other women their age. Oral contraceptives tend to increase blood pressure, too.

Pritikin was diagnosed as having coronary insufficiency, meaning that at least one of his coronary arteries was so blocked with plaque that his heart simply wasn't getting enough blood.

"That was the 1950s, and back then, if you had heart disease, you were told to go home, avoid all exertion, take your pills and basically prepare to die," recalls Pritikin's son, Robert, who took over the Santa Monica

Longevity Center after his father's death in 1985. "Diet was never mentioned, and people would keep on eating bacon and eggs until the day they died, which often came fairly soon."

At the time, doctors believed that once arteries were clogged, there was no going back. The best that could be done was damage control, and that meant medication, usually diuretics to lower blood pressure and nitroglycerin to ease the pain of angina attacks. People with heart disease were also instructed to avoid any physical activity that might place additional stress on their already weakened hearts.

But for Nathan Pritikin, damage control simply wasn't enough. Not content to follow his doctor's advice, he set out to understand what had caused his heart disease and what he could do about it.

Heart-Smart Gets a Start

An inventor by profession, Pritikin had always been intrigued by machines and their inner workings, and the human body was no exception. Years earlier he'd worked on a research project on the incidence of heart disease during World War II. The study found that during the war, deaths from heart disease among civilians dropped dramatically in several European countries, including England, Belgium, Austria, Norway and Sweden.

The results surprised Pritikin. At the time, stress was considered the chief cause of heart disease. Since life during wartime was about as stressful as you could get, why did fewer rather than more people die of heart disease during the war?

When Pritikin re-examined the study, he began to analyze the wartime changes in Europe's food supply. All of the countries in the study had practiced food rationing. Foods like meat, eggs and milk were reserved for soldiers, while civilians had to make do with vegetables, fruits and grains.

Pritikin concluded that something in foods like meat, eggs and dairy products was contributing to heart disease. In fact, he pointed to two possible culprits. One, he believed, was fat. The other was cholesterol, a waxy, fatlike substance found in animal fat.

If fat and cholesterol were the villains convicted of causing heart disease, it would explain why European citizens who'd been forced to switch to a lean, low-cholesterol diet had a far lower incidence of heart attack. The test of this theory? It would make sense that once the war ended and Europe went back to its old eating patterns, heart disease would rise again.

As it turned out, the facts supported Pritikin's theory. Between 1945 and 1958, fatal heart attacks in Europe increased a staggering 700 percent.

Waging War on Fat

Recalling this prior research, Pritikin was convinced that cutting back on dietary fat and cholesterol would improve his heart condition. But his doctors were highly skeptical. After all, they still bought the theory that stress, not diet, was the biggest culprit.

So Nathan Pritikin became his own guinea pig. Over the next nine years, he cut nearly all the fat out of his diet and gave up salt, sugar and caffeine. Against his doctor's advice, he began a walking program, and eventually he began running.

"His doctors thought he was nuts, but they couldn't explain the results," recalls Robert Pritikin. But after 18 months on his new program, Nathan had reduced his total cholesterol from an off-the-charts 280 mg/dl (milligrams per deciliter) to a remarkably low 110.

Encouraged, Pritikin persevered with his diet and exercise program. Tests showed that his heart was not only on the mend but mended. And within a few years, additional testing showed his heart to be remarkably strong, with no evidence of coronary insufficiency.

Pritikin's doctors couldn't say for sure what had happened, since at that time there was no test that showed whether or not a person's arteries were blocked. But all the evidence they had pointed to one incredible conclusion: Pritikin appeared to have cured himself of heart disease, a disease that no one ever recovered from.

Pritikin Goes Public

His next step was to find out whether the diet and exercise program that had produced such dramatic results for him would work for other people with heart disease. In 1975, with the help of a doctor from the local Veterans Administration hospital and of his son, Robert, Pritikin recruited 38 seriously ill heart patients from the VA. He directed half of them to continue with their normal routine, while the others followed the same kind of diet and walking program that had produced such a change in his heart condition.

By the end of the study, the 19 men on the Pritikin diet had improved dramatically. They'd lost weight, lowered their cholesterol and blood pressure readings and were able to exercise longer with less huffing and puffing. Perhaps most amazing was the fact that the chest pain they once felt at the slightest exertion had diminished or disappeared entirely. The control group, meanwhile, stayed the same. The Long Beach Study, as it came to be known, produced the first hard evidence that diet and exercise could be used to treat heart disease.

The medical establishment was far from persuaded, but Pritikin stood firm. Within a year, he'd hired a medical staff and was offering his first month-long course on how to follow the diet and exercise regimen.

The Pritikin Longevity Center was born.

Changes of Hearts

It's been more than 30 years since Nathan Pritikin embarked on his lean, spartan diet. Since then, *cholesterol* has become a household word,

The Pritikin Center: A Laboratory for Change

The Pritikin Longevity Center in Santa Monica, California, is "part hospital, part laboratory, part hotel and part spa," says Nathan Pritikin's son, Robert, who was co-author of the Long Beach Study in 1975 and took over the center after his father's death in 1985.

The center offers no pills and no quick fixes. The full-time staff of cardiologists, nutritionists, psychologists and exercise specialists provides expert guidance on how to change the habits that get us into trouble in the first place: The pack-a-day cigarette habit. The dinner-from-the-drive-through-window habit. The drive-to-the-bank-that's-only-a-block-away habit.

But there's more to the Pritikin approach than breaking bad habits. During a typical two-week stay at one of the two centers (a second one opened in Miami Beach in 1978), you'll begin to form a whole new set of habits revolving around lean, heart-healthy meals, low-fat snacks and daily aerobic exercise.

Your day at Pritikin begins early, with a morning exercise class. But before a single sneaker hits a treadmill in the center's well-appointed gym, you're handed over to a staff physician who's already been briefed on your medical history. After carefully evaluating your physical condition, your doctor assigns you to a class that's geared to your individual fitness level. The goal is for every participant—healthy or sick, athletic or out of shape—to exercise safely within his or her own limits.

After a hearty breakfast of oatmeal, whole-grain bread or cereal and fresh fruit, the first of the day's five or six lectures begins. Cooking demonstrations and more exercise classes alternate with other lectures. You might hear about common heart disease treatments, managing diabetes and preventing cancer through diet, among other topics. In between, you're served Pritikin meals and snacks in a spacious dining room overlooking the ocean.

As it turns out, you'll spend quite a bit of time in the dining room. "We have food available almost all day, usually soup, fresh fruit or cut-up vegetables," says Susan Massaron, a food consultant and cooking instructor at the center. This seems to help participants stick to the program. "The snacks make a big difference: You never get to the point where you're so starved that you'll eat just about anything," says Alan "Bud" Hulsey, a Texas oilman who's been following the program for eight years.

The program also teaches the skills you'll need to make healthy choices when you leave the center. One class, for example, introduces you to some of the nutritious, low-fat foods you'll be looking for in your grocery store, while another offers tips on ordering heart-healthy meals in restaurants.

Despite the many benefits of this program, however, the cost is clearly not within everyone's reach. One week as a resident at one of the centers ranges from about $1,500 up, not including fees for medical programs and services.

In the Words of a Believer

When Dallas oilman Alan "Bud" Hulsey first came to the Pritikin Longevity Center in 1987, learning to eat Pritikin-style was quite an adjustment. "The food was almost inedible at first," he remembers. "I missed salt the most, and I was a big meat-eater."

But Hulsey knew that a lifetime of eating Texas favorites like ribs and hamburgers and fried quail was catching up with him: His weight had climbed to 280 pounds and his cholesterol level was nearly 300 mg/dl (milligrams per deciliter), way beyond the "safe" level of 200 mg/dl or less.

Today, 60 pounds lighter and with a cholesterol level of 170, Bud thinks Pritikin is the best thing that's ever happened to him—and he even likes the food! "Sometimes you have to get creative with it to make it taste good," he says. Here are a few of his secrets.

Add flair without fat. "I've found that you can eat just about anything, no matter how bland it is, if you add some red wine vinegar. It's great in soups. I'll also put salsa in soups that taste a little bland, like pea soup. And whole-grain rice is pretty bland with nothing on it, so I put that in a soup, too. It makes the soup more filling."

Doctor up your spud. "I take the top out of a baked potato—like I used to do when I put butter and bacon and sour cream on them—and saturate it with red wine vinegar, and then put some nonfat yogurt in there. That's really good."

Cut back on meat—where you don't notice it. "My wife will make a stir-fry with vegetables and chicken, and she'll put a whole chicken breast in hers and maybe a third in mine and save the rest to prime the dog food. I can't tell the difference."

Breakfast on Dorothy Hulsey's Healthy Cornbread. It's better than a cheese Danish, Bud claims. "My wife has a recipe for cornbread that has almost no fat or salt or sugar in it. I'll have that with yogurt strained through a strainer so it's like a cheese, and I put a little Equal on it. It's better than a sweet roll."

---

and the fear of fat has spawned an entire industry of fat-free snack foods, frozen entrées and cookbooks. What's more, Nathan Pritikin's "radical" views about diet and heart disease are now supported by a growing mountain of scientific evidence.

After decades of research, scientists now agree that a diet high in fat and cholesterol is a leading risk factor for heart disease. And they also agree that the leading sources of these heart damagers are many of the foods that moms of the 1940s and 1950s wanted their kids to eat, such as eggs, steak, butter, milk, sausage, cheese and fries.

Dorothy Hulsey's Healthy Cornbread
Yield: 24 pieces

Here's the hearty breakfast bread recommended by Bud Hulsey. It's delicious, he says, with a topping of nonfat yogurt cheese. (Both salt and sugar are optional, but the cornbread tastes better if you include them, says Dorothy Hulsey.)

$3^{1}/_{4}$ cups yellow cornmeal
1 tablespoon sugar
1 teaspoon salt
3 egg whites
1 tablespoon oil
1 cup skim milk

Preheat the oven to 350°. Lightly coat a cookie sheet with cooking spray.

In a large bowl, combine the cornmeal, sugar and salt. In a medium bowl, mix the egg whites, oil and milk. Add the wet ingredients to the dry ingredients and stir them together. The mixture should have the consistency of cookie dough. If it's too dry, add a little more milk; if it's too runny, add a little more cornmeal.

Drop the batter by heaping tablespoons on the prepared cookie sheet. Mash each one with a fork as you would a sugar cookie, but don't make them too flat or the cornbread will be too crisp. Bake for 15 to 20 minutes, or until the edges brown.

Yogurt Cheese
Yield: $1^{1}/_{2}$ to 2 cups

This healthy spread has only 34 calories per quarter-cup— and no fat! It's easy to make—if you use the right yogurt. Some brands have additives that keep the liquid from draining off. To make sure your brand will work, take a big spoonful out of the container, leaving a depression. If the hole starts to fill with water within ten minutes, you've got the right yogurt.

4 cups plain nonfat yogurt

Line a strainer with cheesecloth, white paper towels or a coffee filter and place it over a bowl. Spoon in the yogurt and let it drain overnight in the refrigerator.

Eating a fatty diet makes your arteries more likely to clog up with plaque, a sticky mixture of cholesterol and other fatty substances that float around in your bloodstream and eventually stick to the walls of your arteries. The more plaque blocking your arteries, the harder it is for blood to reach your heart, and the greater your risk of having a heart attack.

Experts have known for a long time that eating a low-fat diet is an effective way to prevent this buildup of plaque from happening in the first place. But even the doctors who accepted that fact were surprised to learn that a low-fat diet isn't just a preventive measure: If you already have some plaque clogging up your arteries, switching to a low-fat diet may *reverse* some of the damage that has already been done.

A Pain in the Chest?

Low-fat diets have also been proven to lower blood levels of fibrinogen, a protein needed for blood clotting. Lower fibrinogen levels mean a lower risk of developing a blood clot in one of the coronary arteries. This is critically important, because when an artery is already partially blocked with plaque, a single blood clot can be enough to stop blood flow completely, resulting in what is commonly known as a heart attack.

Other research shows that a very low fat, low cholesterol diet along with regular moderate exercise can also reverse recurrent angina, severe chest pain that signals that the heart isn't getting enough blood.

Best of all, you don't have to wait for years to see the program's benefits. In fact, guests at the Pritikin Longevity Centers usually see positive changes in their test results in a matter of weeks. A study of 4,587 center visitors found that total cholesterol levels dropped by an average of 23 percent after only three weeks on the program. And in most people, high blood pressure and high cholesterol start dropping within the very first week.

Research shows that in as little as six weeks, people on the program have better blood flow to their hearts. "Even within a short amount of time, you're drastically reducing your risk of having a heart attack," says Robert Pritikin.

New Life for Legs

When circulation improves, it's not just the heart that benefits. It's also a great help for people with other types of vascular disease. One such problem is intermittent claudication, in which the blood vessels leading to the legs are so clogged that blood flow is very limited. If you have claudication, you have severe pain in your legs any time you try to walk too far. If you have a severe case, just walking a city block can leave you gasping with pain.

Among the people who check into the Pritikin centers with severe claudication are some who have avoided walking for years, according to Robert Pritikin. Yet even they can benefit from the Pritikin program. One study of a small group of people with claudication found that after 26 days on the program, all were able to walk for at least two hours a day.

Lightening the Load on Your Heart

While the Pritikin program is best known as a weapon against heart disease, it's also a safe, highly effective strategy for weight loss. The Pritikin diet encourages weight loss in several different ways.First, Pritikin meals are ultralow in fat. And as most of us know by now, fat is fattening:

Ounce for ounce, it's got more than twice as many calories as protein or carbohydrates, which are the other two principal components of our diets. Here's the key, according to the Pritikins: If you cut way back on fat intake and eat mostly unrefined complex carbohydrates and lean protein, you can continue eating the same amount of food as you did before and still lose weight, because you're getting a lot fewer calories.

Because you're not depriving yourself of food, the Pritikin Eating Plan is much easier to stick to than a simple calorie-counting diet, according to Diane Grabowski-Nepa, R.D., chief nutritionist at the Pritikin Longevity Center in Santa Monica. "You never have to feel hungry this way," she says. "At the center we've always got snacks available, so when mealtime comes people aren't so hungry that they overeat. As long as you're snacking on fruits and vegetables and not fat-free, calorie-dense cookies or other refined carbohydrates, you can eat as much as you need to and still lose weight."

Also, Pritikin meals are very satisfying because they are based on bulky, high-fiber foods. "Fast food is very highly refined, so it takes a greater number of calories to fill you up," says Grabowski-Nepa. "But if you eat a Pritikin meal, you'll feel full eating only half to two-thirds of the calories you would get if you ate a typical fast food meal."

She speaks from experience: A former junk-food addict, she lost 50 pounds by following the Pritikin Eating Plan. "I felt it was a trustworthy approach, not a game or a

Counting on Complex Carbohydrates

Sure, white macaroni has plenty of carbohydrates. So do white rice, bread made with processed grain and dozens of other "starchy" foods. But these aren't the kinds of carbs that are recommended on the Pritikin Plan.

The problem with these modern, processed foods, according to Robert Pritikin, is that they contain refined and processed carbohydrates that our ancestors never knew. Many foods contain carbohydrates that our bodies absorb much faster than the complex carbs found in whole grains, brown rice and other unprocessed foods.

When you eat white rice, for instance, the refined carbohydrates are quickly changed to sugars that make a beeline for your muscles; the leftover sugar goes to your liver. If you follow your feast with some push-ups, your muscles might burn the extra sugar. But most of us don't exercise enough to do that, so the liver gets too much sugar and rejects the overflow. The excess sugar enters the bloodstream.

Too much blood sugar tilts levels of insulin, the hormone that helps regulate fat absorption. In the end, fat gets trapped in fat cells. So the combination of eating processed carbs and not getting much exercise results in fat gain.

That's why the Pritikin Plan advocates complex carbohydrates. If you eat mostly unrefined, unprocessed carbs and exercise to slow down their absorption, you'll minimize fat storage, according to Robert Pritikin. And less fat means better health.

gimmick, but something I could really do for the rest of my life," she recalls. Nearly 15 years later, she remains fit and trim by following the program and teaching guests at the center how they can make it work for them.

Insulin . . . Or Pritikin?

The Pritikin program is also a proven way to help keep diabetes under control.

Type II, or non-insulin-dependent, diabetes—a condition that affects some 15 million Americans—develops when a person's pancreas stops producing enough of the hormone insulin, which is necessary for converting food into energy. Type II diabetes usually strikes people over 30, unlike Type I (insulin-dependent) diabetes, which is present from childhood. Both types can lead to life-threatening complications such as kidney failure and blindness. Diabetes is also associated with an increased risk of heart disease.

Studies show that the Pritikin diet is an extremely effective weapon against Type II diabetes. In a study of 652 people with this type of diabetes, three weeks on the Pritikin program was enough to make a substantial difference in blood sugar control. By sticking to the Pritikin diet and following a moderate exercise program, 71 percent of those taking oral medication for diabetes and 39 percent of those taking insulin were able to stop taking their medication altogether after consulting with their doctors. They also saw significant drops in their blood pressure and cholesterol levels.

Best of all, when the researchers checked on the group a few years later, the majority had kept their diabetes under control through diet and exercise. And since people with diabetes are at increased risk for heart disease, the Pritikin program was helping to protect them against that complication as well as their ongoing diabetic condition.

If you have diabetes, you should always consult your doctor before making changes in your diet. But once you get the go-ahead, you should be able to follow the standard Pritikin diet with few modifications, according to Grabowski-Nepa.

"If your blood sugar is a little out of control, your doctor might suggest that you initially limit fruit to three or four servings a day and skip any desserts sweetened with fruit juice concentrate. It would also be advantageous to minimize breads, cold cereals and crackers (the calorically dense carbohydrates) in an effort to stabilize blood sugar," says Grabowski-Nepa.

If you have diabetes and need to lose weight, the Pritikin staff suggests limiting bread to two servings a day or less. In place of other servings of bread, choose unprocessed carbohydrates like oatmeal, beans, sweet potatoes, corn, starchy vegetables, whole-wheat pasta, brown rice and other whole grains, they advise. An abundance of fresh vegetables, soups and salads is also emphasized. "This seems to give quicker results in terms of controlling blood sugar," says Grabowski-Nepa.

The Pritikin diet also has some power to prevent diabetes, it seems.

How to Fill Your Tank for Less

One of the benefits of the Pritikin program is that it lets you feel full and satisfied on fewer calories than you're used to eating. Compare these two lunches—one from a drive-through window, the other cooked to Pritikin specs—and see what a fastfood lunch costs you in fat, sodium and calories.

Meal	Calories	Fat (g.)	Sodium (mg.)
McDonald's Lunch			
Chicken McNuggets (6 pieces)	290	16	520
French fries	220	12	110
Chocolate shake	320	2	240
Apple pie	260	15	240
12-ounce Coke	156	0	12
Totals	1,246	45	1,122
Pritikin Lunch			
1 cup black bean soup	130	1	128
Pita pizza made with low-sodium tomato sauce, nonfat ricotta and nonfat Parmesan, zucchini, mushrooms, onions and peppers	160	1	17
Salad made with Romaine lettuce, chick-peas, broccoli, grated carrots and nonfat Italian dressing	237	2.5	61
Totals	527	4.5	206

"Sometimes we see people with high blood sugar who don't even know it," says Grabowski-Nepa. "If we catch them in time and get them on the program, we can usually solve the problem before it starts."

Can It Cancel Cancer?

The link between diet and heart disease is well-established. But a growing body of research suggests that the same diet that protects your heart and blood vessels is also a sound strategy for preventing cancer.

"Everything we know about diet and cancer suggests that a low-fat, high-fiber diet that's rich in fruits and vegetables offers the best protection against cancer," says James Kenney, R.D., Ph.D., nutrition research specialist at the Pritikin Longevity Center in Santa Monica.

"Fat doesn't cause cancer, but high-fat diets do seem to promote some of the most common kinds of cancer," he explains. "Take skin cancer: We know that too much sun exposure is the primary cause, but it's also true that skin cancer seems to occur more often in people who eat higher-fat diets."

Besides increasing the risk of heart disease and diabetes, extra body fat also puts women at a real disadvantage when it comes to breast cancer. Overweight women tend to produce more of the female hormone estradiol, says Dr. Kenney, and higher estradiol levels have been linked to an increased risk of breast cancer.

Picking Your Protectors

Besides keeping fat to a minimum, the Pritikin diet emphasizes fruits and vegetables, which also seem to play a role in protecting us from cancer. "That's the positive side of eating to prevent cancer," says Dr. Kenney. "It's not just a question of avoiding harmful things like fat. Some studies show that eating a few extra servings of fruits and vegetables every day can cut your lifetime risk of cancer by 30 to 50 percent."

To begin with, fruits and vegetables are high in fiber, and a high-fiber diet has been shown to reduce the risk of many types of cancer, especially colon cancer, according to Dr. Kenney. "One study of people with polyps—precancerous growths in the colon—found that in those who ate more fruits and vegetables or wheat bran regularly, the polyps got smaller or sometimes even disappeared," he says.

Fruits and vegetables are also rich in nutrients that may protect against certain types of cancer, says Dr. Kenney. Among the most significant of these are a variety of carotenoids and vitamin C. Also, fruits and vegetables are loaded with other phytochemicals, a group of compounds that are believed to protect against some types of cancer.

One of these is a genistein, a chemical found mainly in legumes like soybeans that appears to inhibit the growth of breast and prostate cancers. Scientists believe that this is one reason that Japanese women and men, who eat a diet rich in soy products, are far less likely than Americans to die of these types of cancer.

Genistein is only one example of the many compounds in fruits and vegetables that may protect us, says Dr. Kenney. "There could be hundreds of them, but it's going to be a long time before science identifies them all and figures out what they do. Until then, the best advice is to eat more fruits and vegetables."

Re-educating Your System

Many people who start following the Pritikin Eating Plan discover an unexpected bonus: smoother digestion.

The credit goes to dietary fiber, the "roughage" found in fruits, vegetables and whole grains. The eating plan provides more than 35 grams of fiber a day, compared to only 10 to 15 grams in the average American diet. All the fiber in Pritikin meals is a natural antidote to constipation, says Dr. Kenney.

If you're not used to eating this much fiber, you may experience some temporary "technical difficulties" with your digestion, such as flatulence. "This is common, especially if you're used to eating a typical American

Pritikin by the Numbers

The Pritikin Longevity Centers have developed a formula for putting their plan into practice. Instead of counting calories or fat grams, you simply keep track of how many servings you eat from each Pritikin food group Here's what you should get every day.

Five or More Servings of Complex Carbs

Unrefined complex carbohydrates are the foundation of the Pritikin Eating Plan. While you should eat a minimum of five servings a day, have more if you're hungry. Whenever possible, choose whole grains like brown rice, oats and barley, as well as whole-grain breads, cereals and pasta. A serving is equal to half a bagel, a slice of bread or a cup of cooked grains or pasta. For packaged foods, read the label: A Pritikin serving is 80 calories' worth.

If whole-grain foods aren't available—the restaurant has only regular pasta, for example—go ahead and have your linguine. Just try to stick to whole grains for the rest of the day.

For variety, substitute a small baked potato or yam or a half-cup of cooked beans for one or more of your daily five. These starchy, low-calorie vegetables provide complex carbohydrates, fiber and nutrients.

Four Servings of Vegetables

At least! One serving equals a cup of salad, a cup of low-sodium vegetable juice or a half-cup of cooked vegetables. Veggies can be steamed, boiled, grilled, microwaved or sautéed in water, wine or fat-free chicken broth. It doesn't matter, says Diane Grabowski-Nepa, R.D., chief nutritionist at the Pritikin Longevity Center in Santa Monica, California. But cook them without butter, oil or salt.

"This is an area where you can go crazy, especially if you're trying to lose weight," says Grabowski-Nepa. "You could eat twice that many servings of vegetables if you wanted to, and the pounds would still come off."

Three Servings of Fruit

Three servings is a minimum. Actually, the sky's the limit unless you are trying to lose weight—then five or six servings is the maximum.

In general, a serving is the amount that fits in your hand: one orange, apple, peach or plum or half a grapefruit or banana. For fruit juice, a serving is a half-cup, but because juices are refined and high in sugar and calories and low in fiber, try to limit yourself to one serving of juice per day.

Two Servings of Nonfat Dairy Products

This is the maximum. Typical single servings are a cup of skim milk, six ounces of nonfat yogurt or two ounces of nonfat cheese. Remember, though, that even nonfat dairy products are high in animal protein. Studies have shown that animal protein stripped of all the fat and cholesterol can still raise your cholesterol level if you eat too much.

Research has also shown that a diet high in animal protein can make your kidneys excrete more calcium, making you vulnerable to osteoporosis and kidney stones, says James Kenney, R.D., Ph.D., nutrition research specialist at the Pritikin center in Santa Monica.

One Serving of Lean Meat, Fish or Poultry

A serving is 3½ ounces cooked portion weight—about the size of your palm and as thick as a deck of cards.

Fitting In Fiber

If you're like the average American, you're used to getting 10 to 15 grams of fiber a day. On the Pritikin Eating Plan, you can expect to get at least 35 to 40 grams a day. Here are some good sources of fiber that fit right into the Pritikin diet.

Food	Serving	Fiber (g.)
Lima beans	½ cup	6.5
Whole-wheat bread	2 slices	5.6
Prunes	½ cup	5.5
Potato, baked, with skin	1	4.9
Pear	1 medium	4.3
Broccoli, cooked	1 cup	4.0
Strawberries	1 cup	3.9
Brussels sprouts	½ cup	3.4
Brown rice, cooked	1 cup	3.3
Green peas	½ cup	3.0
Oatmeal, cooked	1 cup	2.1

diet, which is very low in fiber, and you suddenly double or triple your fiber intake," says Grabowski-Nepa.

If you have problems, try cutting back on high-fiber foods until your symptoms disappear, she suggests. Then reintroduce the foods gradually, one at a time.

It's also helpful to plan to spread your intake of high-fiber foods throughout the day rather than having them all at one meal, says Grabowski-Nepa. "A meal of pea soup, beans and broccoli is bound to cause problems for anybody."

Above all, pay attention to your body; you'll soon figure out which foods cause problems. Eliminate the worst offenders or try Beano, suggests Grabowski-Nepa. Available in drugstores and grocery stores, it's an over-the-counter product that contains an enzyme that helps you digest the part of beans that produces gas. Just add a drop or two of liquid Beano to your first forkful, she says; you won't taste it, but in an hour or two you'll notice the difference.

Less from the Barnyard

Pritikin's wasn't just the *first* low-fat diet; it's also one of the toughest. While other organizations suggest a diet with no more than 30 percent of calories from fat, the Pritikin Eating Plan aims even lower, at about 10 percent or less. Considering that the average American diet is nearly 40 percent fat, the Pritikin approach implies radical change for most people.

"A lot of people are trying to cut back on fat, especially as they get older, but not to the degree we do. It's quite a drastic difference," admits

Label Reading 101

Your healthy diet begins in the grocery store: Keeping fatty, salty foods out of your shopping cart is the first step toward keeping them out of your stomach.

The Nutrition Facts labels on foods will tell you almost everything you need to know to decide whether a food deserves a place in your pantry. But first you need to figure out what percentage of the food's calories come from fat, and that takes a little math work.

Find the number of calories from fat in a serving, then divide this number by the number of calories in a serving to get the percentage of calories from fat. A serving of Quaker Multi-Grain Oatmeal, for instance, gets 10 of its 130 calories from fat, or about 7 percent. (That's different from the Percent Daily Value for fat that's also listed on the label. That is the percentage in a 2,000-calorie daily diet, not the percentage of calories from fat.)

Breads, cereals, crackers and most other packaged foods should get no more than 15 percent of calories from fat.

Protein foods—frozen ground turkey breast patties, chicken breast, canned tuna or low-sodium cold cuts—should get no more than 34 percent of their calories from fat. "That's more fat than we allow for other foods, but since you're only eating 3½ ounces of these foods per day, you're really not getting very much fat," says Diane Grabowski-Nepa, R.D., chief nutritionist at the Pritikin Longevity Center in Santa Monica, California.

Once a product passes the fat test, you need to make sure it isn't loaded with salt. The Pritikin rule: Reject anything that contains more than one milligram of sodium per calorie. Canned soup that has 130 calories per cup, for instance, should contain no more than 130 milligrams of sodium per cup. But it's the average that counts. If a product is slightly higher in sodium than its calorie count and will be added to other foods low in sodium, you can reduce the total sodium of that meal.

Susan Massaron, a food consultant and cooking instructor at the Pritikin Longevity Center in Santa Monica.

Keeping meals Pritikin-lean requires learning to cook differently. "We use no oil or butter, and at first a lot of people can't believe that it's possible to cook that way," says Massaron. "But you can still grill, bake, poach, steam, boil or even sauté in wine or broth. It really opens your horizons when you realize there are so many other ways to prepare things besides frying."

The diet also controls fat intake by limiting the amount of chicken, lean meat and even fish you can eat in a day. The program allows for a 3½-ounce serving of cooked animal protein per day—a piece about the size of a deck of cards. "A piece that size would look pretty skimpy sitting on your plate," admits Massaron. "But if you mix it up in a dish with lots of vegetables and grains, it's very filling and makes it seem like you're getting more meat than you actually are."

You're also limited to two servings a day of skim milk and fat-free cheese or yogurt.

A Minimum of Sodium

Besides cutting back on fat, the Pritikin diet also sets strict limits on salt and sodium intake. While the terms *salt* and *sodium* are often used interchangeably, they are really two different things. Salt is a chemical compound called sodium chloride. According to Dr. Kenney, it is the combination of sodium and chloride in salt that seems to cause most of the negative metabolic effects that we associate with excessive intake—like high blood pressure. Sodium alone doesn't seem to be as dangerous.

Not all experts agree on the exact role of sodium, particularly sodium chloride. Some believe that only a quarter of those with high blood pressure are sensitive to sodium. But others, including Dr. Kenney, think that too much sodium is dangerous for everybody, especially when it's in combination with chloride, as in salt.

The relationship between a high sodium intake and high blood pressure isn't complicated, Dr. Kenney says. "Excess salt makes the body retain water, which increases the volume of your blood," he claims. "And that increases the workload of the heart, because there's more blood to pump." Sodium also triggers the release of a hormone that, in addition to helping the kidneys get rid of excess salt and water, triggers chemical changes in the small arteries. The result is a condition called essential hypertension. Ninety percent of high blood pressure in the United States is diagnosed as essential hypertension, says Dr. Kenney.

"Some people can tolerate more salt than others, but everybody is sensitive to too much in the diet," he says. "Populations like the Eskimos and Masai, who eat a high-fat diet but have no access to salt, just don't get high blood pressure. Their pressures are virtually the same at age 60 as they were at age 20." Populations like the New Guinea Highlanders and Yanomamo Indians of South America eat a low-fat, high-carbohydrate diet—and no salt. In these groups, too, there's no sign of essential hypertension, notes Dr. Kenney.

Too much salt is even more problematic for overweight people, says Dr. Kenney. "If you eat a lot of sugar and fat and you gain weight, your insulin levels go up, and it's hard for the body to get rid of salt when insulin levels are high," he explains. "That's probably one reason that overweight people are more likely to have high blood pressure: They may eat the same amount of salt as anyone else, but they have more trouble getting rid of it."

A high-salt diet may even increase your risk of bone loss, especially as you age. Osteoporosis, the brittle-bone disease that eventually strikes half of all American women, may be worse if you've been on a high-salt diet. "There are studies on humans that clearly demonstrate that a high-salt diet increases the loss of calcium from the bones, so eating too much salt is likely to contribute to osteoporosis," says Dr. Kenney.

How much salt is too much? The body needs only 500 milligrams of salt per day (or 200 milligrams of sodium, since salt is 40 percent sodium by weight). You might easily get that amount of sodium in fresh fruits and vegetables, nonfat dairy products and fish, all of which contain adequate amounts of sodium and chloride, according to Dr. Kenney. But most Americans get at least ten times as much sodium and salt as they need, anywhere from 2,500 to 6,500 milligrams—and that's definitely too much, he says.

"If you stick with the Pritikin guideline of less than four grams of salt (or 1,600 milligrams of sodium) a day, that's low enough to prevent high blood pressure in nearly everyone," he says.

Unfortunately, even though a diet that's low in salt will prevent blood pressure from rising, it can't reverse the damage already done to the small arteries if you have high blood pressure. People with mild to moderate hypertension should still make the effort to get their blood pressure under control and prevent further damage by cutting way back on salt and alcohol and by losing excess body fat, advises Dr. Kenney.

Desalting Your Diet

Most people find the salt and sodium restriction the toughest aspect of the diet, says Massaron. "A lot of people who come here think they're on a low-sodium diet since they've given up putting salt on their food," she notes. "They don't realize that that accounts for only about 15 percent of our sodium intake. The rest comes from processed foods—canned soups and vegetables, frozen entrées, prepared spaghetti sauces and so forth."

If you're used to eating these foods every day, Pritikin food will probably taste bland at first, says Massaron. But don't give up: People find that eventually they truly don't miss the salt."

To weed the salt out of your diet, get into the habit of reading food labels, says Massaron. Frozen vegetables, canned chicken broth, vegetable juice and tomato products usually have salt added, but you can get low- or no-sodium versions. And if you use canned vegetables such as corn or beans, rinsing them with water before cooking will remove some of the added salt, she says. And remember that while food labels list sodium content, you should also be looking at the salt content of foods. Dr. Kenney suggests checking the ingredients list for items such as salt, sea salt and soy sauce. Foods that contain those items may be more harmful to your blood pressure than those that are high in sodium alone, says Dr. Kenney.

Harvesting for Health

The Pritikin diet is generous with rice, bread and pasta. Whenever possible, you should choose unrefined, complex carbohydrates such as oat-

Portable Pritikin: Taking It on the Road

Once you've stocked your pantry and brushed up on your cooking techniques, eating Pritikin at home is easy. But what if you're traveling, or you just want someone else to do the cooking?

Getting a healthy meal in a restaurant isn't impossible, but it does require a little planning, says Susan Massaron, a food consultant and cooking instructor who also develops recipes for the Pritikin Longevity Center in Santa Monica, California. Here are some strategies that work.

Choose an old friend. "If there's a restaurant you go to often, start there," Massaron suggests. "If they know you're a good customer, they'll be more willing to work with you."

Be specific. If you can, talk to the chef or owner about your requirements ahead of time. You'll be likely to get better results than if you just arrive and ask for a meal cooked Pritikin-style.

"You really have to tell them how to cook it for you," says Massaron. Explain that you want your food prepared without salt, butter or oil and without sauce, unless it's a plain tomato or marinara sauce. Specify whether you want it grilled, broiled, steamed or baked, and make sure salads and cooked vegetables come without butter, oil or dressing.

"Keep it simple," says Massaron. "Almost any restaurant can handle a piece of broiled fish, some steamed vegetables and a salad or some pasta with chopped fresh tomatoes and basil and garlic."

Eat before you go. What if someone else is choosing the restaurant and you know that your friend's favorite eatery specializes in deep-fried fare. Try eating before you go, says Massaron. A snack of oatmeal, soup or cut-up vegetables will

meal, brown rice and whole-wheat spaghetti rather than more refined foods like white bread, white rice and regular pasta.

These less refined foods are preferable because they're higher in fiber and nutrients than more refined foods, says Grabowski-Nepa. White rice, for example, is nothing more than brown rice with the husk removed, and it loses much of its nutritional value in the process.

But there are other reasons to favor unrefined complex carbohydrates. People who eat a diet that's high in refined and processed carbohydrates—either sugars or starches—produce more insulin. And high insulin levels have been linked to a greater risk of heart disease, according to the Pritikins. A highly refined diet also tends to increase triglycerides, a type of fat found in the blood. When it comes to heart disease, many experts consider high triglycerides to be just as risky as high cholesterol.

Refined carbohydrates are also less filling than complex carbohydrates, so it's easier to eat them to excess, says Grabowski-Nepa. If you choose to eat unrefined complex carbohydrates, you'll feel more satisfied

take the edge off your appetite, so you're not fighting both hunger and temptation at the restaurant. Then you can pick and choose from the grease-stained menu and be satisfied with something simple like a salad (with either no dressing or a fat-free version) and a baked potato (skip the salt, butter and sour cream).

Bring your own. Speaking of salad, you're not doing your arteries or your waistline any favors if the house dressing is something like full-fat bleu cheese, so Massaron suggests taking some fat-free fixings with you. "I always take a little container of fat-free salad dressing in my purse and order the salad plain," she says. "You can also take some fat-free Parmesan cheese for pasta."

Have a Pritikin pizza. The bring-your-own strategy also works at your local pizza parlor, she says. "Ordinary pizza is loaded with fat because of all the cheese, but if you plan ahead a little, you can have a slice or two without worrying about it," she says. "I stop at the market on my way and pick up a bag of fat-free shredded mozzarella and ask them to put it on my pizza. It's no extra trouble for them: They just open the bag and dump it on. Or you can order a pizza without cheese. It still tastes good."

Book your meal with your flight. Most airlines can arrange to serve passengers a low-fat, low-cholesterol, low-sodium meal if they are given enough notice. The easiest way to get a special meal is to explain your meal preference to your travel agent the next time you're booking a flight, says Diane Grabowski-Nepa, R.D., chief nutritionist at the Pritikin Longevity Center in Santa Monica, California. You can also call the airline the day before your flight. Most require at least 24 hours' notice for special requests. Other good choices include a strict vegetarian meal or a fruit plate.

while consuming fewer calories, which can be a real bonus if weight loss is one of your goals.

Managing Your Sweet Tooth

For anyone on the Pritikin diet, avoiding sugars and other sweeteners can be a difficult task—especially when eating out. But sweets are the most refined carbohydrates of all, which is reason enough to avoid them, according to Dr. Kenney. Sugar has no fiber and no nutrients; it's just a source of empty calories, and the more of it you eat, the less room you'll have in your diet for more nutritious fare.

Also, sugar is both highly refined and calorically dense, so you can eat quite a bit of it and not feel full. "Take a fat-free cake that has 1,200 calories," says Dr. Kenney. "That's as many calories as you'd get in four pounds of oranges or ten pounds of tomatoes. There's no way you could eat more than two or three pounds of oranges—you'd feel stuffed. But many people could eat that little 12-ounce cake in one sitting and still not be full."

Finally, eating sweets stimulates your pancreas to release a flood of insulin, one of the hormones needed to digest carbohydrates. And the more insulin you produce, the more likely you are to store any incoming calories as extra body fat. "All carbohydrates cause insulin secretion, but the more refined they are, the more insulin you produce and the more calories you store as fat," says Dr. Kenney.

That's why even fat-free cookies and desserts can spell disaster for dieters, he says. Most are very high in sugar, which passes through your stomach very quickly and is dumped into your bloodstream. Then your body spends the next hour or two trying to burn off all that sugar. "Meanwhile, you're not burning any fat, so if you're eating this way every day, you're going to have a harder time losing weight than if you eat more unrefined and less processed high-carbohydrate foods," he says.

The Pritikin program does allow some desserts made with apple juice concentrate, says Massaron. "It's very sweet, so you only need to use a tiny bit," she says. But whenever possible, you should try to satisfy your sweet tooth with fresh fruit, especially if you're trying to lose weight.

Making It Stick

"The people who are most successful on the program are the ones who make a million small changes in their lives," says Robert Pritikin—changes in the way they cook, shop, work and socialize. "Put them together and these small changes reinforce your decision to live a healthy life."

He emphasizes that the Pritikin program is a "step-by-step methodology." When you follow the Pritikin program, you take a small step toward better health, get used to the change and then make another step.

"The key is building a safety net that will catch you if you start to slip," says William McCarthy, Ph.D., a behavioral psychologist at the Pritikin Longevity Center in Santa Monica. "By making some simple changes in your home environment and your work environment and your social relationships, you can make it a lot easier on yourself."

That may mean Pritikinizing your kitchen, finding a restaurant that's willing to prepare special meals for you and stashing some healthy snacks in your desk so you won't be tempted by the vending machines at work.

It's also important to create a support system of friends and family who can encourage your efforts to eat healthfully and exercise, such as a spouse who's willing to learn new cooking techniques or a co-worker who will take walks with you on your lunch hour.

"Sooner or later, you're going to wake up in the morning and be tempted to go off your diet," says Pritikin. "But if you've got nothing in your kitchen except healthy food, you end up eating a good breakfast. You don't feel like exercising, but you promised to meet a friend at the gym, so you go. Before you know it, the day is over and you've stuck to the program because you've got all these mechanisms in place to keep you on track." In fact, he says, many people find that it becomes easier to stay on the program than to fall off it.

Around the World with Pritikin

As ethnic restaurants become more and more popular, eating out has gotten a lot more interesting—and for those watching their diets, more confusing. "Ethnic restaurants are like any other restaurants—you can eat well or badly, depending on what you order," says Diane Grabowski-Nepa, R.D., chief nutritionist at the Pritikin Longevity Center in Santa Monica, California. Here are a few strategies for getting a lean, healthy meal wherever your travels take you.

Italian

The fat choice: Fettucine alfredo, lasagna or any other pasta in a cream sauce.

The Pritikin choice: Spaghetti with marinara sauce, chicken or seafood marinara or pasta with a sauce of fresh tomatoes, basil, garlic and balsamic vinegar.

Red flag: Enjoy a portion of Italian bread, but don't order garlic bread, which is slathered with garlic butter.

Chinese

The fat choice: Kung pao chicken or fried appetizers like wontons or shrimp toast.

The Pritikin choice: Vegetable lo mein. Other good choices are chicken with broccoli or Buddha's delight, with plenty of steamed rice.

Red flag: Beware of those bowls of fried noodles on the table—they're loaded with fat. Also go easy on the soy sauce, which is very high in salt.

Mexican

The fat choice: A beef taco in a hard shell, topped with cheese. Also avoid the taco salad, which is made with salty chips, beef and cheese.

The Pritikin choice: Black bean soup or gazpacho or a soft tostada with beans, salsa, lettuce, onions and any other raw vegetable.

Red flag: Tortilla chips. We know they're delicious, but they're also salty and fried in oil or lard. Ask the server to remove them immediately and if possible, replace them with steamed corn tortillas and salsa.

French

The fat choice: Onion soup with cheese and croutons, beef bourguignon or anything in a gravy or cream sauce.

The Pritikin choice: Roasted, poached or broiled fish or chicken, ratatouille, steamed artichokes, steamed vegetables and roasted new potatoes.

Red flag: The dessert cart. If there's no fresh fruit available, skip it—anything else on the menu is probably loaded with chocolate, butter or cream.

Japanese

The fat choice: Anything cooked tempura-style.

The Pritikin choice: Sushi, sashimi or steamed fish, with lots of steamed rice and vegetables.

Red flag: Japanese cooking can be pretty salty. Request low-sodium soy sauce and lemon juice, and be sure to specify no added salt.

9 The Longevity Diet

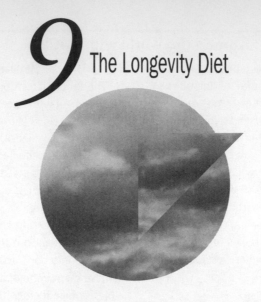

Eating to Stop the Clock

Imagine that you came into this world with a coupon book good for a lifetime's supply of food. No hunting, no gathering, no waiting in line at the grocery store. You could eat whatever you wanted whenever you wanted it, as long as you paid for it with the right number of coupons: a single coupon for a fresh green salad, or a good handful for a hefty slice of cheesecake.

To live a long life, you'd have to make your food coupons last. Eat lightly, and you'd live to be as old as the hills. Squander your coupons on holiday feasts or overindulge in tempting snacks, and you'd eat yourself right into an early grave.

It sounds like science fiction, but this scenario might not be as far-fetched as it seems.

"On a calorie-limiting program, you extend animals' life spans and decrease the incidence of virtually all the diseases of aging," says Roy L. Walford, M.D., professor of pathology at the University of California, Los Angeles, UCLA School of Medicine and a researcher in the field of longevity. "And those diseases that do occur come on at a later age."

While the theory hasn't been formally tested on humans, some researchers believe that with the right low-calorie diet, we too can have more healthy, vital years than we ever dreamed possible.

Of Mice and Men

The idea that a low-calorie diet can prolong life isn't a new one. As early as the 1930s, scientists at Cornell University in Ithaca, New York, found that laboratory mice that ate a very low calorie diet outlived mice that were allowed to eat as much as they wanted.

Since then, researchers have noted very specific differences between the bodies of calorie-restricted mice and those of mice on the all-you-can-eat plan.

As they age, mice fed a low-calorie diet have the cholesterol and blood sugar levels of much younger animals. They see and hear better and are mentally sharper than others their age. Perhaps most important, they have much less risk of developing heart disease, diabetes and cancer—killer diseases that are as lethal to mice as they are to humans.

Monkeying Around with Life Span

There's no denying that a low-calorie, super-nutritious diet works wonders in mice, but the fact is, these critters are no bigger than your hand. How do scientists know that the diet would have the same results in big lugs like ourselves?

To help bridge the gap, some longevity scientists are focusing their attention higher on the evolutionary ladder. Since 1987, researchers at the National Institute on Aging in Bethesda, Maryland, have been studying the effects of a low-calorie, high-nutrient diet in two of our closest animal cousins, rhesus and squirrel monkeys.

"Monkeys are a lot closer to people on the evolutionary scale than rats," says George Roth, Ph.D., of the Gerontology Research Center at the National Institute on Aging and one of the scientists leading the study. "If it were to work in monkeys, this would bode well for the possibility that it might have beneficial effects in people as well."

Because monkeys have a much longer life span than rodents (three decades versus two or three years, at best), it will take quite a while to find out whether the low-calorie diet actually helps them live longer, notes Dr. Roth. But researchers are hopeful because so far, monkeys on the diet show many of the same short-term changes that calorie-restricted mice do. If it turns out that the diet also increases the monkeys' life spans, scientists will be a giant step closer to finding out whether it will work for humans, too.

Biosphere: The Human Laboratory

Animal studies are intriguing. But scientists agree that the best way to test the Longevity Diet is with humans in a controlled, laboratory-type setting. Only in such a setting can they keep track of exactly what and how much the study participants are eating.

Of course, that kind of close scrutiny is a lot easier with rats or mon-

Living Lean in the Arizona Desert

When scientists designed the Biosphere, a sealed steel and concrete structure in the Arizona desert, studying the effects of a low-calorie diet wasn't what they had in mind. Their goal was to find out whether it was possible for humans to create, live in and run a self-sustaining community, complete with nearly 4,000 different plant and animal species.

The eight scientists living in the Biosphere grew their own food, recycled their own waste and kept the three-acre facility up and running, which was no mean feat: Except for sunlight and electricity, Biosphere was completely cut off from the outside world.

The Biosphere scientists expected to eat about 2,500 calories a day. But when they weren't able to produce as much food as originally planned, the team's physician—longevity researcher Roy L. Walford, M.D., professor of pathology at the University of California, Los Angeles, UCLA School of Medicine—recognized it as a once-in-a-lifetime opportunity to put his theories about calorie restriction to the test.

"It was a stroke of luck that I happened to be the team's physician," remembers Dr. Walford. "A regular nu-

tritionist would have panicked and had food brought in."

On an average day, each team member consumed about 1,800 calories—not many, considering how much physical labor was involved in maintaining the Biosphere. But what the menu lacked in quantity, it made up in quality: Meals were composed mostly of the fresh fruits, vegetables and grains the team grew, plus occasional small portions of meat, fish and eggs. To make sure they were getting enough of all required nutrients, the team planned their meals with the help of a computer program developed by Dr. Walford and took vitamin and mineral supplements as needed.

Everyone on the team was of average weight before the study began. After six months on the diet, all had trimmed down considerably. The four female scientists weighed an average of 119 pounds, with 15 percent body fat (down from 134 pounds and 24 percent body fat before the study). The men averaged a lean 136 pounds and 8 percent body fat, down from 163 pounds and 16 percent body fat. They also lowered their blood pressure, cholesterol and blood sugar levels.

---

keys than with people. As recently as a few years ago, such an experiment seemed downright impossible. Then came Biosphere.

Biosphere was a totally self-contained environment with its own sealed-in atmosphere and food sources. The eight-member Biosphere team went on a low-calorie diet under the guidance of Dr. Walford. This "experiment" was a scientist's dream: a group of human subjects who couldn't cheat on the diet even if they wanted to. After only six months, the Biospherians had lost weight and reduced their blood pressure and cholesterol levels, and they had better blood sugar control—the same kinds of changes scientists have seen in calorie-restricted animals.

Of course, it's too soon to tell if the Biospherians will live longer as a result of eating this way, should they decide to stay on the diet for the rest of their lives. But these results are impressive all by themselves, says Dr. Walford, since being lean and lowering your blood pressure and cholesterol levels are great ways to improve your health, regardless of your age.

A Question of Quality

The diet that produced these impressive results in the Biosphere team wasn't just lower in calories than the average diet, it was also much more nutritious. The diet was nutrient-dense: Every calorie was packed with vitamins, minerals and other important nutrients.

The Biospherians' diet consisted mainly of whole grains, beans and fresh fruits and vegetables. Their meals were rounded out with small portions of eggs, fish, lean meat and nonfat dairy products.

Most significantly, their diet was free of nutritionally bankrupt foods—it didn't include potato chips, sweets or soft drinks or anything fried, buttered or otherwise high in fat. Every food on the menu was rich in vitamins, minerals or both, and meals were carefully planned to make sure the team got enough of all essential nutrients. So even though they ate significantly fewer calories than the average American, they were actually a lot better nourished than most of us.

It's impossible to overestimate the importance of good nutrition on a low-calorie diet, says Dr. Walford. You're not doing yourself any favors by cutting calories if it means shortchanging yourself on vital nutrients. He believes that when it comes to disease prevention and longevity, the nutritional quality of the diet is at least as important as its low calorie count.

The Okinawan Experience

Aside from the experiment with the Biospherians, it's hard to find examples of people who have eaten nutritious low-calorie diets long enough to reap the rewards. In places with an abundant supply of good food, like North America, calorie intake is too high. In less developed countries where people consume fewer calories, the food supply tends to be poor, and nutritional deficiencies are common.

One exception to this rule is the Japanese island of Okinawa, where the traditional diet is pretty close to the high-nutrition/low-calorie diet espoused by Dr. Walford. Okinawans eat about 30 percent fewer calories than other Japanese (and maybe half as many as Americans do). Their diet is heavily weighted with fresh fruit, vegetables, fish and meat and includes very little salt and sugar.

Researchers suspect that this spare, nutritious diet has something to do with why so many Okinawans live for 100 years or more. In fact, this island has more centenarians than any other Japanese island.

And Okinawans don't just live longer than other Japanese; they also enjoy superior health. They have 30 to 40 percent less risk of developing cancer, heart disease, high blood pressure, diabetes and senility.

What the Diet Can Do for You

Of all the diet's potential benefits, probably the most exciting is the possibility of preventing degenerative diseases like heart disease, diabetes and cancer—illnesses that have reached epidemic proportions in Western countries. Whether or not it can actually slow the aging process, if the Longevity Diet can help us sidestep these killer diseases, our odds of living to a ripe old age are greatly improved. Here are some ways that this diet can help you beat major health problems.

Halt Heart Disease

This killer cuts short more lives than any other ailment. Living a longer, healthier life means finding a way to stave off the disease itself as well as the chest pain and shortness of breath that so often accompany it. Research suggests that following a nutrient-rich, low-calorie diet may be an effective way to prevent both heart disease and its complications.

First, the Longevity Diet can effectively control cholesterol levels, according to Dr. Walford.

With regard to cholesterol, the eight Biospherians weren't in bad shape to begin with: They had an average total cholesterol level of 191 mg/dl (milligrams per deciliter), which is within the healthy range specified in U.S. government guidelines. But after six months on a nutrient-rich, low-calorie diet, that number plummeted to a very low 123 mg/dl—a level rarely seen in this country except among strict vegetarians.

Second, because the Longevity Diet helps pare off excess pounds, it can help lower high blood pressure. After only six months on the diet, the Biosphere team's average blood pressure readings dropped from an already low 109/74 to 89/58.

Deter Diabetes

If you keep your weight under control, you are less likely to develop diabetes. Medical tests showed that the Longevity Diet had a very positive effect on the Biosphere team's blood sugar levels. Since high blood sugar is one of the most common indicators of diabetes, and levels even moderately higher than average put you at increased risk of developing the disease, the diet had an important payoff.

The experience of the Biosphere team agrees with the findings in animal studies. Researchers report that monkeys that have eaten a low-calorie diet for several years use insulin, the hormone that regulates blood sugar, more efficiently than monkeys on an ordinary diet, thus making them less likely to develop diabetes.

Survival of the Thinnest

In the past, most experts believed that being too thin—like being too heavy—brought with it certain health risks. Today, that idea has been rejected by a number of scientists.

The problem, says Roy L. Walford, M.D., professor of pathology at the University of California, Los Angeles, UCLA School of Medicine, is that many of the "unhealthy thin" subjects in the old studies were cigarette smokers, who tend to weigh less than nonsmokers but are at greater risk of premature death from heart disease, cancer and other diseases. More recent studies that have taken this into account have found that the thinnest nonsmoking subjects live the longest and run the least risk of disease.

The idea that you can add years to your life simply by controlling your weight is good news—unless you're the type who gains weight just from looking at food. But even if your genes make being thin virtually impossible, you can still benefit from a moderate weight loss, says Dr. Walford. The key, he says, is to keep your weight below your set-point—the weight you'd naturally stabilize at without trying to control it.

"We've studied mice that are genetically very obese, and when we put them on a calorie-restricted diet they were still mildly obese, but they lived a great deal longer," he says. "It's not a question of being ultra-thin but of being thin compared to what you would be if you were not dieting.

"You don't get the extension of life span simply by doing exercise to reduce body weight," says Dr. Walford. "You have to do it by limitation of calories. You can't do it by other means because only limitation of calories induces specific biochemical and metabolic changes that retard aging."

Cut Your Cancer Risk

Longevity researchers also claim that the high-quality, low-calorie diet may protect us from certain types of cancer. Colon, stomach, breast and prostate cancers are believed to be influenced by what we eat, and eating a very nutritious, low-calorie diet appears to be the best way to keep them at bay, according to Dr. Walford.

Again, evidence comes from animal studies, and researchers have yet to prove the same effect in humans. But research data show that a lower-calorie diet seems to have the unique potential of lowering the incidence of leukemia, or cancer of the white blood cells. This is particularly striking when you consider the fact that no other dietary factors—fat intake or how many vitamins or minerals you get in your diet—appear to have any bearing on leukemia risk.

Scientists aren't sure exactly how a low-calorie diet can help prevent cancer, but they do have several theories, says Dr. Walford. One is that the diet slows the rate of cell division in many body tissues. Animal studies show that a lower-calorie diet increases the rate at which old or damaged liver cells die off and new ones are produced, which may prevent potentially cancerous cells from surviving and multiplying.

A low-calorie diet also seems to prevent certain types of damage to DNA, the material in every cell that's essential for sending chemically coded messages that dictate how cells grow, behave and change, says Dr. Walford. When DNA is damaged, abnormal cells are produced, which may set the stage for cancer. Cells taken from rats fed a low-calorie diet also seem to be better at repairing DNA damage when it does occur. Researchers believe that both of these factors may play a role in protecting calorie-restricted animals from cancer.

Dr. Walford also notes that a low-calorie diet increases the body's own intrinsic antioxidant defense system. The diet lessens damage from free radicals, harmful particles produced during normal metabolism that, if left unchecked, cause cellular damage that some researchers believe sets the stage for cancer, according to Dr. Walford.

The abundance of vitamins and minerals in a low-calorie, nutrient-dense diet may also protect us against cancer.

With its emphasis on fresh fruits and vegetables, the Longevity Diet is particularly rich in vitamins C, E and beta-carotene—the so-called antioxidant nutrients that have made so many health headlines in recent years. The antioxidants' claim to fame is their ability to disarm free radicals.

The Longevity Diet is also high in fiber—the indigestible part of plant-based foods like fruits, vegetables and whole-grain products. A high-fiber diet has been associated with a lower risk of several types of cancer, especially colon cancer.

Eat Less, Live Longer?

Taken together, heart disease, cancer and diabetes account for the vast majority of deaths in Western countries. So if the high-nutrition, low-calorie diet can help us sidestep these killer diseases, it's an excellent bet that it will add years to our lives.

But the longevity benefits of the diet may go beyond disease prevention, according to Dr. Walford. He believes that eating this way may actually slow the aging process.

Also, if your health is improved, it stands to reason that you'll have more energy and a better attitude, points out Elson Haas, M.D., medical director of the Preventive Medical Center of Marin in San Rafael, California, and author of *Staying Healthy with Nutrition*. Fewer worries mean less stress, and you get the benefit of positive emotions.

Looking at the details of laboratory studies of mice, it's clear why researchers think that people on a calorie-restricted diet might be able to outlive their plumper peers. When researchers take mouse species with a maximum life span of 38 months and put them on a restricted diet at an early age, the mice live almost 50 percent longer—an astounding 55 months. This is the equivalent of a human being living to the age of 160 or 170, says Dr. Walford.

Exactly how a low-calorie diet prolongs life is not completely clear, but it's pretty obvious that if you eat fewer calories, you will have less body fat, and excess fat is associated with numerous health problems. Another theory is that a low-calorie diet decreases the production of free radicals, which have been implicated in the development of heart disease and cancer and are also believed to play a role in age-related changes such as age spots, wrinkles and cataracts.

How Long Can You Live?

Dr. Walford is convinced that if the diet's effect on humans is anything like its effect on other species, it could help us live well past the 100-year mark. And a few people, with the right combination of diet and genes, could live 120 years or longer.

While our genetic makeup would naturally be a factor, Dr. Walford believes that the right diet will maximize anybody's potential life span, regardless of genetics.

When researchers tested the restricted diet on different types of mice—some naturally short-lived, some from parents with longer life spans—they *all* lived significantly longer than expected. "The probability is good that you will live-longer eating this way than you otherwise would," Dr. Walford concludes.

What You Can Expect from the Longevity Diet

To find out what it's like to start on the Longevity Diet, one of our editors experienced it for a week. Here are some observations, along with some advice for anyone who's ready to start.

• Expect to make an effort. Unlike simply cutting your fat intake or steering clear of junk food, eating this way really feels like being on a diet. You'll probably find yourself thinking about food a lot more than usual, even foods you haven't craved in years.

• Try keeping a list of everything you eat, noting calories and vitamin and mineral content. Add it all up late in the afternoon and use this to plan your evening meal so you can make up for any nutrients you've missed that day.

• A nutrition book is a must. Make sure it gives nutrition information for all common foods. Don't count on much help from nutrition labeling, since you'll be eating fresh produce, fish and lean meat, all sold without labels.

• If you're stumped for meal ideas, get a copy of *The Anti-Aging Plan: Strategies and Recipes for Extending Your Healthy Years,* by Roy L. Walford, M.D., professor of pathology at the University of California, Los Angeles, UCLA School of Medicine, and his daughter Lisa, who provided some simple but surprisingly tasty recipes.

• If you've got a sweet tooth, keep plenty of fresh fruit around. If you occasionally crave the intense sweetness of jelly beans or bubble gum, the natural sweetness of a pear or a slice of pineapple might not satisfy you at first. But after a week or so, it does get easier.

Researchers agree that results also depend on how early or late in life you start the diet. In all studies, the animals who started eating a restricted diet early in life—either before or shortly after reaching adulthood—lived the longest.

But it's never too late to start, says Dr. Walford.

"If you're already 50, you're never going to be 40 again," he says. "But if you start following the diet at 50 and stick with it for ten years, your physiologic age might be more like 55 instead of 60. You'll still get old, but it will take you longer to get there."

Increasing Your "Health Span"

Of course, most of us aren't interested in merely staying alive longer if it means more years of illness, disability and all of the negative changes that we associate with old age. What we really want is more healthy, active years. And according to Dr. Walford, following a low-calorie, nutrient-dense diet gives us our best shot at attaining that (see "Try a Low-Cal Day" on page 166.)

In animal studies, this type of diet has been shown to stave off many of the changes that usually come along with aging, he says.

Mice on a restricted diet, for example, were much less likely to develop cataracts than mice of the same age on the standard diet. "There's a loss of a particular protein in cataracts, and it's not lost in calorie-restricted mice," says Dr. Walford. "It's quite a remarkable finding."

Elderly mice on the low-calorie diet also stay mentally sharper than others their age. In one study, three-year-old calorie-restricted mice were able to run through a maze—the standard rodent intelligence test—just as quickly as mice who were a fraction of their age.

How to Do It

If you'd like to try the Longevity Diet, you've got a couple of options, according to Dr. Walford.

If you're the headstrong type, you can jump right in, taking care to select nutrient-packed foods and keeping a careful watch on your calories from day one. If you'd rather ease into it, you can start by eliminating junk food and improving the nutritional quality of your diet. Once you've gotten the hang of planning nutrient-dense meals, you can start keeping track of your calorie intake and cutting back if necessary.

Either way, putting together a nutritious low-calorie diet will take some careful planning, especially at the beginning. To make sure your choices meet or exceed the daily requirements for vitamins, minerals and fiber, you'll need to invest in a good nutrition book that gives both the Daily Value (DV) recommendations and the nutrient and calorie content of a wide variety of foods. (If you have a computer, a number of companies produce nutrition software that puts this information at your fingertips.)

For the most part, you'll want to stick to basics like fresh fruits and vegetables, whole grains, beans and moderate portions of lean fish or meat. But even within these food groups, you'll soon find that some foods are better nutritional bargains than others, and you'll want to include them in your meals whenever possible.

Making Your Calories Count

When you're keeping a lid on calories, whatever you do eat has to be top quality. There's no room for dead wood on this diet: Any food that doesn't make a substantial contribution to your body's daily nutritional needs is off the menu.

Sweet treats, fast-food burgers and other highly processed foods are the most obvious offenders. High in calories and virtually devoid of nutritional value, they're indulgences that you just can't afford on a limited calorie budget.

But it's not only junk food that you'll need to watch out for. Even relatively healthy foods like regular pasta and white rice aren't the best choices for someone on this type of diet. Most pasta is made from semolina, a type of refined flour from which fiber and vitamins have been removed, and white rice has been stripped of its bran, the most nutritious part of the grain. So be sure to substitute whole-wheat pasta and brown rice, which contain the same number of calories as their refined cousins but supply a whole lot more nutrition for each calorie.

The rule about choosing less refined food applies to just about every food in your grocery store. In general, the more a food has been tinkered with by human hands, the more fat, salt and sweeteners have probably been

A Few Words of Caution

One of the goals of the Longevity Diet is moderate weight loss—between a half-pound and a pound per week. While this is safe for most healthy people, low-calorie diets aren't for everybody.

• People with diabetes should always consult a physician before changing their eating habits.

• Pregnant women should not be on the diet unless it's okayed by a doctor.

• Calorie restriction isn't recommended for children or teenagers who haven't reached their full adult stature. By all means, feed your kids this natural, nutrient-dense diet, counsels Roy L. Walford, M.D., professor of pathology at the University of California, Los Angeles, UCLA School of Medicine—just let them eat as much of these nutritious foods as they want.

• You also need to make sure you're not losing too much, too soon. You should modify the diet or see a doctor if you lose more than 20 to 25 percent of your body weight. (If you're already fairly slim, even this could be too much.) And if you're a woman and you notice changes in your menstrual period, it could mean you're losing weight too rapidly.

(continued on page 168)

Try a Low-Cal Day

The Longevity Diet may be a challenge if you're used to eating whenever you're hungry. But if you want to test it, here's a menu with less than 1,200 calories from the anti-aging plan developed by Roy L. Walford, M.D., professor of pathology at the University of California, Los Angeles, UCLA School of Medicine.

Breakfast 1 slice toasted nonfat whole-wheat bread (60 calories)

Poached egg (80 calories)

8 ounces orange juice (112 calories)

Coffee or tea

Lunch 1 Stuffed Pepper (384 calories)

4 ounces nonfat yogurt with 1 teaspoon all-fruit jam or honey (60 calories)

Dinner 2-ounce lean pork chop, broiled with ½ cup unsweetened applesauce (130 calories)

½ cup mashed potatoes with 1 tablespoon cottage cheese (80 calories)

1 stalk steamed broccoli (60 calories)

Snack 1 large Tropical Dream Bar (70 calories)

8 ounces skim milk (85 calories)

Tropical Dream Bars

Yield: 24 small or 12 large bars

1 **egg**
1 **egg white**
½ **cup honey**
½ **cup evaporated skim milk**
1 **teaspoon vanilla**
1 **cup whole-wheat pastry flour**
1 **cup rolled oats**
½ **cup nonfat dry milk**
½ **cup wheat germ, lightly toasted**
   Dash of salt
½ **cup unsweetened shredded coconut**
¼ **cup finely chopped dried papaya**
¼ **cup finely chopped dried pineapple**

Preheat the oven to 350°. Coat an 8" × 8" baking pan with canola oil cooking spray.

In a large bowl, using a wire whisk, blend the egg, egg white, honey, evaporated milk and vanilla.

In a medium bowl, mix the flour, oats, nonfat dry milk, wheat germ and salt. Add to the wet ingredients and stir until barely moistened. Add the coconut, papaya and pineapple.

Spread the batter evenly in the prepared pan; do not pack down. Bake for 7 minutes. Let cool completely before cutting into the desired number of bars.

....

Stuffed Peppers
Yield: 8 peppers

Rice	2	cups chicken or vegetable broth
	1	cup brown rice
	3	cloves garlic, minced
	1	teaspoon dried oregano
	$^{1}/_{2}$	teaspoon black pepper
Peppers	8	large green or red bell peppers
Stuffing	$^{1}/_{2}$	teaspoon olive oil
	3	cloves garlic, minced
	1	pound ground turkey or 10 ounces firm tofu, cubed
	4	medium tomatoes, chopped
	2	cups frozen corn kernels, thawed
	1	can (8 ounces) kidney beans or $^{1}/_{2}$ cup dried kidney beans, soaked and cooked
	4	sheets (4" × 2") nori, cut into thin strips
	2	teaspoons dried oregano
	2	teaspoons dried tarragon
	1	teaspoon black pepper or $^{1}/_{2}$ teaspoon red pepper
	1	cup low-fat or nonfat cottage cheese

Preheat the oven to 350°F. Coat an 8" × 8" baking dish with canola oil cooking spray.

To make the rice: In a 2-quart saucepan, bring the broth to a boil. Add the rice, garlic, oregano and pepper. Reduce the heat, cover and simmer for 40 minutes.

To prepare the peppers: Carefully cut out the stems and the surrounding $^{1}/_{2}$" or so of the peppers. Set the lids aside. Carefully remove the inner whitish membranes and the seeds. Rinse with cold water to remove remaining seeds.

To make the stuffing: Heat the oil in a medium skillet over low heat. Add the garlic and turkey or tofu, stirring lightly to cook evenly. If using turkey, add the tomatoes while the meat is still slightly pink and tender; if using tofu, add the tomatoes when the tofu is warmed through. Cook over low heat for 5 minutes. Add the corn, beans, nori, oregano, tarragon and pepper. Simmer for 3 minutes.

Add the cooked rice and remove from the heat. Mix the cottage cheese into the stuffing.

Fill each pepper to the top and replace the lids. Carefully place the peppers side by side in the prepared baking dish and bake for 30 minutes.

Note: This dish is extremely easy to freeze. Simply place the peppers in a freezer-safe dish or individual plastic freezer bags. To reheat, thaw the peppers in the refrigerator overnight, then heat in the microwave or in a covered baking dish in a 350° oven.

....

added to it, and the more nutrients have probably been lost in the process.

Take the humble spud. A plain old potato, baked in its skin, has 270 calories and almost no fat. It's loaded with fiber and potassium. It also gives you almost half the DV of vitamin C and has hefty amounts of B vitamins. In comparison, a McDonald's-size portion of french fries has almost as many calories, more than ten times the fat and only a fraction of the vitamins.

How Low Can You Go?

Once you improve the quality of the food you eat, you're ready to start thinking about quantity. Exactly how much you should eat to get the maximum benefit from this diet depends on your metabolism—and that's determined by a number of different factors, including your age and sex, how much you exercise and even what kind of diet you ate as a child.

To find the right calorie level for you, Dr. Walford recommends trying to determine your setpoint—what you'd weigh if you ate normally and didn't worry about calories. The goal is to take in enough calories so that your weight stabilizes at 10 to 20 percent below that number. This is the weight that, according to Dr. Walford's research, is associated with the best health and the longest life.

If the needle on the scale always seems to gravitate toward 130 pounds, for example, try to lose very slowly until you reach 117 pounds. Then gradually increase your calorie intake so you remain at that weight.

If all of this sounds a little abstract, just limit yourself to around 1,800 calories a day, suggests Dr. Walford. If you start losing weight too quickly at this level—say, more than a pound a week—you can eat a little more. On the other hand, if after a few weeks your weight hasn't budged, you may have to reduce the number of calories a little more.

Satisfying Your Stomach

Eating until you're full sounds simple enough. But if you're like most people, your first question has nothing to do with calories and setpoints. You want to know if you'll be hungry on this diet.

The short answer: Not as hungry as you think.

Of course, if you're used to eating twice as many calories as the Longevity Diet provides, you're sure to feel a little hungry at first, says Dr. Walford. But thanks to the type of foods the diet features—whole, unprocessed, natural foods—your appetite may be easier to control than you think.

Studies show that refined sugars in the diet stimulate appetite, says Dr. Walford. "Some research indicates that people who eat a very refined diet take in about 25 percent more calories than people who eat a more natural diet," he says.

If you're really hungry, of course, you may simply be eating too few calories. In that case, you can eat more, as long as you stick to nutrient-rich foods.

"The goal is not to starve yourself," says Dr. Walford. "If you're really hungry, you can allow yourself more food, as long as you stick to nutrient-dense natural foods. You'll still lose weight, and you'll be much healthier than if you filled up on processed foods."

The Supplement Question

If your goal is to get as many essential nutrients as possible while eating abstemiously, supplements may seem like the ultimate solution—an easy way to get large doses of vitamins and minerals without consuming a single calorie.

Indeed, the right supplements can be a valuable addition to the Longevity Diet, according to Dr. Walford. Unless you're incredibly careful, chances are good that a very low calorie diet will occasionally fail to give you quite enough of every single nutrient every single day, he says, and supplements can provide valuable insurance against the occasional nutritional shortfall.

That said, it's important to think of supplements as a prudent addition to a nutritious diet, not as a replacement for one. "It's appealing to think that you can eat a less than optimal diet and make up the difference with supplements, but it doesn't work that way," says Dr. Walford. "There's good evidence that supplements may be protective against disease, but you still have to eat a nutrient-dense diet."

In his book *The 120-Year Diet*, Dr. Walford devotes particular attention to the antioxidant nutrients: vitamins C and E, beta-carotene and selenium. Due to some controversial studies that question the benefits of beta-carotene, however, Dr. Walford recommends supplementing only vitamins C and E and selenium. If you choose to take supplements, the following ranges represent safe doses for these nutrients, according to Dr. Walford.

Vitamin C: 500 to 2,000 milligrams, taken in two or three doses during the day. Amounts over 1,200 milligrams daily may cause diarrhea in some people.

Vitamin E: 200 to 300 international units in the form of d-alpha tocopherol. People who are taking anticoagulants or have had strokes or bleeding problems should get a doctor's okay before taking vitamin E supplements in any amount.

Selenium: 100 to 200 micrograms. It's best to talk to your doctor, however, before taking more than 100 micrograms a day.

10 The Raw Foods Diet

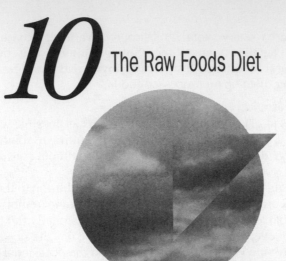

Eating Nature's Way

It's as simple as nutrition gets. Fresh fruits and vegetables eaten just the way nature delivers them: Fresh, whole, unprocessed—and raw.

At first glance it seems like the ultimate lazy person's diet, invented by someone with an abiding antipathy for dishwashing, kitchen appliances and slaving over a hot stove. But according to those who opt to eat all of their meals uncooked, a diet based on raw fruits and vegetables has more going for it than convenience. It's just nutrition the way nature intended it.

"Every other species eats food in its natural state, without cooking or processing of any kind," says James Lennon, executive director of the American Natural Hygiene Society, a Tampa, Florida, organization that promotes a diet emphasizing uncooked foods. "It seems sensible that we should do the same."

Proponents maintain that a diet of uncooked foods offers a cornucopia of health benefits—better digestion, a stronger immune system, an end to weight problems and greater energy and vitality. Some even believe that it can help the body defend itself from the onslaughts of serious illnesses like diabetes, chronic fatigue syndrome and cancer.

Even medical professionals who don't eat a raw foods diet themselves concede that raw foods can be highly nutritious. "For sheer nutrient content, you can't beat it, as long as you eat a good variety of foods," says Elson Haas, M.D., medical director of the Preventive Medical Center of Marin in San Rafael, California, and author of *Staying Healthy with Nutrition*.

The Lure of "Living Food"

The raw foods diet is the antithesis of the highly processed, fruit- and vegetable-deficient diet that most Americans are eating. It's essentially a strict vegetarian diet that eliminates all foods of animal origin, including meat, fish, eggs and dairy products. Because they require cooking, grains and grain products like bread and pasta are also absent from the menu. That leaves mostly fruits and vegetables and their juices, as well as nuts, seeds and sprouts.

For some people—no one knows how many—eating a mostly raw diet is a way of life, chosen for a combination of health and philosophical reasons.

"There is a belief that the food is 'alive,' electromagnetically, measurably alive, and eating it contributes to your vitality," says Morgan Martin, N.D., a naturopathic physician and professor of nutrition at Bastyr University in Seattle. "It's not an idea that's been demonstrated in scientific terms. It's more of a philosophy about food and its function in the body."

Scientists have known for years that raw fruits and vegetables are rich in enzymes—protein molecules that kick off chemical reactions, including those that happen during digestion. Raw foodists believe that the rich enzyme content of fresh fruits and vegetables improves digestion and the absorption of nutrients.

Because enzymes are heat-sensitive, cooking food destroys them before the food even makes it to the dinner table, making them both less nutritious and harder to digest properly than uncooked food, according to proponents.

"Raw food contains both oxygen and enzymes, which are necessary to fully digest vitamins, minerals and proteins," says Brian Clement, director of the Hippocrates Health Institute, a clinic in West Palm Beach, Florida, that promotes a diet consisting mainly of raw fruits, vegetables and sprouts. "When you cook a food to about 115°, all the enzymes and oxygen leave, so the nutrients in the food aren't completely absorbed."

The idea that the enzymes in raw produce are important for good nutrition is highly controversial. "We can't even say for sure that raw foods are more digestible because of those enzymes, because the enzymes are not necessarily digestive enzymes," notes Dr. Martin. But even those who don't buy this theory agree that a well-planned raw foods diet can be extremely nutritious.

No-Bake Bread

Of all the foods that you're likely to miss on a raw diet, bread tops the list. If you find yourself craving a sandwich, try this simple, wholesome no-bake bread, made of sprouts and warmed in an oven on very low heat.

....

4–6 cups wheat and/or rye sprouts
1 teaspoon caraway seeds

Oil a baking sheet.

Grind the sprouts or blend them in a food processor with a little water. Add the caraway seeds.

Press the dough into a small, flat loaf and place it on the prepared baking sheet. Heat in a 105° oven 12 to 20 hours. The bread is done when it becomes crisp.

....

A Jungle of Nutrients

It goes without saying that a diet comprised of raw foods is a radical departure from the way most of us are used to eating. "In this country, we have an almost endless variety of foods available to us, but most of what we choose to eat is of poor quality—high in calories and in some cases almost devoid of nutrients," says Dr. Martin. "On a raw diet you're very restricted in what you can eat, but every food you do eat is highly nutritious."

While most Americans struggle to eat five servings of fruits and vegetables a day—the minimum recommended by most nutritionists—raw foodists can easily get that many servings in a single meal, adding up to a diet that's extraordinarily high in vitamins, minerals and fiber.

Eating fruits and vegetables raw also means that you get more of certain nutrients that are destroyed in cooking. Raw broccoli, for example, is an excellent source of vitamin C, but once it's steamed, boiled or microwaved, it loses up to 30 percent of its vitamin C.

A number of studies suggest that all the extra nutrients you get from raw produce may have a profound effect on long-term health. Studies have found that people with high levels of vitamin C in their blood tend to have lower total cholesterol readings. Just as important, they have higher levels of HDL (high-density lipoprotein, the "good" cholesterol), giving them a real advantage in preventing heart disease.

Epidemiological studies show a reduced risk of several different cancers in people who eat a diet rich in vitamin C and beta-carotene—both found in abundance in raw fruits and vegetables.

Research has also focused on the anti-cancer properties of glutathione, a little-known compound found in fruits and vegetables. A large study conducted by the National Cancer Institute in Bethesda, Maryland, and the Centers for Disease Control and Prevention in Atlanta found that a diet rich in glutathione was associated with a lower incidence of cancer of the mouth or pharynx (windpipe). Glutathione is found in many foods, but so far only the glutathione found in raw vegetables and fruits seems to be protective against cancer.

Nutrients to Watch

At the same time, those on a raw diet need to do some careful planning to make sure they're getting enough protein, which fruits and vegetables do not contain in great abundance.

The best protein sources on a raw diet are sprouts—the small, tender shoots that emerge from the seed when a grain or bean plant begins to germinate. Sprouts are easy to grow and contribute valuable protein to salads and other raw dishes.

Another nutrient that you'll need to round out a raw foods diet is vitamin B_{12}, which is found only in foods of animal origin like meat, eggs and dairy products. If you eat a raw foods diet only a few weeks or months of the year, B_{12} isn't something you'll need to worry about, since most people have enough stored B_{12} to last for several years. But if you eat a raw diet for longer than that, you may be at risk of a B_{12} deficiency and should talk to your doctor about testing, dietary management or supplementation, says Dr. Martin.

Pregnancy and breastfeeding also increase your need for B_{12}. And since a B_{12} deficiency can have serious consequences for your baby's future health, your doctor may recommend dietary changes or a supplement to make sure you're getting enough.

Focus on Fiber

Another advantage of a raw diet is that it's loaded with fiber. Fiber isn't a nutrient per se—in fact, it's indigestible and just passes through your digestive tract. But the *way* it passes through is exactly what makes it so valuable. Fiber is responsible for escorting wastes through your intestines and out of your body.

"It's been shown pretty clearly that there's a lining to most people's colons that is fairly putrid," says Dr. Martin. "And because we absorb all of our nutrients through that lining, some residues of that putrefying matter are absorbed into the blood." Loaded with fiber, a raw foods diet can help flush out any wastes that may have accumulated in the colon.

If you're used to eating a standard American diet, all the fiber in a raw diet will take a little getting used to. Expect some minor unpleasant side effects like cramping and gas, especially in the beginning days of the diet, says Dr. Haas.

Making It Work

If you'd like to try a raw diet, here are a few guidelines to keep in mind.

Ease into it. People who adopt a raw foods diet at the Hippocrates Health Institute are encouraged to change their diets gradually over a period of six months to a year. How long it takes depends on what your diet was like in the first place, says Clement. "If you eat a typical American diet, with

Sprouting at Home

An essential part of a balanced raw diet, sprouts are rich in vitamins, minerals and high-quality protein. To grow sprouts easily at home, you'll need some seeds (available at natural food stores) and a quart or half-gallon glass jar with a wide mouth. (A quart jar is much easier to handle and usually adequate, unless you're sprouting enough for a big family.) You'll also need cheesecloth or wire mesh to cover the jar and a strong rubber band to hold it in place.

Put the appropriate amount of seeds (see below) in the jar, then fill it halfway with water. Cover the mouth of the jar with the cheesecloth or wire mesh and secure it with the rubber band. Place the jar on a countertop out of direct sunlight and let the sprouts soak for the required length of time (see below).

After soaking the sprouts, invert the jar in a sink or basin, tilting it at a 45-degree angle to let the water drain. Propping it up in a dish drainer works well. Leave the jar in that position as your seeds are sprouting, which may take anywhere from one to six days, depending on the type of seeds.

During this time, rinse the sprouts twice a day. Hold the covered jar under running water and fill it to overflowing, then invert it as before to drain.

Once the sprouts are ready for harvesting, some varieties will have to be hulled. (Pea, lentil and grain sprouts are the exceptions.) To remove the hulls, take the sprouts from the jar and place them in a sink that's half-filled with cool water. Stir the water gently to loosen the hulls. Rinse the sprouts in a colander before using.

Seed	Amount	Soaking Time	Sprouting Time	Notes
Almonds (shelled)	1 cup	12 hours	1 day	Don't actually sprout—just swell up; no hull to remove.
Cabbage	⅓ cup	4–6 hours	4–5 days	Remove hulls after harvesting.
Corn	1 cup	12 hours	2–3 days	Use sweet corn; remove hulls after harvesting.
Green peas (whole)	1 cup	12 hours	2–3 days	Don't require hulling.
Lentils	1 cup	12 hours	3–5 days	Don't require hulling.
Oats	1 cup	12 hours	2–3 days	Use whole "sprouting" oats; can be made into breads.
Pumpkin	1 cup	8 hours	1 day	Don't actually sprout—just swell up; no hull to remove.
Sunflower	2 cups	8 hours	1–3 days	Remove hulls before soaking.
Wheat	1 cup	12 hours	2–3 days	Don't require hulling; can be made into breads.

meat and sugars and dairy products and processed foods, you might start by eating meat six days a week instead of every day," he suggests. "Allowing yourself a transitional period makes the change easier, both physically psychologically."

Try it in the summer. If you're trying an uncooked diet for the first time, you'll probably find it more appealing in warm weather, says Dr. Martin, who sometimes follows the diet in the spring and summer months. "It also works well in a tropical climate, where the growing season is longer and you have a greater variety of fresh produce available year-round," she says.

Eat heartily. Most people are surprised by the sheer quantity of food they have to eat on an uncooked diet, says Dr. Martin. "The foods we're accustomed to are much more concentrated: Meat, sugar, dairy products and even grains are much higher in calories than an equivalent amount of vegetables, so we feel satisfied on less food. Take those foods out of the diet, and you have to eat a lot more just to get enough calories."

Break it down. Another way to add variety to the diet is by juicing or grating vegetables. This may also make raw vegetables easier to digest.

"The nutrients in a raw carrot are bound up in cellulose—the indigestible, fibrous part of the carrot that passes right through the digestive tract," explains Dr. Martin. "If the carrot is lightly steamed, the cellulose breaks down, so the nutrients are more available."

Cooking isn't the only way to accomplish this, adds Ronald Cridland, M.D., of the Health Promotion Clinic in Rohnert Park, California. For those on a raw food diet, juicing, grating or simply chewing very well will also help break down the cellulose so the nutrients will be more available, he says.

Start sprouting. Sprouts are sold at food co-ops, natural food stores and even supermarkets in some parts of the country. If you can't find them in your area, sprouts are easy to grow at home, even if you live in a small apartment.

Choose organic. "The more fruits and vegetables you eat, the more important it is to buy ones that are organically grown," says Dr. Martin. She warns that many commercially grown fruits and vegetables are sprayed with pesticides that could contribute to rising cancer rates. If you buy organic or grow your own, you don't have to worry about that risk.

11 Fasting

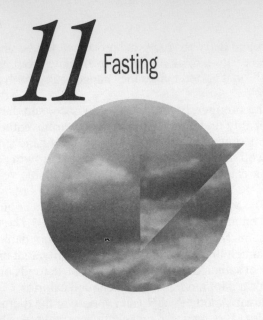

The Fast Track to Good Health

Imagine what would happen if factories never shut down to let the cleaning crews in. Waste paper would pile up to the ceiling. Garbage would rot in the hallways. And productivity would steadily grind to a halt.

The same thing happens to your body after years of shoveling in pizza, fries, burgers and cola, say some doctors. If you don't stop to let the "cleaning crews" in, your arteries clog, your organs malfunction, and your body eventually quits. The quickest way to clean up, they say, is to fast.

"Fasting rests your body from the heavy amount of work that is required for digestion," explains naturopathic physician Steven Bailey, N.D., director of the Northwest Naturopathic Clinic in Portland, Oregon. According to theory, "it speeds up the breakdown of fat cells so you can release and eliminate stored wastes and generate new cells," he says.

You Are What You Don't Eat

Although it sounds like a New Age therapy, fasting is one of the oldest "cures" in human history. Defined simply, fasting just means going without food and consuming only water for as long as your body has the nutritional reserves to function properly. Devout people of almost every religion have fasted throughout history to promote mental, physical and spiritual health. And Hippocrates, the father of Western medicine, regularly prescribed fasting as a cure for disease.

Today, a handful of doctors across the country are reviving this ancient healing weapon to combat modern diseases. They ask people to fast for varying amounts of time—anywhere from 3 to 30 days—and sometimes the fasting produces remarkable results. These doctors believe that fasting can be an important part of a healthy lifestyle and lead to a long, healthy life—as long as people who fast also maintain a well-balanced, plant-based diet when they aren't fasting.

"There's nothing in the science of aging as well-documented for expanding the life span of laboratory animals as fasting. Humans are not designed to function properly with nutritional excess, especially excesses of fat, protein and glucose," maintains fasting advocate Joel Fuhrman, M.D., a nutritional medicine specialist, director of the Amwell Health Center in Belle Mead, New Jersey, and author of *Fasting—and Eating—for Health*. "This is something the whole nation doesn't understand. They think more is better. But excess can be just as destructive as deficiency."

Clean Your Plate!

Looking back, it's little wonder where we got that idea. We were admonished by our parents to clean our plates and reminded of the "starving children in China" who didn't have the heaps of rich food that filled our plates. Politicians promised us a "chicken in every pot" as a pledge to give us a better life. Abundance conjures images of good times, good friends and good living. Fasting, on the other hand, suggests hunger strikers, shipwrecked sailors and spiritual seekers suffering for humanity.

Yet according to fasting supporters, it's the abundance, not the sparseness of food that's ultimately doing us in. Dr. Fuhrman believes that the typical high-fat, high-protein diet is crippling us with osteoporosis, arthritis, atherosclerosis, heart disease and diabetes. It's suppressing our immune systems and putting us in the grave with cancer and heart attacks, he says.

Ideally, we should never have to fast. We should live in such a healthy environment that we wouldn't accumulate metabolic waste, adds Alan Goldhamer, D.C., director of the Center for Conservative Therapy in Penngrove, California. But we don't. Especially today, when people are getting sick from diseases of excess, fasting is the ultimate approach, he says.

Polly Doesn't Want a Cracker

If you need proof that fasting is the simplest, most natural way to heal yourself, just look at the animal kingdom, say fasting proponents.

Are You Starving?

One surefire way to get a fasting expert's dander up is to mistakenly refer to a fasting period as a starvation diet. They are two very different processes, says fasting advocate Joel Fuhrman, M.D., a nutritional medicine specialist, director of the Amwell Health Center in Belle Mead, New Jersey, and author of *Fasting—and Eating—for Health*. And there is nothing healthy about starving!

By definition, fasting is refraining from food while your nutritional reserves are high enough to sustain your normal functions. As soon as those reserves hit zero, you begin starving. You need to break your fast before your body starts digging into vital tissues for its energy.

For most people, that point doesn't begin until 40 days or more have gone by, says Dr. Fuhrman. But you should definitely see a professional to both supervise extended fasts and to teach you what signs and symptoms you should be on the alert for when you're conducting shorter fasts at home.

How do you know when your dog is sick? He doesn't eat. Why doesn't he eat? Because he's healing, explains Herbert M. Shelton, an early international fasting authority who guided people through more than 30,000 fasts. In his book *The Science and Fine Art of Fasting*, Shelton notes that animals instinctively go into seclusion and fast when they are injured or ill. If we would pay attention, we would notice that we do the same thing, he says.

When you're sick with the flu, you automatically drink lots of liquids, relax and let your body do the rest, says Dr. Fuhrman. You don't even have an interest in food. It's a natural reaction. Fasting experts just take it to the next step: If it works for small ailments, they suggest that maybe it will also work for large ones. It just takes a longer fast. But doctors are quick to point out that fasting may actually be harmful or even life-threatening if you have some kinds of health problems.

A Working Vacation for Your Body

Although these theories are largely discounted by the mainstream medical community, fasting proponents believe that fasting works by giving your body a much-needed break from processing the incessant flow of food it gets every day. Your body can take a breather, heal overworked cells and regenerate so that you can process nutrients even more effectively when the dinner bell sounds again, they say.

The liver plays a key role in fasting because it chemically changes the toxins that are being released from the cells of your body and allows them to be excreted more readily. The toxins, say fasting experts, include chemicals, pesticides and toxic by-products that result from taking in too many nutrients—although this has not been definitely proven in studies. Also, advocates of fasting say that the fast gives your body the chance to break down and metabolize all the fat that it has been saving for a rainy day.

"Autolyzation," or self-digestion, can take place only during a fast, says Dr. Fuhrman. During this process, the body consumes its superfluous tissue, such as fat, blood vessel plaque (the goop that blocks your arteries and causes heart disease) and diseased cells. Fasting advocates say the autolyzation process conserves rather than breaks down vital tissues.

Whether this actually occurs is not proven, but those who fast believe that the whole process produces the youthful effects Ponce de León searched for during all those years that he pursued the famed Fountain of Youth. "During a fast, your body speeds up the reclaiming of dying cells and their waste products and uses it for new cell growth. Fasting restores physiologic youth to your body," says Dr. Bailey.

Who Qualifies as an Expert?

As you may have guessed, the curricula of mainstream medical schools usually don't include Fasting 101 — or any other fasting courses, for that matter. Doctors who use fasting as a therapy have to seek special training. If you go to one of these doctors seeking advice, you need to be sure the one you choose is properly certified.

The organization that certifies these doctors is a group of health professionals dedicated to natural medicine and known as the International Association of Hygienic Physicians. To qualify for certification, health-care professionals must complete a six-month residency with a physician who has already been certified. The professionals they certify as experts on fasting — meaning that they are qualified to help you do it — include medical doctors, chiropractors, osteopathic doctors and naturopathic doctors.

Running on Empty

If these arguments have you thinking that you might want to become a fledgling faster, you may be wondering "What will keep me going for three or more days with nothing to eat? How will I survive when I'm used to refueling three or more times a day?"

To rescue your hungry body from complete deprivation, you have a supply pack in the form of fat, muscle and stored carbohydrates. During a fast, your body uses an intricate system of converting stored materials, such as fat, into energy while sparing vital tissues, such as organs. In fact, the vast majority of your cells live off the energy they get from your fatty tissue supplies.

Only your brain and red blood cells need pure glucose—a simple sugar that your body usually gets from carbohydrates—to function. Your liver stores some glucose, but it generally runs dry after the first day of a fast. Then your brain and blood start pulling operating power by drawing on special energy-providing proteins called amino acids that are found in your muscles. The amino acids are converted to glucose, temporarily making up for the lack of food. So if you're going to do an extended fast, you should be prepared to lose a little muscle.

After two to three days of fasting, your body realizes that if it wants to have something left to flex when the fast is done, it had better start producing an alternative source of energy. So the liver starts to break down fat, producing glucose-substitute chemicals called ketones. Once ketone production swings into high gear, the blood and brain use these compounds instead of glucose for power. The process is called ketogenesis, and it's one of our basic survival mechanisms.

"Ketones are beneficial when you're fasting because they preserve the body's protein stores," says Trevor Salloum, N.D., a fasting specialist in Kelowna, British Columbia.

An accumulation of too many ketones in the blood, however, can be dangerous. This condition, called ketosis, can lead to your body's becoming too acidic, which can be fatal. That's why it's important to always fast under medical supervision so that your doctor can monitor your condition.

Juicing Up

For people who don't like the prospect of total deprivation, even for a few days, some doctors provide the option of going on a modified fast. On this kind of regimen, you don't eat food, but you can drink fruit juice, vegetable juice or herb tea. That way you're giving your digestive system a much-needed break, but you're still providing fuel for your body.

Other advocates see juice fasting as a first step for people who can't handle water fasting right away. "Water fasts are the best, but a lot of people are just too 'toxic' to have a successful water fast," says Dr. Bailey. "So we have them work up to it and cleanse their bodies with a few juice fasts first."

Although experts say both juice and water fasts can be powerful healing tools, orthodox fasters believe water fasts are the better of the two.

"As soon as you add calories, you change the physiological process of fasting," explains Ronald Cridland, M.D., of the Health Promotion Clinic in Rohnert Park, California. It's his view that if you are juice fasting, "you continue to produce insulin. But water fasting creates a catabolic state, where the body is breaking down and absorbing excess tissues, which is useful for shrinking tumors and getting rid of excess weight. That doesn't mean juice diets aren't beneficial. They are. But water fasting is the modality that allows the body to heal itself to the maximum capacity." A doctor experienced in fasting can tell you which method is right for you.

Getting Past Hunger

So what stops many people from trying this ancient prescription for healing? That gnawing sensation in the pit of the stomach that has been blamed for everything from the French Revolution to the Third Reich.

Hunger. Herbert Hoover called it the mother of anarchy. Not surprisingly, it's often the death of fasting. Yet experts insist that although people use hunger as an excuse, hunger isn't the problem—withdrawal is.

If you find that you're absolutely miserable after missing just a meal or two, it's a signal that you really need to fast, says Dr. Fuhrman. Some people immediately begin to experience headaches, confusion, abdominal cramping and weakness when they start fasting. "This is the body going through withdrawal while it is detoxifying," Dr. Fuhrman maintains. "Only people who have been eating the rich American diet get these symptoms, because their bodies are accustomed to excessive levels of fat and protein." He notes that discomfort is relatively rare if you have been eating a natural, plant-based diet for at least two weeks before your fast. Other doctors disagree, however, saying that anyone can have these reactions. "Most people have withdrawal symptoms when they go on water fasts, even if they've been eating well," according to Elson Haas, M.D., medical director of the Preventive Medical Center of Marin in San Rafael, California, and author of *Staying Healthy with Nutrition*.

When you are truly hungry, say fasting experts, you feel it in your throat, like thirst. And it's natural for your mouth to water. Sure, you want food, but when you're used to fasting, you don't get sharp pangs of hunger or other kinds of discomfort. Hunger should be pleasant, say those who are experienced with fasting.

Warning: When Not to Try This at Home

If you're going to go for more than two to three days without food or if you're fasting for the first time, you need a doctor's supervision, says fasting advocate Joel Fuhrman, M.D., a nutritional medicine specialist, director of the Amwell Health Center in Belle Mead, New Jersey, and author of *Fasting—and Eating—for Health*.

He likens fasting to childbirth. "Most women could have a baby without a doctor there and be just fine," says Dr. Fuhrman. "But there are one or two instances out of a hundred where either the baby or the mother might have some trouble and need a physician. The same is true with fasting."

There are also some people who simply should not fast because of existing health conditions, say fasting experts. These conditions include severe anemia, Type I (insulin-dependent) diabetes, cancer, epilepsy, eating disorders, AIDS, pregnancy and nursing, liver or kidney disease and tuberculosis. And a doctor will not let you fast if you have the condition known as MCAD (medium-chain acyl-CoA dehydrogenase) deficiency, because it's an enzyme defect that prevents the body from changing fatty acids into energy. And if you are on any medication, you must see a doctor before going on even a short fast.

If You're Going to Try It

After you've had a checkup and a doctor has given you the go-ahead for a two- to three-day solo fast, the following tips will help you forge a painless path for going foodless.

Take some time off. The biggest mistake people make when they fast is not getting enough rest, say fasting experts. "Fasting is a vacation so your body can restore normalcy. It can't do that if you are under the stresses of normal life. Most of your fast should be spent resting or sleeping," says fasting advocate Joel Fuhrman, M.D., a nutritional medicine specialist, director of the Amwell Health Center in Belle Mead, New Jersey, and author of *Fasting—and Eating—for Health*.

But if you can't get away from work and you want to do a quick fast, you can try doing it on a weekend, says Dr. Fuhrman. Start Friday morning and fast until Sunday at dinnertime, easing back into the work week with a small meal of fruit on Sunday evening.

You can also simply go on a juice fast for a few days, advises Elson Haas, M.D., medical director of the Preventive Medical Center of Marin in San Rafael, California, and author of *Staying Healthy with Nutrition*. That way you will have the cleansing benefits of fasting plus the energy to continue most of your normal activities.

Make it easy come, easy go. Just as you wouldn't shift in and out of Park while cruising down the freeway, you shouldn't just dive in and out of a fast, say experts. "We have people get away from heavy foods like proteins, starches and sugars and start eating fresh fruits and vegetables a few days before a fast," says William Esser, N.D., D.C., founder of Esser's Health Ranch in Lake Worth, Florida. He suggests breaking the fast with fruit and vegetable juice before moving on to solid foods.

Have water, water everywhere. Going off food does *not* mean that you go off water, doctors remind fasters. They recommend that you drink at least one quart, preferably two, of pure, unchlorinated water daily during a fast. Since fasts are mildly dehydrating, doctors say you should also avoid hot showers and sunbathing, which promote dehydration because your skin dries out faster as your body heats up.

Hit the library. One of the biggest complaints fasters have is boredom. Since you're taking a break from your normal routine when you're fasting, it's a great time to catch up on your reading and to watch all those videos you've been dying to see.

Don't underdo it. While you shouldn't be running marathons when you're fasting, you're not waiting for rigor mortis to set in, either. Some stretching or gentle yoga is just what the doctors order to help you prevent stiff muscles, particularly if you're spending a lot of time in bed during the fast.

Avoid Tylenol. Because your liver has extra work to do when you're fasting, it can't process the pain reliever acetaminophen (Tylenol) as efficiently as it normally would, according to Dr. Fuhrman. For this reason, you should never take any medicine containing acetaminophen during a fast, he says. It's potentially toxic.

The Healing Power of Fasting

When it comes to healing disease with fasting, an old Jewish proverb takes the same line as fasting advocates: "He that eats till he is sick must fast till he is well." But today's proponents go even further: They say that if you want to stay well, you also have to change your diet after you fast.

Fortunately, even if you love hot dogs, hamburgers and potato chips, a good fast will clean your palate so that you'll be able to appreciate the subtle flavors of whole, natural foods, says Dr. Fuhrman. "Your senses are heightened by fasting, and you aren't able to tolerate the overwhelming sweetness, saltiness and spiciness of American foods."

"Once people's bodies are clean, their bowels move well, their energy is better, and they are more likely to stick with the right habits," adds Dr. Cridland. "But if they go back to their old ways of eating, they'll have all their old problems back."

That said, here are the conditions that doctors who use fasting believe it can heal.

Lick Addiction

"Fasting helps people eliminate habits such as the use of tobacco, coffee and alcohol," says Dr. Goldhamer. "It's remarkable how by the second or third day, many smokers literally exhibit no physiological cravings."

Although there are many theories as to how fasting breaks addiction, Dr. Cridland believes it's a matter of giving people a clean slate to start over with. "For people with addictive behaviors, taking the time to clean out their bodies makes it much easier for them to stop smoking or get off drugs, alcohol or caffeine," he says.

Put the Brakes on Aging

No matter what theory of aging you consider—and there are several— fasting is a surefire way to slow down the entire aging process, says Dr. Fuhrman.

At the most fundamental level, aging begins with our cells in a process that Dr. Haas calls cell suffocation, which is caused by a buildup of waste and plain old wear and tear. We age either because our cells have accumulated so much waste that they cease to function properly or because long-time use and overuse simply wear the cells out, says Dr. Fuhrman. In his view, fasting counteracts both of these processes by giving cells a rest and allowing them to regenerate.

Alleviate Rheumatoid Arthritis

Although millions of Americans are afflicted with rheumatoid arthritis (RA) it's a mystery why these people have it and others don't. The pain, stiffness and joint deterioration of RA are caused by harmful substances that damage the silklike sheaths that surround your joints. It's as if your body set out to wreck its own joints, causing pain and fatigue. Fasting has been shown to help—in some cases enormously, according to Dr. Fuhrman.

"It's well-documented that fasting takes away the pain of rheumatoid arthritis. That's not even controversial," says Dr. Fuhrman. "The controversial part is that a lot of patients have their arthritis come back when they start eating again."

Believing that it's food sensitivity that often triggers rheumatoid arthritis, Dr. Fuhrman recommends a very slow reintroduction of food after a fast. "We only give people with rheumatoid arthritis one new food every three days after a fast," he says. "That way, you can tell which foods they do fine with and which ones they have a reaction to." In Dr. Fuhrman's view, "there's no way to do that without a fast."

In one study on fasting, food and rheumatoid arthritis, researchers explored the effects of fasting on 53 people who had the disease. Twenty-seven of them fasted for seven to ten days and then gradually went on a lacto-vegetarian diet, meaning they ate no meat or dairy products. The other 26 were told to rest but did not fast. The study showed that the 27 who fasted had significant improvement in swollen joints, joint pain, grip strength, infection-fighting white blood cell counts and morning stiffness when compared to those who did not fast. The fasters were still feeling the benefits a year later.

At least one small study has suggested that the anti-arthritis effects of fasting disappear shortly after the fast concludes, regardless of whether people go back to eating burgers or bean sprouts. But Dr. Fuhrman points out that most studies have shown that relief from the symptoms of rheumatoid arthritis usually continues after a fast if a healthy, plant-based diet is adopted.

Attack Your Asthma

"Fasting is magical against asthma. I think people with asthma all over the world should come and take part in a fasting program," says Dr. Fuhrman.

To illustrate his point, Dr. Fuhrman cites one of his most severe cases, a woman who used steroid inhalers and prednisone—strong medications that help people who have frequent asthma attacks. Even though she used the medication, she was frequently hospitalized because she was unable to breathe, according to Dr. Fuhrman. "She followed a strict diet for a couple of years and did a little better, although she was still on steroid inhalers and prednisone periodically. Finally, I convinced her to fast. In 6 to 7 days, we had weaned her off her medications. She fasted for 21 days. Now she takes aerobics classes, and she can sleep through the night. She lives normally."

Other doctors have also reported high success rates with asthma. "We're tracking a large number of people right now who have come in to have their asthma treated," says Dr. Goldhamer. "Asthma tends to respond quite consistently to fasting, and we generally can dramatically reduce or eliminate the need for routine medication."

Shrink Benign Tumors

Fasting is a safe and effective treatment for noncancerous tumors, says Dr. Fuhrman. Benign tumors such as those found in the breasts and ovaries, fibroid tumors (benign tumors in and around the uterus) and polyps (potentially precancerous growths that occur in places like the colon) are absorbed and disposed of like other bodily waste during a fast, he says. But this absorption and disposal process works only if you first shed excess body fat, Dr. Fuhrman concludes. Otherwise your body will draw on your fat stores for the entire fast without ever getting to the tumor.

The only evidence of this process is from individual case histories—what researchers call anecdotal evidence—and not all advocates agree that fasting alone is therapeutic. Lifestyle changes have an impact, too, they point out. Nevertheless, some fasting proponents offer examples of cases where benign tumors and polyps were healed.

In one striking case reported by Dr. Goldhamer, a 36-year-old woman came to see him about symptoms she was having, including pelvic pain and breast tenderness—all unrelated to her menstrual cycle. After a battery of tests, he diagnosed a cyst on her left ovary. He put her on a fast for 15 days. She complained of pelvic pain throughout the duration of the fast, but when it was over, the ovarian cyst was gone, as was all of her discomfort.

In another case, Dr. Bailey was treating a woman who had benign breast cysts that had become progressively worse for ten years. "After her first fast, she had significant relief from pain and significant reduction in the cyst size," says Dr. Bailey. "After three to four years of multiple fasts and changes in diet and lifestyle, mammography showed she was cyst-free."

Just don't confuse benign tumors with cancerous growths, warns Dr. Fuhrman. Only your doctor can make a sure diagnosis, so any time you're in doubt, be sure to talk to your physician. "Cancerous growths are unpredictable, and people with cancer should not fast," Dr Fuhrman says.

Kick Cardiovascular Disease

Extensive research has shown that heart disease can be slowly reversed by using aggressive nutritional regimens like strict vegetarian diets, says Dr. Fuhrman. But he believes that fasting can produce rapid improvement in someone who is having chest pain and needs immediate relief from cardiovascular problems.

"I've had miraculous results with fasting and heart disease because fasting accelerates the rate of regression you would get from a strict diet alone," says Dr. Fuhrman. "In four to five days, chest pains go away. People have been able to go out and play tennis and golf and live a normal life. Of course, they need to change their eating habits radically after a fast, or there is no point in fasting."

"Fasting is a significant physiological rest for someone with cardiovascular disease," adds Dr. Cridland. As he sees it, fasting works primarily

Fast Philosophy

by decreasing the workload of the heart. "You are ridding the body of excess fluid, lowering blood pressure and metabolizing fat and choles- terol." Studies show that your blood also becomes thinner during a fast, so your immediate risk of heart at- tack or stroke is greatly reduced, Dr. Cridland and Dr. Fuhrman agree.

One of Dr. Cridland's most no- table cases was a man with badly blocked arteries and severe angina— crushing chest pain that radiates to the left arm, neck, jaw and shoulder. "This fellow had to stop twice on his way from the parking lot into work to rest and take nitroglycerin," re- calls Dr. Cridland. His condition was so poor that he wasn't even a candi- date for bypass surgery. But with fasting, he improved, according to Dr. Cridland. "He did a 21-day fast with us, and his problem resolved."

Of course, this is an extreme case. All symptoms of heart disease should be checked and treated by your doctor. Fasting works best as a preventive measure.

Wipe Out Chronic Infections

"Fasting has a very powerful immune-enhancing effect," says Dr. Cridland. It gives the body a chance to increase lymphokines, which as- sist the white blood cells in fighting infection. Fasting also increases T- lymphocytes, which are involved in resolving viruses, and increases phagocytic ability, which is the ability of the immune system to eat ab- normal cells or bacteria floating around in the body. "We get significant improvement in people with chronic immune deficiency diseases with fasting," Dr. Cridland says.

Doctors who use water and/or juice fasting say that it can help people who have chronic fatigue syndrome, which can cause months or even years of drowsiness, fever and achy muscles. It may also help those who carry the Epstein-Barr virus, which causes mononucleosis, with symptoms such as sore throat, fever and fatigue that can last for weeks. Fasting also helps with candida infections, such as the burning, itching yeast infections that women get, according to doctors who are proponents of fasting. All of these are diseases that involve impaired immunity.

Do Away with Type II Diabetes

Fasting experts are quick to caution that people with Type I (insulin-dependent) diabetes should *not* fast. And they further warn that people with Type II (non-insulin-dependent) diabetes should fast only under the close supervision of a doctor. But with these cautions in mind, proponents of fasting praise the method as one of the best ways to control Type II diabetes during its initial stages.

Dr. Fuhrman uses a lengthy dietary process for people with Type II diabetes, first using a strict plant-based diet, then putting them on a prolonged fast. He says that he can get 95 percent of people with diabetes off their medication and control their blood sugar better than they can control it with periodic injections of insulin.

Fasting is not heavily researched in diabetes treatment. Various studies have shown its worth in improving people's blood sugar levels for up to four months following a fast. But remember, if you have any form of diabetes, don't ever attempt fasting except under a doctor's supervision.

Clear Up Colitis

"Fasting is particularly helpful for people who have digestive disorders of all types because it gives the digestive system a chance to rest and heal itself," says naturopathic physician William Esser, N.D., D.C., founder of Esser's Health Ranch in Lake Worth, Florida.

As evidence of fasting's digestion-restoring powers, Dr. Fuhrman describes

Straight from the Faster's Mouth

Lou Bancala didn't like thinking about open-heart surgery. The idea of having his chest sawed open scared him. In fact, so did everything about the surgery, including the risks associated with the procedure. Yet surgery is exactly what Bancala, a Towaco, New Jersey, sandwich shop owner in his early fifties, was facing.

Having already tried angioplasty and diet to clear the blockage in a major artery, he feared there might not be any alternative to surgery. Then he found out about fasting.

"I was taking aspirin and blood thinners every day, plus Valium because I was a nervous wreck," says Bancala. He already exercised and ate a very low fat diet, so at least he had a good start on beating the condition. Bancala went to see fasting advocate Joel Fuhrman, M.D., a nutritional medicine specialist, director of the Amwell Health Center in Belle Mead, New Jersey, and author of *Fasting— and Eating—for Health*. Dr. Fuhrman thought Bancala could possibly reverse his condition if he tried fasting.

Bancala fasted for 16 days without much discomfort. He had no headaches, cramps or nausea; he experienced only a coated tongue and did a lot of mental wall climbing. "The hardest part was the boredom," recalls Bancala.

In the end, he lost 35 pounds—and best of all, his chest pains stopped. Preliminary scans showed partial reversal of the blockage. "I feel as good as I have in 20 years," says Bancala.

the case of a man he saw who had a history of severe ulcerative colitis, which is marked by inflammation in the colon and repeated daily bouts of bloody diarrhea.

This man came to Dr. Fuhrman after several gastroenterologists suggested removing his colon to treat the condition. He had already fasted once in the hospital but was given intravenous nutrition, so it wasn't a pure fast. After weaning him off his medications, Dr. Fuhrman put him on a two-week fast. When the fast was finished, the inflammation was gone. Three months later, he was still symptom-free, according to Dr. Fuhrman.

Head Off Headaches

Headaches are your body's way of telling you that it's had enough, says Dr. Fuhrman, who believes we could all save ourselves a bundle on pain relievers if we'd just take a break from our feeding schedule.

According to Dr. Fuhrman, the main cause of headaches is the retention of toxins within the central nervous system. These toxins not only make your nerves overly sensitive to stimulants like light and noise, but as the body tries to rid itself of these toxins, the result can be a flood of chemicals like nitric oxide that irritate your body's tissues and cause headaches, he says.

Dr. Fuhrman cautions people that if they're going to fast to rid themselves of headaches, they'd better be prepared to feel worse before they feel better. Since fasting causes the rapid release of toxins, which is what he says causes headaches to begin with, you're not going to get relief until your system is clear.

Lower High Blood Pressure

"We found that fasting normalizes high blood pressure in a matter of a week or two," says Dr. Goldhamer, who is currently studying the effects of water fasting on 150 people with high blood pressure. "It also helps people make the transition to healthful eating and living so their high blood pressure doesn't return," he says.

Fasting can help even when diet and medication fail, says Dr. Fuhrman, pointing to the case of one woman who was particularly resistant to treatment. She was in her sixties and had a blood pressure reading of 210/110, well above the normal limit of 140/90. Although she was taking three different medications, they couldn't control her elevated blood pressure. Even after three months on a strict low-fat vegetarian diet—plus her medications—her blood pressure was still high at 190/105.

Then she tried fasting. Immediately after a 16-day fast, her blood pressure was 127/67. After two weeks it was higher but still in the acceptable range at 140/80.

If you're going to fast for your high blood pressure, however, experts warn that you should take it slowly. Going off your blood pressure medication suddenly can be very dangerous. Be sure to talk to your doctor before making any changes.

Overcome Overweight

While not everyone agrees, most fasting proponents, like Dr. Fuhrman, Dr. Cridland and Dr. Salloum, generally don't recommend fasting as the first line of defense against obesity because it slows your metabolic rate for four to seven weeks afterward. The problem then is that unless you're committed to converting to a new way of eating, you'll gain the weight back with a vengeance.

Despite its potential pitfalls, fasting can be used as a springboard to help people who are very overweight lose a lot of weight initially. After they're out of immediate danger, other approaches come into play. Most doctors would recommend a healthful dietary regimen, regular exercise and adequate sleep to maintain slow and steady weight loss.

Pamper Your Prostate

When writing about the myriad benefits of fasting, Herbert Shelton included prostate enlargement as one of the ills that fasting could treat. But he also reported that the improvement was rarely permanent. Most of the men who saw improvement, Shelton reported, returned to the lifestyle that, in his view, initially caused prostate enlargement. If you're going to fast to reduce your prostate to a size that doesn't cause discomfort and difficulty— which Shelton says will take only a few days—you must follow up with lifestyle changes. He advises men to avoid overeating, overworking, sexual excess, anxiety and chemicals like coffee, tea, tobacco and alcohol.

Fast as a Cure-All

Like asthma, sinusitis and allergies generally clear right up with fasting, says Dr. Fuhrman. In fact, he's seen patients whose sinus congestion disappeared when they were on a detoxification diet in preparation for a fast rather than actually fasting. But Dr. Fuhrman warns people with respiratory problems that their conditions will quickly return unless they keep eating a natural, plant-based diet.

Concerned about pollutants in your environment or pesticides in your food? Go on a fast, says Dr. Salloum. "A fast is a good way to clean the body of environmental toxins like PCBs (polychlorinated biphenyls). Studies have shown that when people fast, they release and eliminate the poisons from the foods they eat and the air they breathe that are stored in their fat cells."

Advocates believe that the benefits of fasting are so numerous that there are almost no limits. It's claimed that fasting can help clear up skin conditions like acne and eczema. It's also said to help with tinnitus (chronic ringing in the ears), vertigo (dizziness), glaucoma and fibromyalgia (recurrent achiness and fatigue throughout the body). Proponents also claim that fasting helps with cervical dysplasia (the growth of abnormal cells on the cervix), thyroid disorders, connective tissue disorders like tendinitis and chronic aches and pains of all kinds.

How Not to Eat

If you're considering fasting for a medical condition, advocates agree that the only way to do it is with the guidance of a medical professional. If you're just interested in improving your general health, you should still get the green light from your doctor. But fasting experts generally consider short fasts safe to do solo as long as you're generally in good health.

Plan your fast the way you would a party. Give yourself time to prepare, time for the event and time to recover. Most fasting experts agree that you'll be most successful if you follow these recommendations.

Before the fast. If you're a meat-and-potatoes eater, you should switch to vegetarian foods a few weeks before you fast. If you smoke and/or drink alcohol or caffeinated drinks, you should also stop a few weeks before you fast. If you're already a healthy-living vegetarian, eat lighter fare, with more emphasis on fresh fruits and vegetables. Then, a few days before the fast, limit the amount of sugars, starches and fatty foods you eat, say the experts.

During the fast. Once you start fasting, make bed rest your first priority. Doctors say the biggest mistake fasters make is not getting enough rest. And drink plenty of water. Drink at least four —and preferably eight— eight-ounce glasses a day to make sure that your body is getting enough water to operate, says Dr. Fuhrman.

After the fast. Breaking your fast doesn't mean feasting. You should reintroduce your body to food with fruit or vegetable juice or a small portion of an easily digested fruit or vegetable like watermelon or steamed zucchini. Too much food at once can cause stomach cramps or even lead to ulcers. During a fast, your digestive juices decline, and they'll need some time to get back up to speed, says Dr. Fuhrman.

A Slow Return from Fasting

When people fast, especially for the first time, they often make the mistake of breaking their fast too quickly, say fasting experts. One reason: They may be frightened by the physical changes they are undergoing.

"This is why you should work with a trained professional," says Dr. Goldhamer. "Often people mistake symptoms of healing for health problems."

But Dr. Goldhamer notes that the opposite can also be true; real health problems can emerge that can't be remedied with fasting. "Other people get in trouble because they think everything is part of healing and do not recognize real problems," he says.

What are the reactions you can expect to have during a fast? Most people experience only a few—possibly a coated tongue, tiredness or headaches. For others the responses to food deprivation include vomiting, dizziness, dark urine, body odor, insomnia, aching limbs and fainting. Experts say that if a fast is done properly, with plenty of bed rest and water intake, most of these symptoms will disappear a day or two after beginning a fast, says Dr. Fuhrman. If they don't, of course, your doctor should hear about it, which is one big reason that you should consult with a physician before you begin.

There's no doubt about it, says Dr. Goldhamer, "fasting can be very difficult and very intense, but I haven't seen anything else that has such a profound impact on health."

The benefits are twofold, in Dr. Goldhamer's view. First, fasting helps people relieve many common health problems. "And second and most important," he adds, "it helps them make the transition to a healthier lifestyle."

A Long, Long Time until Dinner

Angus Barbieri of Tayport, Fife, Scotland, holds the record for the longest fast: He went 382 days without solid food. It wasn't a pure water fast, of course, but from June 1965 to July 1966, Barbieri subsisted only on tea, coffee, water, soda water and vitamins.

Barbieri's goal was weight reduction, and the fast certainly worked. His weight dropped from a whopping 472 pounds to a lean 178.

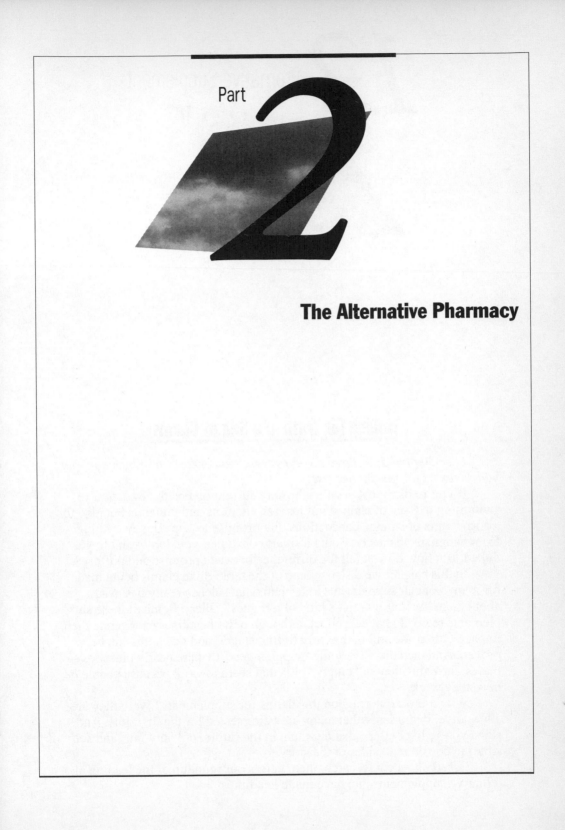

Part

2

The Alternative Pharmacy

12 Alternative Supplements

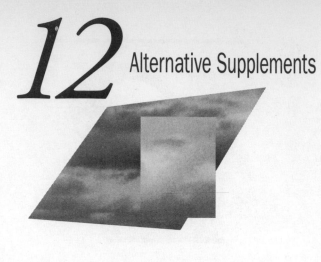

Trolling for Truth in a Sea of Claims

Lose 30 pounds in three days! Prevent cancer forever! Flush out your body's toxins for instant energy!

If you're like most people who stay current on health news, you're swimming in a sea of claims, not just for vitamins and minerals but also for a cornucopia of strange concoctions that promise to wipe out everything from hangnails to cancer. Being a smart consumer, you don't want to get duped. But how do you tell the difference between promise and puffery?

In this chapter we discuss some of the tabloidlike claims being made for many popular supplements today and what science really has to say about them. As you'll see, it's kind of a rogues' gallery. Some of these supplements really do have an effect, although news headlines exaggerate their impact. Others are still in the early testing stages, and no claims can be proven. And then there are some "supplements" that are nearly placebos—that is, the equivalent of "empty" pills that seem to work because people *believe* they work.

Why are we reporting on the claims for supplements? Well, they are alternative, in the sense that many are being tested for the first time. And since you're likely to read about them in the future, it's only fair (and sensible) to consider all sides of the story.

Based on recent research, then, here's our roundup of the leading alternative supplements that have made headlines.

Man Sheds 300 Pounds Overnight! Awakes a Hunk!

Amino Acids

Like good Madison Avenue mavens, manufacturers of amino acids love to play to their customers' dreams. "BIG MUSCLES! FAST!" they shout. Some body builders and wannabe strongmen down their powders and liquids in hopes of trading body fat for sheer muscle. Unfortunately, what most people end up shedding is money.

Amino acids—22 have been identified in the body—are the stuff from which protein is made. As Mom always said, you need protein to grow big and strong. But most of us eat good amino acid sources like chicken, tuna and beans, and there are scant few cases of protein deficiency in the United States. So do we really need protein supplements?

"Not unless you're spending two or three hours in the gym working on competitive muscle building," says Richard Gerson, Ph.D., president of the consulting firm Gerson Goodson, Inc., executive director of Peak Performance Learning Center, both in Clearwater, Florida, and author of *The Right Vitamins*. "Although most of them prefer to supplement their diets with protein drinks and tablets, even body builders can get all the amino acids they need from food," he says.

Other folks, however, will insist that amino acids such as L-carnitine, branched-chain amino acids, L-lysine, L-glutamine and L-arginine are the cat's meow for peak performance. And such amino acid supplements continue to be top sellers at many health food counters.

All Hype, No Hulk

L-arginine is one of the most hyped aminos for those who want more bulk for their buck. Since L-arginine stimulates the pituitary gland to make more growth hormone, a substance that actually does burn fat and build muscle, the premise is that more L-arginine will stimulate more growth hormone. Unfortunately, nobody knows if that's true. Plus, experts doubt that the small amounts available in supplements will burn anything but the money in your pocket.

Some researchers have suggested that L-arginine will work if you combine it with another amino acid, L-lysine, but there's no proof of that, either.

If you still insist on trying one or both, proponents recommend keeping daily doses under 1.5 grams of each for safety reasons. Experts suspect that long-term use of higher doses may create an amino acid imbalance in some people. And there's anecdotal evidence that excess L-arginine—along with too little L-lysine—promotes herpes outbreaks in people prone to cold sores, so you might want to take them in equal doses, say proponents.

Other amino acids that are sometimes recommended include L-glutamine and the branched-chain types like L-leucine, L-isoleucine and L-valine. Studies show that these supplements may help people who have been

Tryptophan Troubles

If you're like a lot of people, a couple of hours of tossing and turning sends you to the kitchen for a glass of warm milk. Not so long ago, you would have been able to reach for a bedside bottle of tryptophan—milk's soporific ingredient—and pop yourself into Dreamland.

Tryptophan is an amino acid that is converted into the sleep-regulating chemical serotonin in the brain. For 20 years, Americans who had a problem with slumberless nights bought it over the counter to help them get some rest. Then an accident happened.

In 1989, a bad batch of tryptophan crossed the sea from Japan and fell into the unsuspecting hands of consumers abroad. The contaminated supplements caused an outbreak of a rare, incurable blood disorder called eosinophilia-myalgia syndrome. Fifteen hundred people were reported affected, and at least 38 died. Many still have to deal with the aftermath, ranging from severe joint pain and fatigue to scarring of the skin and internal organs.

Although tryptophan was thought by many to be a remedy for ailments such as depression and premenstrual syndrome, the Food and Drug Administration deemed it unsafe and banned its sale. If you want to get tryptophan from foods, the best sources besides warm moo juice are meat and fish.

injured or who are under tremendous stress get back on their feet again. But they won't give healthy people a leg up in the gym or a better body at the beach.

Help for Walkers, Not Hoisters

One amino that might show some promise is L-carnitine. This is the amino acid that taxis fat into the cell's mitochondria, small components in the cell plasma that act like energy-producing furnaces. Theoretically, the more L-carnitine you have, the more fat will be transported and burned. But again, the benefits of carnitine are not the fat-burning miracles promised on the labels of body-building products. It's possible that they improve endurance in speed walkers, but that's the only benefit that's been shown.

In one study, researchers found that race walkers who were given four grams of L-carnitine every day for two weeks experienced an increase in their max VO_2—the maximum rate at which the body can use oxygen—of 6 percent. In a two-hour treadmill session, however, the walkers didn't lower the amount of lactic acid (the stuff that causes muscle soreness) they produced, nor did they burn any more fat because of L-carnitine. "Practically speaking, this is a high amount of L-carnitine and fairly expensive," notes Elson Haas, M.D., medical director of the Preventive Medical Center of Marin in San Rafael, California, and author of *Staying Healthy with Nutrition.*

The amount of L-carnitine needed for optimal health is not known, and experts generally don't recommend supplements. And it's important to note that L-carnitine and D-carnitine are not the same thing and do not have the same effects. L-carnitine is an active nutrient, whereas synthetic D-carnitine may actually interfere with the *L* form.

Healing the Muscle between Your Ears

In the wonderful claims department, people who promote amino acids also say that they heal the "muscle" between your ears. And it's true that some doctors commonly use amino acids—including glycine, tyrosine and phenylalanine—to treat depression, addiction, stress and mental conditions like schizophrenia.

Amino acids fuel the brain's message network. If you envision your brain as a city block, with each tiny cell being a house, imagine that each house depends on "mail carriers" from the nervous system. These carriers, called neurotransmitters, fax messages like "Hey, the stomach's hungry" to the right places so that you can react appropriately. By helping in the production of neurotransmitters, amino acids provide the juice that helps the fax system run properly.

"Sometimes, for reasons we don't really know, the amino acids we need to get a message across are missing," says James Heffley, Ph.D., a biochemist and nutrition adviser in Austin, Texas. "Once we get that amino acid in there, the brain starts doing the right thing again, and sometimes we can stop supplementing the amino acid."

"I use them to treat depression, alcoholism, drug addiction and heavy smoking," says Harry Panjwani, M.D., a psychiatrist in private practice in Ridgewood, New Jersey, who frequently treats patients with amino acid supplements. "But you need to use them selectively and with a doctor's supervision."

Some Lip Service

Getting enough amino acids may also help you have stronger arms and more kissable lips, say researchers.

Studies show that L-lysine suppresses the growth of the herpes simplex virus, the germ that causes those burning, itchy, angry lip blisters to which some people are prone.

L-lysine may also help give you a leg up in maintaining strong, healthy bones, a study shows. When women took calcium and 800 milligrams of L-lysine every day, the amino acid supplement helped increase the women's absorption of calcium by 20 percent.

If you think you're a candidate for supplements, studies suggest that amounts between 2,000 and 3,000 milligrams daily are usually most effective, says Mark A. McCune, M.D., chief of dermatology at Humana Hospital in Overland Park, Kansas, and assistant clinical professor of dermatology at the University of Kansas School of Medicine in Kansas City. "Some people might find that 1,000 milligrams is enough. But in my experience, most people require the higher amounts," he adds. Dr. McCune also notes that he does not recommend L-lysine for children under 16.

Remember, if you're going to supplement amino acids, you should clear it with your doctor. "Amino acids are more demanding in their balance than vitamins and minerals," says Dr. Heffley. He notes that scientists are still unsure of maximum safe dosages, and amino acids have the potential to interfere with the absorption of each other, so you should approach them with caution.

Aspirin

Tree Bark Rids Body of Myriad Ills!

Does that headline sound like pure hype? Well, a substance once derived from tree bark is currently one of our leading medicines, used to prevent a legion of common ailments, including muscle pain, heart disease, stroke, even memory loss and a type of cancer. If you haven't already guessed, it's the chalky little pill found in almost everyone's medicine cabinet—aspirin.

Although technically a drug, not a nutritional supplement, aspirin used to be derived from a chemical called salicin, which was obtained from the bark of the white willow tree. Now it's made from oils and other ingredients that aren't quite as natural as tree bark. The lowly aspirin has more than 50 million regular users in the United States, some who take it for general aches and pains and others who use it as a daily supplement.

When aspirin is taken as a supplement, it's most commonly used to prevent cardiovascular diseases like heart attack and stroke. Both of these problems have a similar origin: A blood clot blocks a blood vessel that's already been narrowed by cholesterol and other harmful substances that collect on artery walls, restricting blood flow. Aspirin prevents this from happening by thinning your blood and keeping the platelets—disc-shaped blood components—from sticking together.

The bitter white pills can also lessen the severity of any heart attack you might have, say researchers. In a study of 2,114 people who came into a hospital in Worcester, Massachusetts, because of heart attack, 65 percent of those who reported taking aspirin (332 people) had small, less serious cardiac events compared with 49 percent of those who didn't take aspirin.

Help for Your Head

You already know that aspirin is great for headaches. But it can also help people who have brain damage following a stroke, says John S. Meyer, M.D., professor of neurology at Baylor College of Medicine in Houston, who works in the cerebral blood flow laboratory of the Veterans Affairs Medical Center, also in Houston.

"If doctors put these people on anti-clotting drugs like aspirin, and you control risk factors like hypertension, smoking and cholesterol, they recover," says Dr. Meyer. "Their brain function improves."

Although more research needs to be done, some investigators believe that aspirin also has potential for protecting against Alzheimer's disease.

In a preliminary study at Johns Hopkins University in Baltimore, researchers compared the medication histories of 50 pairs of twins. In each pair, at least one of the twins had developed Alzheimer's disease. The study suggested that those who had a history of taking aspirin or other anti-inflammatory drugs had a significantly lower chance of developing Alzheimer's than those who got along without the medication. Although experts are not yet ready to give the go-ahead and say that everyone should take aspirin as an Alzheimer's prevention measure, they think this study provides a promising lead.

A Cancer Conquest

It's way too early to say for sure, but aspirin may even be able to help prevent colorectal cancer, say researchers.

In a study that compared over 1,500 people without cancer with 490 people with cancer of the colon, 340 with cancer of the rectum and 212 with precancerous growths known as polyps, researchers found that the risk of developing colorectal cancer was lower among people who frequently took aspirin.

Another study seconded these findings. In the study, 157 people who had colorectal polyps were compared with 480 people who did not. Researchers found that those who took aspirin or a similar anti-inflammatory drug once a day or more had more than a 60 percent lower risk of having polyps than those who did not take the drugs.

How aspirin works against colorectal cancer is still unclear, but researchers are optimistic about these early findings.

White Knight, Dark Knight

If you have the green light from your doctor to take this two-cent wonder pill as a supplement, remember not to overdo it. Experts generally recommend limiting the daily dosage to 81 to 160 milligrams—one-quarter to one-half of a standard 325-milligram tablet.

Although everyone tends to think of aspirin as a white knight, waging war on invaders of good health, aspirin has its dark side, too. It can cause problems with stomach irritation or ulcers, allergies and Reye's syndrome, a serious neurological condition that can occur in children who are given aspirin. It can also prolong a bout of gout, the painful episodes that some people get when deposits of uric acid build up in the joints of the big toe, ankle or knee.

Bee Power Builds Human Dynamos!

Bee Pollen and Propolis

For years, health enthusiasts have harbored a strange reverence for the beehive and its products, and headlines that hype the busy bee's regenerative power keep the rumors constantly buzzing. Honey is a staple of folklore medicine, and royal jelly—the milky substance that makes the queen bee such a prolific mom—is rumored by some to stop aging and cure cancer. (For more about royal jelly, see page 230.)

You can add two more miracle products from our buzzing friends to that list—bee pollen and propolis.

Tests of Flower Power

The next time you see a bee flitting around your flower bed, have some respect for those furry little legs as well as that nasty stinger. The dust that falls off his legs may reduce allergies—if you begin with a small dose and gradually increase your intake over time, says Dr. Haas. But there are claims that bee pollen heals other conditions as well, including but not limited to viral infections, fatigue, skin problems, premenstrual syndrome, hot flashes, headaches, heart palpitations, impotence, overweight, arthritis, stress, cancer, infertility, colon problems and prostate enlargement.

Of course, you'd need more than you could gather from that one bee, but you get the idea. Bee pollen proponents swear by supplements made from this powder, believing that it's a nutritional powerhouse—jam-packed with all the vitamins from A to K, 27 different minerals, 22 amino acids and 18 enzymes, as well as DNA and plant hormones.

But you'd have to take an awful lot of bee pollen to get significant levels of these nutrients, says Dr. Haas. And unfortunately, there is absolutely no scientific evidence that bee pollen does anything more than make good honey. At best, doctors believe that it *may* be good for allergies.

"Bee pollen has been very helpful for many people with allergies," says Michael Janson, M.D., director of the Center for Preventive Medicine in Barnstable, Massachusetts, and author of *The Vitamin Revolution in Health Care*, "although there is not enough scientific documentation to support some of the exaggerated claims."

The rationale for using pollen for allergies is the same one that people use for immunization: Take a small dose of what ails you, and your body will build up forces to reckon with it. In this case, you'd be taking allergens—that is, the actual substances that cause the allergies in many people. Doctors warn, however, that in the case of pollen, it can backfire and, in an extreme case, you may just end up with an anaphylactic reaction—a potentially life-threatening, throat-constricting allergic reaction.

"Life-threatening allergic reactions have occurred in a few patients who have taken bee pollen," says Martin Valentine, M.D., Johns Hopkins professor of medicine at the Maryland Asthma and Allergy Center in Baltimore. "I would hesitate to recommend these supplements unless research can show that they are safe for everyone."

Propolis: The Bees' Knees

Another supposed "miracle" from the hive is propolis—literally "defenses before a town"—which is the resin that bees pick up from the buds of trees and flowers. They use propolis to caulk cracks and crevices in their hives, making them almost sterile.

Propolis proponents say that this sticky stuff is not only dripping with droves of nutrients such as B vitamins, minerals and bioflavonoids but also supposedly contains a natural antibiotic called galangin that makes it an immunological wonder. Some even go so far as to call it a natural penicillin.

Unfortunately, all the buzz about propolis's miraculous powers is scientifically unsubstantiated, and doctors say that research needs to be done before they can recommend it for anything.

If you decide to try a product from the bees' knees anyway, just tread carefully, say the experts—and they remind people that an allergy to bee pollen, although rare, can be life-threatening.

Be particularly wary if you have asthma or diabetes, says Dr. Haas. People with asthma should not use bee products, because they contain allergens that can make your asthma worse. And people with diabetes should check with their doctors before taking any supplements like bee pollen or propolis that contain natural sugars.

Beer Declared the Elixir of Life!

Brewer's Yeast

Isn't that just the headline that every beer-lover would love to read?

While it's too bad that it's not true—beer's obviously no elixir—the sudsy stuff isn't all bad, either.

In fact, one of the ingredients that are used in the brewing process (although you can't get it from drinking beer) may perform a host of duties that can help to make life more pleasurable. Some studies show that brewer's yeast might help regulate blood sugar, treat some symptoms of diabetes, improve skin, put a stop to diarrhea and maybe, just maybe, repel ticks and fleas.

Brewer's yeast is made up of the pulverized yeast cells that brewers use to leaven their product. It's one of the best sources of the B-complex vitamins thiamin, riboflavin, niacin, vitamin B_6, pantothenic acid, biotin and folic acid. It also has trace minerals like chromium and selenium, plus protein.

Unfortunately, overzealous brewer's yeast boosters have credited it with everything except bringing back the dead, so it's been hard to separate truth from fiction. By the sheer virtue of its nutritional value, however, it's a good supplement, says Dr. Gerson.

Although people with diabetes should always check with a doctor before taking any supplements, studies show that brewer's yeast not only helps prevent diabetes in people who have problems processing blood sugar or who have a family history of diabetes, it also can help reduce symptoms in people who already have diabetes. Experts say that brewer's yeast probably works so well because of its high levels of chromium, a mineral that's been shown to increase glucose tolerance. Two tablespoons of the stuff packs a heaping 190 micrograms of chromium, which is more than the Daily Value of 120 micrograms.

Help for You and Fido, Too

On top of keeping your blood sugar in check, brewer's yeast offers a plethora of potential benefits for every member of your family—maybe even those with four legs and a tail, say some experts.

If strong antibiotics have you trotting to the bathroom with a case of the runs, a group of British doctors would have you reach for brewer's yeast tablets rather than an expensive diarrhea medication. They say brewer's yeast probably works by encouraging the regrowth of good bacteria in the bowel, and it may even work when medication falls flat.

Other people use the supplement to give them better skin and hair—a benefit that hasn't been proven but that many swear is real and which could work for some people, says Dr. Gerson. "It's effective in people who are deficient in B-complex vitamins, because those nutrients are good for the hair and skin," he says.

Where do Fido and Tabby fit in? Although no researcher has proven the benefits for furry friends, some animal lovers say that slipping brewer's yeast into their pets' evening chow can help keep fleas and ticks at bay.

"The research has been done, and there's absolutely no evidence that it has any effect at all," says Michael W. Dryden, D.V.M., Ph.D., assistant professor of pathology and microbiology at Kansas State University College of Veterinary Medicine in Manhattan, Kansas. "Still there are lots of people who swear that it works. So if someone says it works for their pets, I don't discourage it. The B vitamins are good for the dog!"

So should everyone start digging in?

"It's nothing magical," says Dr. Gerson. "But if people are concerned about getting these vitamins and minerals, then sure, brewer's yeast is a fine supplement."

You can buy brewer's yeast as tablets, powder or flakes. Doctors recommend not exceeding the daily dosage suggested on the label. And Dr. Haas notes that some people are allergic to yeast, so be sure to talk to your doctor if that's a concern for you. Some health food stores also carry brewer's yeast wafers made specifically for pets.

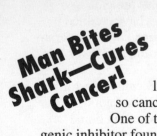

Man Bites Shark—Cures Cancer!

Cartilage

Sharks have super immune and disease-fighting systems. They rarely get cancer. And some folks believe that if we take a little of whatever makes sharks so cancer resistant, we won't get cancer either.

One of the compounds that sharks possess is the anti-angiogenic inhibitor found in the fish's cartilage. This inhibitor, which is now being hailed as the secret cancer-fighting ingredient, allegedly prevents the formation of new blood vessels in the body.

Advocates say it works like this. Tumors cannot grow without a network of blood vessels to feed them nutrients and remove their metabolic waste. Cut off this blood supply, and the tumors will shrivel and die. Although much more research needs to be done, shark cartilage advocates believe that human beings can benefit from the same chemical that halts blood vessel production and consequently, tumor growth.

Although experts don't know the name of this substance yet, William Lane, Ph.D., a biochemist, independent consultant in marine resources and co-author of *Sharks Don't Get Cancer: How Shark Cartilage Could Save Your Life*, believes that it won't be long before it's identified. Dr. Lane currently has a hand in conducting clinical trials, approved by the Food and Drug Administration (FDA), to test the effectiveness of shark cartilage against advanced prostate cancer and Kaposi's sarcoma, one of the cancers that frequently strike people with late-stage AIDS. Other FDA-approved trials on shark cartilage involve breast, colon and liver cancers. But it's hard to say when the research will prove conclusive. "If early indications of the FDA trials are positive," notes Dr. Lane, "and if the theories are true, it could be an exciting breakthrough."

"There's not much I can say at this point," says Michael M. Rothkopf, M.D., a physician in private practice in Livingston, New Jersey, who is also conducting FDA studies on shark cartilage. "We need to see how it works in people."

Dr. Rothkopf has been seeing people in the last stages of terminal cancer and conducting tests to measure tumor growth or shrinkage, pain, survival and quality of life. So far, some people have been telling him that they feel better and are more active, but there's much more work to be done, he observes.

The American Cancer Society supports FDA-approved clinical trials of alternative cancer therapies such as shark cartilage and encourages cancer patients to participate in these trials. They caution against the use of shark cartilage supplements at this time, however, and suggest you talk to your doctor first.

Taking a Bite Out of Arthritis, Psoriasis and More

If shark cartilage lives up to its promises, it may also be able to take a shark-size bite out of a few other diseases that plague millions of people, such as rheumatoid arthritis, psoriasis, fibroid tumors and sight-threatening diseases like macular degeneration and diabetic retinopathy.

"All of these conditions rely on the generation of new blood vessels to progress," says Dr. Lane. "If you stop that from happening, you'll stop these diseases."

But even though preliminary evidence suggests that shark cartilage may turn out to be tomorrow's wonder drug, only time and controlled studies will tell for sure. And in the meantime, experts warn against taking the shark cartilage that's available at your local health food store.

Dr. Lane suggests that there are more sharks on land than there are in the water. "So many of the products being sold as shark cartilage are mostly sugar or milk powder," he says. "Even if they have shark cartilage in them, the 35-pill bottles they're selling don't contain enough to do anyone much good. You need therapeutic dosages of a specially formulated product."

Plus, shark cartilage can be downright dangerous if you have certain health conditions that require you to build new blood vessels, says Dr. Rothkopf.

"People who are pregnant should *not* take shark cartilage," he warns. "You also should avoid it if you've had a recent heart attack or surgery or have flesh or skeletal wounds that are healing." He adds that shark cartilage is a good source of dietary calcium and should not be taken by anyone who already has high blood calcium levels.

The bottom line for now: Leave the shark cartilage to the sharks and the doctors who study them.

Modern-Day Superman Repels Bullets with Heart!

Coenzyme Q_{10}

To hear proponents tell it, coenzyme Q_{10}—an old supplement with a space-age name—is to a weak heart as spinach is to Popeye. Take enough of the stuff, and you'll have a strong, strapping heart muscle ready to take on the world.

This reputation has made coenzyme Q_{10} (called coQ_{10} for short) one of the top-selling supplements. But many cardiologists don't believe the claims, and a great many of them have never even heard of using it for cardiac care.

One of ten types of coQ enzymes found in the body, coQ_{10}'s primary job is helping to convert the food we eat into energy. Although our bodies make much of the coQ_{10} we need to function, we also get it from our diets, particularly by eating oily fish, whole grains or organ meats. While all experts recognize coQ_{10} as important, some researchers believe that the nutrient should be promoted to vitamin status, because we may run into serious health problems if we don't have enough of it.

That's where the debate about the role of coQ_{10} starts.

Keeping the Ticker Ticking

Despite the skepticism of many cardiologists, there's one pool of researchers who believe that coQ_{10} improves heart function by enhancing pumping action and electrical activity and lowering blood pressure. Specifically, some believe that many cases of heart failure and cardiomyopathy (disease of the heart muscle) are the direct result of a deficiency of coQ_{10} and that supplementation can both prevent and treat these ailments. These researchers point to several studies to reinforce their point.

In one Italian multicenter study, 2,664 people with heart failure were given between 50 and 150 milligrams of coQ_{10} every day for three months. Researchers found that their symptoms improved in a wide range of areas, including insomnia, enlargement of the liver, breathing trouble and heart palpitations. More than half of them improved in at least three areas.

In another study that spanned eight years, investigators at the University of Texas Medical Branch in Galveston gave 424 people with various forms of heart disease coQ_{10} supplements ranging from 75 to 600 milligrams every day, then recorded the results. They found significant improvement in heart function. Most notably, at the beginning of the study most patients were taking between one and five heart medications, but by the study's end, 43 percent of them were well enough to stop taking one, two or three of their heart drugs.

Another study by the same researchers showed that this aspiring nutrient may also be able to deflate high blood pressure. When 109 people who were taking high blood pressure medication were given an average of 225 milligrams of coQ_{10} daily, 51 percent of them came off one, two or three of their medications after about four and a half months.

Promise or Puffery?

Critics remain unconvinced, calling for better-controlled studies before they'll jump on the coQ_{10} bandwagon.

"They may be right," says Jay Cohn, M.D., a cardiologist at the University of Minnesota Medical School in Minneapolis and editor of the *Journal of Cardiac Failure*. "But we need more research. CoQ_{10} seems to have a favorable effect, but we haven't seen anything dramatic."

Dr. Cohn feels that whether or not coQ_{10} is effective in heart disease treatment and prevention will remain a mystery until scientifically controlled studies are conducted—meaning studies in which some people are given the supplement, some are given dummy pills and neither the researchers nor the participants know who is taking which.

"If those kinds of studies are done and coenzyme Q_{10} proves to be effective, then we'll all recommend it," says Dr. Cohn. Until then, he adds, there's no proof that the supplements people are getting from their health food stores will do anything but cost them money.

On the other hand, doctors who have noted the benefits of coQ_{10} see no harm in trying it, whether or not the medical establishment is skeptical. "CoQ_{10} is not a strong, toxic drug," notes Dr. Haas. "This nutrient clearly supports improved function," he says, adding that its preventive use may be better than its power to "cure" people who have heart disease. Since it's a nontoxic, possibly helpful nutrient, he sees no reason to dismiss it.

Meddling with Genes Erases Years!

DNA/RNA

Are your old nucleic acids getting a little worn around the edges? Are you ready for a new batch of DNA (deoxyribonucleic acid) and RNA (ribonucleic acid) to get you on your feet again? Some researchers maintain that "restocking" our supply of genetic coding—with DNA/RNA pills—may be just what the doctor ordered to stimulate immunity and slow aging. But the practice of

Youth in Advertising

As Robert Frost penned in his classic poem on the fleeting beauty of youth, "Nature's first green is gold, her hardest hue to hold. Her early leaf's a flower, but only so an hour . . . . Nothing gold can stay."

Well, now it seems that golden youth can spring eternal. There's a hormone called dehydroepiandosterone (or the more pronounceable DHEA) that is produced by human adrenal glands. This hormone, available on a limited basis, has been tested in studies.

In fact, DHEA became a big hit following a study in La Jolla, California, in which researchers gave 30 middle-aged to elderly people either DHEA or a dummy pill, then recorded the results.

The people who took the hormone felt better. A lot better. Researchers found that women in the study reported an 84 percent increase in their sense of well-being, which was defined by soundness of sleep, joint comfort, mobility and ability to cope. The men's sense of well-being increased 67 percent.

This study adds to the encouraging data collected by laboratory researchers. When older animals are given DHEA, results suggest that the hormone helps boost immunity and helps protect them from heart disease and cancer. They also lose weight without losing their appetite.

DHEA supporters believe that the hormone supplements work simply by replacing what's lost over time. DHEA levels peak in people at about age 25 and decline thereafter. Hence, the conclusion drawn by some researchers is that DHEA is intimately linked to aging and age-related disease.

But other experts warn that we don't know enough about this "fountain of youth" to take a dive into it. DHEA is not considered an approved drug by the Food and Drug Administration, but it is available with a prescription through some pharmacies that have a compounding license.

The odd thing, however, is that you'll also see supplements parading as DHEA at a few health food stores. That's because a substance called DHEA that comes from Mexican wild yams is sold as a kind of newfound youth serum. And it's *this* DHEA—which is different from the actual dehydroepiandosterone—that is marketed as a life-prolonging supplement.

"The real DHEA is derived from wild yams but modified in the laboratory," says Michael Janson, M.D., director of the Center for Preventive Medicine in Barnstable, Massachusetts, and author of *The Vitamin Revolution in Health Care.* "The yam supplements sold as DHEA are not converted in the body, and there is no evidence that they are effective at raising DHEA levels."

DNA/RNA supplementation has been widely panned by medical science. Since there is no proof, only speculation, to support claims for DNA/RNA, many people are simply listening to proponents in the supplement industry. Makers of supplements have been infusing everything from nutritional supplements to face creams with these life-giving molecules and marketing the nucleic acids through health food stores. Not surprisingly, they often claim miraculous results.

The bottom line from experts, however, is that we need much more research before we can justify using them in anything. Besides, if you're interested in these acids, you can get them from food sources, say experts. Just one tablespoon of brewer's yeast packs a heaping 1.5 grams of RNA. Fish, nuts, wheat germ, bran, eggs and meats are all rich sources of either DNA and RNA or precursors of these molecules that convert to nucleic acids in our bodies.

We should also pamper the genetic material we already have, say some experts. Key nutrients for keeping your genes strong and healthy include the B vitamins folic acid, vitamin B_6, pantothenic acid, riboflavin, biotin and choline. Other gene-boosters are vitamin C and the minerals zinc, magnesium, manganese, chromium and selenium.

If you're going to try supplementing your gene pool anyway, proponents suggest not exceeding 1.5 grams daily. Also, if you have a tendency to develop gout, you should see your doctor before trying any nucleic supplements. They produce excessive uric acid in the body, which may trigger a gout attack.

Enzymes

Man Eats Brick, Asks for Seconds!

We don't need to tell you that there's no pill that will let you digest brick. But for people who feel as though they've swallowed a brick after eating foods like beans or cheese, there is help. It comes in the form of two kinds of digestive enzyme supplements, one that helps ease gas problems and another that improves digestion of dairy products.

Don't Gas Up

The first of these enzymes is sold as a gas-buster named Beano. Considering beans' gaseous reputation, that's an appropriate brand name for the digestive enzyme known as alpha-galactosidase. Studies show that Beano may be able to decrease gastrointestinal disturbances like flatulence and possibly diarrhea as well.

Here's how it works: Legumes like beans and peas—and cruciferous vegetables like cauliflower and cabbage—all contain hard-to-digest sugars that are converted into the gases carbon dioxide, hydrogen and methane by bacteria inside your intestines. Eat these foods regularly, and you have three choices—explode, float away or (the only real option) get rid of the gas. Beano gives you a fourth choice—break down those sugars before they hit your gut. And that's exactly what it does.

In one study, participants tested the enzyme to the limit by downing a combustible chili made from navy, pinto and kidney beans, broccoli, cabbage, cauliflower and onions, with a side order of cornbread and water. The number of flatulence episodes in the group that used Beano was significantly lower than the number among those who ate the meal plain, without the enzymatic quencher.

Beano comes as drops or pills. If you choose the drops, add five drops to your first bite of food. You can add a few more if needed. If you have pills, just take one to three before you eat. But don't try to add the drops to foods when you cook, because high temperatures kill the active enzymes.

Although Beano is safe for most people, it alters the way you process sugar, so if you have diabetes, you should check with your doctor before taking it. You also need to get your doctor's advice on Beano if you have galactosemia, a condition that results in an adverse reaction to milk and all foods containing the enzyme galactose. Also, since Beano is made from mold, you may have an allergic reaction if you are sensitive to mold or penicillin. Doctors advise that you not use Beano if you have such allergies.

Note: If after you start using Beano, you find yourself blaming the dog because it really is the dog, you can buy digestive enzymes for Fido, too. The product is called Curtail Drops and is sold by some veterinarians.

A Way to Welcome Milk

If milk leaves you feeling as bloated as the animal it came from, you've probably switched to nondairy substitutes. But there may be another route if your system won't tolerate milk or milk products: Some experts suggest using lactase if you know you're lactose-intolerant.

The lactase enzyme, commercially available in products such as Lactaid and Dairy Ease, is what helps us digest lactose, the sugar found in milk. If our bodies aren't making enough of this enzyme—a problem shared by a whopping 70 percent of the world's population—we're considered lactose-intolerant. That's a shorthand way of saying that milk products give us digestive woes, including cramping, bloating and diarrhea.

Studies show that about 6,000 international units of lactase, which is the amount found in the recommended dosage (two tablets) of most supplements, is enough to dramatically improve the digestion of about 20 grams of lactose, the amount found in 14 ounces of milk. If you have lactose intolerance, that means that the supplement helps you tolerate the equivalent of a tall glass of milk. The best advice is to follow the directions on the box. Or you can buy milk with the lactase already added.

A Rose a Day Keeps Arthritis Away!

Evening Primrose Oil (GLA)

Some studies have given new meaning to the phrase "stop to smell the roses." Maybe, just maybe, say some researchers, you should be stopping to eat those roses as well—but only if they're evening primroses.

While all the hype around evening primrose oil may prove to be just that—hype—proponents say its benefits are as prolific as the fragrant flowers. Primrose oil is credited with fighting a slew of ailments, including arthritis, ulcerative colitis (inflammation of the colon), diabetes, psoriasis, eczema, breast pain, premenstrual syndrome, heart disease and even cancer.

Advocates also have history on their side. Native Americans used the oil from these bright yellow night bloomers for a host of problems. And the early English deemed evening primrose oil "the King's cure-all."

There just aren't enough studies to prove any of it. And some of the research on the oil suggests that too much for too long can be bad for you. But proponents agree that there is some compelling evidence for potential future use.

Chasing Inflammation Away with GLA

The secret of primrose's potential is in its seeds, which contain the oil. In that oil is a substance called gamma-linolenic acid, also known as GLA.

Once GLA gets into your system, it encourages the production of hormonelike substances called prostaglandins that help you maintain healthy blood vessels, a sound gastrointestinal tract and stable blood sugar. Another of their primary functions is fighting inflammation.

The most compelling evidence for the effectiveness of GLA has been seen in its use against the inflamed, painful joints caused by arthritis.

In one study, 37 people who had rheumatoid arthritis and inflammation of the joints (synovitis) were given either 1.4 grams of GLA or an equal amount of cottonseed oil in a dummy pill. (To increase the amount of GLA, researchers in this study used borage seed oil, with 18 to 25 percent GLA, not the more commonly known evening primrose oil, which is about 8 to 14 percent GLA.) After 24 weeks, those taking the cottonseed oil weren't any better off, but roughly 30 to 40 percent of those who received the GLA had reductions in symptoms of swollen joints and joint tenderness. Many also found that their grip improved, another signal that arthritis symptoms were diminishing.

There's just one slight problem: The dosages of GLA used in this study are much higher than any doctor would allow. Although only minor side effects such as soft stools and belching have been reported so far, scientists are concerned that high doses of GLA over the long term might produce cell-damaging molecules called free radicals, with the result that the therapy could do more harm than good.

"There's some concern that high levels of dihomogamma-linolenic acid (DGLA), which is what GLA becomes in the body, may be positively associated with a risk for heart disease," says Bruce Holub, Ph.D., professor of nutrition in the Department of Nutritional Sciences at the University of Guelph in Ontario. Until we know more, he cautions against overuse of primrose oil or any other supplement containing excessive amounts of GLA.

Skin, Stools, Sugar and Stress

Advocates of evening primrose also believe the flower's oils are good for psoriasis, ulcerative colitis, eczema, heart disease, diabetes, breast pain and cancer, among other problems and ailments.

With regard to skin irritations such as psoriasis and eczema, clinical results have been sketchy at best, says Dr. Holub. "As with most proclaimed health benefits for GLA, it's an area of controversy and inconsistent science," he says.

In a study of primrose oil's effect on ulcerative colitis, British researchers found that 43 people taking the oil had significant improvement in their stool consistency for the six months during treatment and for three months afterward. But the oil didn't relieve other colitis symptoms, such as frequent bowel movements and rectal bleeding.

Although there has been some evidence that GLA may allay the breast pain that's sometimes brought on by monthly hormonal changes, research hasn't been conclusive.

As far as heart disease, diabetes and cancer are concerned, some investigators believe that GLA may trigger reactions in the body to combat these diseases. But much, much more work needs to be done, say researchers, before they can even speculate.

For now, the word from experts is, take time to smell the roses, but leave the oil for further research. In the meantime, you can make sure your body gets a healthy dose of GLA by eating foods like fish, nuts and oils, which contain linoleic acid, a substance that converts to GLA in your body. Dr. Holub estimates that the average American consumes a healthy 17 grams of linoleic acid daily.

Woman Celebrates 131st, Credits "Good Muffins"!

Fiber Supplements

By now, everyone's heard the hype on fiber. While it won't guarantee you a slot in the centenarians' club, many of the claims about fiber's beneficial effect on conditions like high cholesterol, diabetes, constipation and even colon cancer are well-founded. Studies also offer impressive proof of fiber's ability to protect us from heart disease, fatal heart attack and overweight. In fact, it's too bad the rage for oat bran has simmered down and the fiber fad has fizzled, because people still aren't getting enough of the rough stuff, experts say.

What makes fiber so special is not what you get out of it but what it gets out of you. As fiber makes its way through your digestive tract, it doesn't break down like most foods. Instead it fills you up, slows down food absorption and speeds waste removal.

Taking Two to Tangle

There are two types of fiber that you should be concerned about getting: soluble and insoluble.

Soluble fiber does what its name implies. It soaks up water, giving foods like kidney beans a gummy quality. For people who want a natural supplement that provides this kind of fiber, oat bran is available at most health and natural food stores. And if you take a supplement containing psyllium, you get mostly soluble fiber.

Insoluble fibers, unlike the soluble kind, don't soak up water. Instead they give foods like cauliflower and popcorn their toughness. Insoluble fibers go by the names cellulose, hemicellulose and lignin.

What Fiber Does for You

If you're looking to reap all of fiber's benefits, you need to get enough of both types, say the experts. Soluble fiber zaps cholesterol by binding with cholesterol-containing acids, sweeping them out of the body with the rest of the waste. In so doing, it lowers cholesterol and helps prevent heart disease.

Soluble fiber also forms a gel in the gastrointestinal tract, which slows down the absorption of food and helps control the rise in blood sugar that people with diabetes normally have after a meal, say experts.

Although both types help protect against colon cancer, insoluble fiber plays the starring role by adding bulk to stools and flushing harmful waste out of the colon quickly, says Diane Grabowski-Nepa, R.D., chief nutritionist at the Pritikin Longevity Center in Santa Monica, California.

Both types of fiber can also reduce digestive disorders related to constipation. "If your stools are dense and moving quickly, then naturally constipation isn't a problem," says Grabowski-Nepa. But moving all of this fiber also gives you the benefit of exercising your intestines, she explains. That in turn prevents the intestinal walls from becoming weak and forming small bulges that can become inflamed—a painful condition that's called diverticulitis.

As a bonus, high-fiber foods fill you up and stay in your stomach longer, which makes it much easier for you to lose weight, says Grabowski-Nepa.

Fill 'er Up

For optimal health, the American Dietetic Association would like to see everyone get between 20 and 35 grams of fiber every day. Because most of us eat too many highly processed foods like white bread and doughnuts instead of whole-grain foods, we fall way short, getting about 11 to 12 grams.

Supplements like oat bran, wheat bran and psyllium (also sold under the brand name Metamucil) can help you get the daily measure you need, according to Grabowski-Nepa, and they give you both kinds of fiber. She notes two cautions, however: Choose a sugar-free brand whenever possible and be careful not to overuse any fiber supplement.

"No supplements are as good as eating foods," says Grabowski-Nepa. "But if you're just not getting enough fiber, they're better than nothing."

Pressed fiber pills, which are generally just crushed psyllium seeds, are not good choices, according to Grabowski-Nepa, because the dosages are usually pretty small, and the pills may not be as effective. "If you want

Go Garlic!

Doctors, researchers and herbalists have long been fascinated by the apparent healing powers of multi-cloved, pungent garlic, and research has highlighted some of garlic's beneficial properties. Among other things, garlic may help lower cholesterol levels, protecting your heart and blood vessels. Studies also suggest that it may help to lower blood pressure and dissolve blood clots.

The problem, of course, is garlic's notorious odor. While many people love garlic in any form and often use it in cooking, you might prefer to get it in deodorized supplement form. Many brands of garlic supplements are sold in health food stores and drugstores.

If you opt for capsules because you want to evade the odor, choose a carefully dried product that says "enteric-coated" on the label, advises Varro E. Tyler, Ph.D., professor of pharmacognosy at Purdue University School of Pharmacy in West Lafayette, Indiana. "This means the supplement has an acid-resistant coating that keeps the enzymes in garlic from being destroyed in the stomach. This way, the enzymes don't release the active odoriferous agent until the garlic reaches the small intestine, where the agent can be absorbed very quickly, almost without odor."

a really complete supplement, doctors recommend Metamucil as one of the best for soluble fiber," she adds. Wheat bran is an excellent source of insoluble fiber.

Fiber Cautions

If you're going to use supplements, especially the sprinkle-on kind, you'd better make like a sponge and start sucking up the water, says Grabowski-Nepa. Otherwise you may end up with exactly what you're trying to avoid—blockage.

"The fiber can have a reverse effect and create a plug in the intestinal tract," warns Grabowski-Nepa. If you add psyllium or oat bran as a supplement to your meals, you should drink eight glasses (eight ounces each) of water a day. "Make sure you have a cup of water for every two teaspoons of fiber you add to your diet," she says.

Just because fiber supplements can be helpful for adults, however, doesn't mean that you should give them to children, according to Grabowski-Nepa. While swapping fat for fiber can be an effective way to help grownups shed some weight and improve their health, experts say that there's no need to sprinkle supplements like oat bran on Junior's breakfast cereal. "Too much fiber can cause young children's intestinal tracts to act too quickly, so they lose the absorption of certain nutrients," says Grabowski-Nepa. "Children don't need added fiber. Just make sure that they eat natural foods like fruits and vegetables and have whole foods rather than processed flour products."

Whale-Eating Eskimos Live Hundreds of Years!

Fish Oil

There are a lot of fish (and fishy claims!) in the supplement sea, but when it comes to heart disease, getting more fish oil—either by eating fish or popping supplements—just might be the catch of the day. This good oil may also help alleviate a school of other ailments, including diabetes, kidney problems, arthritis and possibly cancer. Some experts say that the oil can even help make healthier babies.

But even a well-studied supplement like fish oil is subject to its share of controversy.

As you've probably heard, if you're fishing for a healthy heart, studies show that you'll benefit from omega-3 fatty acids, commonly known as fish oil. Omega-3's are a type of good-for-you polyunsaturated fats, specifically the tongue-twisting eicosapentaenoic acid (EPA) and docosahexaenoic acid (DHA), that you can get from eating fatty cold-water fish like salmon or taking a fish oil supplement. They make blood less likely to clot. And with more omega-3's in your system, your blood vessels are less likely to constrict. Fish oil also helps the body flush out blood fats called triglycerides, which can be harmful at high levels.

The benefits of fish oil? According to one study, eating just one serving of fatty fish a week can cut your risk of heart attack by 50 to 70 percent!

But other studies about fish oil tend to be contradictory. At Harvard, for instance, researchers reviewing the cases of 1,356 people—some with high blood pressure and some healthy—found that they needed much more fish oil than they could get from eating three ounces of a fatty fish like mackerel once a week. To help lower blood pressure significantly, the people in the study needed three grams, or about three ounces of mackerel, per day.

Also, some studies have found that the people helped most by fish oil supplements are those with high blood pressure, high cholesterol and hardening of the arteries (atherosclerosis). The more serious their condition, the more pronounced the results of taking fish oil. People with mild cases of high blood pressure don't seem to receive the same benefits.

"That's not to say fish oil won't help people with milder high blood pressure," says Lawrence Appel, M.D., assistant professor and medical epidemiologist at Johns Hopkins University School of Medicine in Baltimore. "People with more severe cases just have more room for improvement."

As a fish oil investigator, however, Dr. Appel doesn't endorse fish oil supplementation as a protector of cardiac health. He isn't convinced of its effectiveness or practicality.

"The practicality of someone taking six to ten fish oil capsules a day is pretty small. Plus, we don't know the long-term consequences of taking large doses of fish oil every day," he says. "Not to mention that we don't know how effective fish oil is by itself. Is it the oil, or do people who eat fish and take supplements have healthier lifestyles?"

More Head and Chest Protection

Still, the effectiveness of fish oil supplements continues to intrigue researchers. Although more work needs to be done, scientists are studying fish oil's effectiveness in making heart attacks less severe. And they're asking some other questions as well. Will fish oil reduce the rate of restenosis—the renarrowing of the heart arteries—among people who have had angioplasty? Will it alleviate angina, the chest pain caused by heart disease? Can it reduce the risk of stroke?

After observing that eating seafood seems to reduce heart attack risk in humans, researchers at the Stritch School of Medicine at Loyola University of Chicago in Maywood, Illinois, studied the effect of fish oil supplements on heart attacks in animals. They found that giving daily doses of omega-3's significantly reduced the severity of heart attack among the animals that were studied.

If fish oil can help keep heart arteries open after they've been widened by angioplasty, it will be a major benefit for people who have had the procedure. After reviewing cases of angioplasty—a procedure in which crucial arteries are expanded with surgically inserted "balloons"—researchers found that people who had been supplementing with fish oil were significantly less likely to have re-stenosis than those who did not take supplements.

Very large doses of fish oil may also wipe out angina. When researchers gave 39 people with coronary artery disease ten grams of either fish oil supplements or olive oil every day for 12 weeks, they found that those who received the fish oil had 41 percent fewer angina attacks than those who received olive oil. Plus, those taking the fish oil also needed less medication for their angina than those not receiving it.

Your heart isn't the only organ that appears to benefit from plaque-free, uncongested arteries. Your brain may, too. In a 25-year Netherlands study of 552 men, researchers found that those who ate at least three-quarters of an ounce of fish a day—a little less than a third of a can of tuna—had half as many strokes as men who ate less fish less often.

Tuna against Tumors

Aside from taking the punch out of our nation's number one killer—heart disease—fish oil supplements may help take on another public health enemy. There's some evidence that fish oil might be able to help prevent two kinds of cancer—colon and breast—according to two studies.

In one study, researchers selected people with a history of colorectal polyps (precancerous growths) to find out how they responded to supplementation with fish oil. The study showed that doses of as little as 2.5 grams of fish oil a day could prevent the abnormal cell proliferation that is associated with the risk of polyps and with colon cancer risk.

Another study focused on the omega-3's found in fish oil. Specifically, researchers investigated the effect of omega-3's on breast cancer. Their study showed that animals fed omega-3's from fish before being injected with human breast cancer cells ended up having smaller breast tumors and fewer cancer cells spread to the lungs than those who were given a placebo dose of corn oil.

Fishy Fingers

Researchers are also seeing if fish oil supplements may give people with arthritis stronger, less achy hands.

So far the results have been promising, although the number of supplements needed to produce such results is very high. In a Danish study of 51 patients with rheumatoid arthritis, researchers found that those given 3.6 grams—the amount in three to four over-the-counter 1,000-milligram capsules—of omega-3's a day had significant improvements in stiffness and joint tenderness compared with those who were not given any fish oil.

Researchers at Albany Medical College in New York seconded those findings in a study of 66 people taking nonsteroidal anti-inflammatory medication for rheumatoid arthritis. After giving them either fish oil supplements or corn oil, the investigators found that those receiving fish oil had significantly less joint pain and morning stiffness than those taking corn oil.

"Not only did researchers find that omega-3 fish oil gave people benefits on top of their normal arthritis medications, but they often did better on just the fish oil," says Dr. Holub. Again, though, the problem is the dose: "You're talking 15 to 20 over-the-counter capsules a day, and that's too much," Dr. Holub notes. "A lot of fish oil over time can cause the unhealthy LDL (low-density lipoprotein) cholesterol to rise." But according to Dr. Holub, other cardiovascular risk factors, such as high blood pressure, blood platelet stickiness and high triglycerides, may be reduced by fish oil.

Keeping Your Kidneys Afloat

Studies suggest that fortifying your diet with more fish or fish oil supplements may also help cast away kidney problems.

In one study at the Mayo Clinic in Rochester, Minnesota, scientists found that fish oil supplements slowed the steady decline of kidney function among people who have a kidney disease called IgA nephropathy. Characterized by protein and blood in the urine, high blood pressure and fluid retention, IgA nephropathy often results in kidney failure.

The researchers gave 106 people with this disease either 12 grams of fish oil or a dummy capsule of olive oil. After two years, kidney function had deteriorated significantly in only 6 percent of the people taking fish oil, compared with 33 percent of those who received the olive oil. Four years later, 10 percent of those receiving fish oil had kidney failure compared with 40 percent of those not receiving fish oil.

Another study hints that fish oil may be key in keeping diabetes—another kidney-threatening disease—at bay. Studying the eating habits and blood samples of 666 people over age 40, researchers discovered that those who ate salmon every day had a 50 percent lower chance of having glucose intolerance than those who ate fish less frequently. These findings relate to diabetes because people who have glucose intolerance have bodies that can't process sugar, a condition that often signals diabetes. Since fish oil can raise blood sugar, however, people who already have diabetes should supplement omega-3's only under a doctor's supervision.

Building Better Babies

Finally, fish oil may help pregnant women have healthier pregnancies—and babies.

According to a study of 47 women in the third trimester of pregnancy, 24 who took 2.7 grams of omega-3 fatty acids daily had lower levels of thromboxane A_2 (TxA_2). This compound is associated with pregnancy-induced high blood pressure and preeclampsia, a condition of high blood pressure and excess protein in the urine that can occur during pregnancy. With less TxA_2 in the system, researchers concluded, there was less danger of these complications. The women who did not take omega-3's had more TxA_2 than those who took the oil, the study showed.

These fish-eating benefits also seem to be passed on to the babies. In the Faeroe Islands north of the United Kingdom, investigators compared the sizes of 1,022 babies and found that the more frequently the moms ate fish while pregnant, the larger and longer their babies were. Scientists speculate that fish oil may work by increasing blood flow into the placenta, thereby upping the amount of nutrients the growing baby gets.

But doctors put in a word of caution as well. Fish oil supplements may not be appropriate during pregnancy, so consult your doctor about taking them if you're pregnant.

Also, you shouldn't take fish oil capsules if you're allergic to any kind of fish. And that means *any kind*. Manufacturers of supplements aren't required to specify on the label what kind of fish they're using.

Dr. Haas also adds that if, after consulting your doctor, you decide to use fish oil to treat a specific condition like arthritis, it's best to use fish oil supplements. Although in his opinion adding fish to your diet probably won't provide therapeutic effects, he feels that a good diet that includes fish should help you maintain overall health.

Little Japanese Fans Cure Memory Loss!

Ginkgo

One of the hottest-selling supplements in Europe is an ancient staple from Chinese medicine called ginkgo, an extract of the pretty, fan-shaped leaves of the Asian ginkgo biloba tree. Fans of these little fans say that the extract can relieve many ailments that time inflicts on us, particularly the ills caused by decreased blood flow to all parts of the body, including the brain and extremities. Among the problems that ginkgo is said to cure are short-term memory loss, vertigo (dizziness), hearing loss and the ringing in the ears known as tinnitus.

Ginkgo is believed to be effective in a concentrated extract form, not in leaf form. So drinking a tea or similar herbal concoction made from leaves probably won't give you the possible benefits of the extract. Ginkgo extract is available in the United States and is labeled as a food or dietary supplement.

Scientists warn people not to fall prey to excessive claims made by ginkgo manufacturers, particularly claims about the miracle "age-reversing" powers of their product. But they concur that ginkgo does appear to be useful for increasing cerebral blood flow in older people.

Opening Channels of Communication

How does ginkgo improve brain circulation? Its secret lies with flavonoids and terpenoids, powerful compounds with enormous ability to mop up cell-damaging free radicals.

Scientists believe that ginkgo's most important terpenoids are ginkgolides. These have potent antioxidant power, so they can prevent free radicals from damaging blood vessels in the brain. Ginkgolides also suppress a blood-clot-promoting substance in the body called platelet activating factor (PAF). By fighting PAF, ginkgo helps keep the blood pumping through your gray matter.

"I use it all the time for older people, and I've seen some significant improvements in many of them," says Dr. Janson. "However, it doesn't work for everybody and should not be considered a miracle cure, although there is scientific documentation for its value," he says.

Fanning Away Stress

In one small animal study, researchers found that ginkgo also seems to be able to counteract the decreased mental capacity that comes with stress.

In an experiment with both young and old rats—some 4 months old and some 20 months old—ginkgo supplementation suppressed the effects of stress, and the rats were better able to perform tasks that delivered food rewards. Although it worked in both the younger and the older rats, it was particularly effective in improving the reaction time and performance of the older rats.

Much more work needs to be done, researchers say. Still, they're optimistic that ginkgo may be able to counteract the effects of stressful events, such as the death of a loved one or a divorce, in people's lives.

Supplementation with ginkgo is generally safe, according to Dr. Haas, although some people have reported experiencing restlessness or digestive upset while taking the herb. Also, since ginkgo affects blood clotting (because it suppresses PAF), be sure to check with your doctor if you're currently taking aspirin or another anti-clotting drug or if you have a clotting disorder.

Inositol

Wonder Drug Lowers Cholesterol, Makes Great Hair!

Sandwiched somewhere between choline and riboflavin, you'll find inositol on the ingredient label of many multivitamin supplements. You can also buy inositol by itself in supplement form. Some say it will lower cholesterol. Others say it will give you good hair or a thinner figure. Actually, it's just another supplement that may do some people good, but of which most of us get enough from our daily diets.

Inositol, which is part of the B-vitamin complex, is found in so many plants and animals that most of us get about a gram a day without even thinking about it, says Dr. Holub. "Plus, our kidneys make about four grams every day," he says.

Inositol stays busy in the body keeping membranes healthy, helping to produce substances like prostaglandins and shuttling fat from place to place. Experts say it's particularly good for bone marrow, eye tissue and the intestines. It may also contribute to healthy hair growth. Although studies have shown that inositol may help lower triglycerides, its effects on the blood are minimal, says Dr. Holub.

Some studies indicate that inositol supplementation may be a promising treatment for mental health conditions like panic disorder and depression, but again, more research is needed.

Babies and Diabetes

The two groups of people who probably benefit most from inositol supplementation are babies born prematurely and people with diabetes, although neither pregnant women nor anyone with diabetes should take supplements without a doctor's supervision.

Babies need inositol, and Mother Nature enabled human moms to supply it, says Dr. Holub. Mother's milk contains 100 to 200 milligrams of inositol per quart, he says. But mothers who are bottle-feeding their babies should check with their doctors about the inositol count in the formula they use, says Dr. Holub, as not all formula brands are created equal.

If you have diabetes, you may have a legitimate reason to supplement inositol, say experts. People with diabetes tend to have low levels of inositol in their nerve tissue, and some researchers believe that inositol supplementation can lessen the symptoms of diabetic neuropathy, a common complication that causes the hands and feet to tingle and turn numb, as if they'd fallen asleep.

Coffee Concerns

While experts see no reason for healthy adults to supplement inositol, you should be aware that too many cups of coffee can cause your inositol levels to dip. If you can't give up your daily jolts of java, experts advise eating more inositol-packed foods like cantaloupe, whole grains and citrus fruits (except lemons).

If you think you might benefit from taking inositol, talk to your doctor and follow his recommendation for supplementation. And be aware that doses as high as two grams may cause diarrhea.

"Good Germ" Stops Attack of Marauding Yeast Infection!

Lactobacillus acidophilus

Like so many nutritional supplements, acidophilus gets a lot of hype. It's also enormously popular. A survey by *Whole Foods*, a magazine for natural food retailers, found that between 33 and 40 percent of natural food store customers bought acidophilus supplements each year during a three-year test period.

That may be because this is one supplement that seems to live up to its hype. Acidophilus—better known as the friendly type of bacteria that is found in yogurt—has been found to not only prevent yeast infections but also to boost immunity, stop diarrhea associated with antibiotic use and help people digest milk products. It may even help fight gastrointestinal cancer.

Lactobacillus acidophilus (its full name) occurs naturally in our bodies, and we also get it from dairy products like milk and yogurt, as long as they contain live or active cultures (which should be specified on the label). Sometimes, however, the number of good bacteria in our bodies falls, and the bad bacteria start taking over. That's especially common when people take long courses of antibiotics, which are good for wiping out bad bugs but also kill the good ones.

A Yeast Squelcher

Acidophilus can also replace diamonds as a woman's best friend if she's prone to itchy, burning yeast infections.

In a study on the yogurt-yeast connection, researchers gave yogurt with acidophilus to 13 infection-prone women every day for six months. Subsequently, the women had no yogurt for the next six months. Researchers found that the women fared far better with yogurt than without it. The group reported only 4 yeast infections during their yogurt-eating period, compared to a whopping 32 infections during the period when they weren't eating yogurt.

Because *L. acidophilus* stimulates the production of disease-fighting cells and helps keep the digestive tract so healthy, it may even prevent gastrointestinal cancer, says Georges Halpern, M.D., Ph.D., adjunct professor of medicine in the Department of Internal Medicine at the University of California, Davis. "More research is needed, but it definitely looks like it should help," he says.

Sounds good, right? But should you run out and buy acidophilus supplements if you're healthy?

"Generally, you can get enough acidophilus in your diet just by eating yogurt with live cultures," says Dr. Janson. "But if you're taking antibiotics or hormone therapy or have trouble with yeast infections, you may benefit from supplements."

Wanted: Dead or Alive

Scientists have traditionally thought that acidophilus cultures were like mob informants: They can't do anyone any good if they're dead. More recently, however, there's been a change of thought.

"Studies have found that if you take between 5 and 20 billion 'killed' acidophilus a day, you can prevent the adhesion of a number of disease-causing bacteria to your intestinal tract," says Dr. Halpern. "So killed acidophilus may be as useful as yogurt."

So you may be getting some benefits whether you're taking acidophilus powder supplements from your local health food store or eating yogurt with live *L. acidophilus* cultures. If you're unsure whether your brand contains these critters, check the label.

If acidophilus in all forms is good for you, that could put a seal of approval on frozen yogurt. While freezing itself doesn't affect the bacteria, in some cases the cultures are killed during the pasteurization process before the yogurt is frozen. But because of the growing consumer interest in "active cultures," some companies now add them after pasteurization. The only way to be sure you're getting acidophilus benefits from frozen yogurt is to contact the maker and ask.

Make Friends with Milk

If you're someone who loves ice cream, cheese and milk, but you suffer from bloating, gas and diarrhea when you eat them, acidophilus can help you enjoy these tasty treats again.

Lactose intolerance is what happens when your body doesn't have enough of the enzyme lactase, which is needed to break down the lactose, or sugar, in dairy foods. (For more on lactose intolerance, see "when Milk's No Natural" on page 312.) Acidophilus comes to the rescue by breaking down the lactose before it can get to your gut.

To get on better terms with dairy, experts say you can buy acidophilus in powder form and sprinkle it in your regular milk or take an acidophilus supplement. Some health food stores also carry flavored drinks that contain acidophilus.

Lecithin (Choline)

If you can remember the name of a granule supplement called lecithin, researchers say that you may also be able to remember lots of other little things that we all tend to forget, like where your car keys are and the name of the new co-worker you met five minutes ago.

In a small, unpublished but hope-inspiring study, researchers gave 117 people the equivalent of two tablespoons of lecithin a day for three weeks. The people in the study began showing significant improvement in their ability to remember names and retrieve misplaced items. Although the largest gains were made by the younger members of the group—ages 35 to 50—folks who were 65 to 80 also showed significant improvement.

Another study showed similar results. Researchers found that when they gave 41 healthy people ages 50 through 80 two tablespoons of lecithin a day for five weeks, those people had fewer memory lapses (like misplacing things) than people who were receiving a fake powder. In fact, the people receiving lecithin dropped from 35 memory lapses a week to just 19 while taking the supplement.

The secret ingredient hidden in lecithin is phosphotidylcholine, commonly called choline. It's actually a building block for another chemical in your brain called acetylcholine, which transmits messages from one nerve cell to another. Our bodies make some choline. We also get some in our morning oatmeal, and we get a bite of it when we eat soybeans, kale, cabbage, egg yolks or peanuts. But scientists suspect that some of us aren't getting enough or that we may need more. They're quick to warn, however, that they don't know exactly who needs it and how much, or if too much is harmful. So talk to your doctor before taking lecithin.

Experts don't generally recommend taking pure choline supplements. The pure form breaks down in your intestines to form a fishy-smelling chemical that works its way through your system and gives new meaning to the term *morning breath*.

If you're troubled by frequent bouts of forgetfulness—most of us do misplace car keys and forget names in our hectic everyday lives—you may want to think about taking lecithin, suggests Dr. Haas. The supplement is available in liquid, granule and capsule form without a prescription at most pharmacies and natural food stores. The FDA has found that, while there are no guarantees that lecithin will help you remember anything, supplements in the range of 13.5 grams or two tablespoons a day are safe.

Gathering Globs of Cholesterol

As an emulsifying agent, lecithin is used in chocolate bars to keep the fat from separating. While that doesn't give you license to go on a Godiva binge for the sake of getting your choline, this fat-gluing action seems to help lower both cholesterol and blood pressure in people taking lecithin supplements, say researchers.

"I don't advocate that everyone start mixing lecithin into their orange juice in the morning, but there is evidence that choline causes cholesterol to emulsify," says Dr. Janson. "This may help reduce the negative effect of high cholesterol," he adds. In other words, once the cholesterol is gathered up, the body can flush it before it sticks to the artery walls.

85-Year-Old Woman "De-ages," Attends Prom!

Melatonin

Dracula, Ponce de León and practically every man and woman over the age of 45 have one thing in common—the quest for eternal youth.

As yet, nobody's found a way to achieve it, so the chances of grannies getting a second shot at their proms are still as slim as a prom-dress shoulder strap. There is a possibility, however, that melatonin gives all of us a crack at being not so old—at least by conventional standards.

Some researchers believe that they've found the "clock" in our bodies that causes aging and also a way to grab the hands of that clock and turn them back.

The key, they say, is a nocturnal hormone called melatonin. It's produced in the brain by the pea-size pineal gland, which works zealously when we're young children but is already slowing down by the time we reach our teens. By age 45, we're producing only half the amount of melatonin that we did as children. By 80, we're producing half of that. The result? Age-related physical decline, say the researchers.

Cells and Missiles

Every breath we take generates a veritable onslaught of highly reactive molecules called free radicals that home in on our healthy cells like heat-seeking missiles, wreaking havoc on our membranes and damaging our DNA. This process, known as oxidation, is blamed for lots of diseases, including cancer and heart disease.

Our body fights this constant oxidation onslaught with the compounds commonly known as antioxidants, such as vitamins C and E and beta-carotene. And now some researchers believe that melatonin is the Sherman tank of antioxidants, because while most antioxidants are limited to protecting just certain cells in certain parts of the body, melatonin can go anywhere, says Russell Reiter, D.Med., Ph.D., professor of neuroendocrinology at the University of Texas Health Science Center in San Antonio. "At the correct levels, it can even help stave off the damaging effects of radiation," says Dr. Reiter.

To study its cell-protecting effects, Dr. Reiter and his colleagues took one blood sample from a group of people during the day, when melatonin levels were naturally low, then gave them melatonin. The researchers took another sample two hours later, when the blood levels were high again. They isolated the white blood cells in both samples and zapped them with radiation. The high-melatonin samples had 66 percent less damage than those without melatonin.

"It acts like an internal lead apron," says Dr. Reiter. Doctors may someday recommend it as a preventive measure before getting an x-ray or mammogram, but more studies must be done to determine what might be an appropriate dose.

Dr. Reiter also has tested melatonin protection against cancer-causing herbicides and chemicals in rats and has found consistent protection against DNA damage.

Although more research needs to be done, the potential benefits of melatonin are sweeping, says Dr. Reiter. "Nothing is going to make a 70-year-old person 45 again, but the implication is that if you can keep up your natural defenses, like those provided by melatonin, you can possibly slow down physical degeneration and some of the diseases we associate with it, like cancer."

Rock-a-Bye Melatonin

One thing scientists will say with confidence right now is that melatonin—often called the hormone of darkness—will probably replace sleeping pills and sheep as safe, effective treatment for sleep problems. "It may not work for everyone, though; probably just for people who have dysfunctional biorhythms," says Dr. Haas.

Melatonin's primary job is keeping your circadian rhythms in sync with your environment. When the sun goes down and we hit the sheets, our melatonin levels rise, lulling us into slumber. When the sun peeks through the curtains, they dip, waking us to a new day. If we're not making enough of this soporific hormone, we may end up with poor sleep or insomnia.

Since our melatonin levels drop as our age climbs, by the time we reach our golden years, the supply is pretty short. Scientists think this is why so many elderly people are plagued by sleepless nights.

In one study, a group of elderly people with insomnia were able to fall asleep and sleep soundly through the night when given as little as one or two milligrams of melatonin two hours before bedtime. When they stopped taking melatonin, their sleep deteriorated.

Melatonin also has been used successfully for children who have sleep problems because of neurological disorders like attention deficit disorder, mental retardation and autism. And it has proven to be a successful sleep-inducing treatment for people who are blind. It may also help reset your body clock. Here's how.

Why Geese Don't Go East

If you're a frequent traveler, you know the trauma of crossing time zones. Your body might be in Toledo, but your head's still in Los Angeles.

A pinch of melatonin can help you "catch up," say experts.

"Melatonin is very good for jet lag," says Dr. Reiter, "because it can readjust your internal body clock."

Say you're flying from San Diego to Boston. It may be midnight when you arrive on the East Coast, but your body, still thinking it's only nine o'clock, would rather stay up with Letterman than get some shuteye. One to three milligrams of melatonin can speed up your acclimation and help you get to sleep, suggests Dr. Haas. "Clearly, using melatonin for jet lag and re-setting the body clock is its best use," he says.

Couldn't Hurt a Mouse

Because melatonin is not technically a drug, it isn't subject to strict FDA regulation. In fact, you can buy melatonin at your health food store—a level of convenience that makes some people nervous.

"We definitely need to find out more about it," concedes Dr. Reiter, "like how safe it is to take while pregnant." But so far, he's very impressed with its safety record.

"I've had researchers tell me that this is the least toxic molecule they've seen. Scientists haven't been able to come up with a dosage lethal enough to make a mouse sick, let alone kill one."

If you consider yourself a candidate for melatonin, it's best to check with your doctor, and small doses are sufficient, say the experts.

"If you have trouble sleeping, a milligram or less at bedtime is all you need," says Dr. Reiter. Dr. Haas points out that up to three milligrams is safe and may be needed to get some of the desired effects. Since melatonin appears to be safe, you can easily try it for a week with your doctor's approval, and if you get some benefits, continue to use it, says Dr. Haas.

140-Year-Old Yogi Reveals, "It's the Mushrooms!"

Mushroom Extracts

Talk about a charmed reputation. They were the food of spiritual enlightenment for American Indians. The way to psychedelia for 1960s flower children. Plants of immortality in Asian countries. And great umbrella-shaped homes for pixies and gnomes throughout the ages.

They're mushrooms. And Americans, believing that they may have the power to lower cholesterol, normalize blood pressure, treat arthritis, shrink tumors and even fight AIDS, are embracing them not just as tasty treats but also as nutritional supplements.

But hey, we all know the rule: If things sound too good to be true, they usually are. So you probably won't be surprised to learn that mushrooms won't make you immortal. Studies show, however, that there are compounds in some mushrooms that may be able to fight disease and boost immunity.

Super Shiitakes

One of the best-known medicinal mushrooms is the shiitake. It's widely used in Japan as a stimulant, liver tonic and stroke preventive. Over the years, Japanese researchers have demonstrated that the shiitake can help reduce cholesterol and blood pressure and suppress the growth of HIV (the virus that causes AIDS) and tumors.

Unfortunately, the mushroom is not well-studied in the United States, although Western scientists do recognize a potential healing component in shiitakes that seems to have definite disease-fighting power. It's called lentinan.

Lentinan stimulates the immune system, including the production of antibodies, white blood cells and an immune system chemical called interferon. This chemical has battled it out with tumors in laboratory mice. Lentinan has been shown to inhibit the growth of tumors in these animals, and in some cases it halts metastasis (the bodywide spread of cancer) and extends life.

In other studies, shiitake extracts have flexed their muscles against viruses, including HIV and the herpes simplex type 1 virus, which causes cold sores.

Unfortunately, no one is sure if eating the mushrooms or even taking mushroom extract supplements will do any good. When scientists test shiitake extract, they administer it intravenously, and researchers have found oral supplements less effective.

"You have to be very careful with mushroom supplements," warns Kenneth Jones, author of *Shiitake: The Healing Mushroom.* "So many of these companies are selling such minuscule amounts of the extract, it's practically a placebo."

Fungi Kung Fu against Cancer

The reishi and maitake mushrooms are two other fungi for which researchers are cheering in their fight against cancer and viruses.

Like the shiitake, reishi extract—known as *G. lucidum*—has shown immune-enhancing ability and may curb the growth of tumors, according to proponents. They also believe that reishis can help to fight a host of ailments, including high blood pressure, allergies, asthma, fatigue, arthritis, high cholesterol, dizziness, liver problems and congestion.

The maitake mushroom—known as the dancing mushroom in Japan—has made headlines here and abroad for battling tumors. It's also won publicity for its prowess against HIV.

In laboratory studies, an extract from the maitake called glucan was able to prevent HIV from killing T-cells, which are crucial immune system cells. Unfortunately, the processing system used to create the extract compound made it toxic, so no further studies were conducted.

"Although some clinical studies are being done on the effectiveness of these mushrooms against various diseases, there just isn't a lot of money for

Jetson-Style Dining? Not Yet!

Remember the sumptuous meals the Jetson clan used to dine on? A handful of multicolored pills. Breakfast, lunch, dinner and snacks, down the hatch. We laughed then. But as we pile up vitamins, minerals, phytochemicals, amino acids, fiber and the rest, you have to wonder if we're not coming ever closer to joining the ranks of George, Jane, Judy and Elroy Jetson.

"We're not even close," assures James Heffley, Ph.D., a biochemist and nutrition adviser in Austin, Texas. "We're just now at the point where we can say that we know there are additional substances in foods besides nutrients that are beneficial. And it's almost a certainty that we don't know all the things that are good for us. It wasn't that long ago that we assumed that only the omega-6 fatty acids were essential and didn't consider omega-3 fatty acids in foods to be important."

Although Dr. Heffley believes that supplements can improve our health, he says that relying on supplements to prop up a lousy diet is a mistake. And it's extremely important and always best to try to get your nutrients from foods, adds Elson Haas, M.D., medical director of the Preventive Medical Center of Marin in San Rafael, California, and author of *Staying Healthy with Nutrition*.

herbal research," says Jones. "Researchers are probably years from knowing clinically how effective these substances really are."

Kombucha: The Mushroom That Isn't

Body builders, Asian medicine enthusiasts and miracle seekers are all sipping tea and singing the praises of a marvelous "mushroom" that isn't a mushroom at all—kombucha.

Known as the tea mushroom, kombucha is actually a mixture of bacteria and yeasts that is fermented in a black ciderlike tea for eight to ten days. The kombucha fungus forms as a floating, lily-pad-like disc on the top of the liquid, which is then strained for drinking. Although this fungal beverage is more like a tea than a supplement, most people who drink it do so not for the taste but for what they believe are the health benefits.

Kombucha advocates say that this fungal fluid, which you brew at home, is great for everything—gout, low energy, wrinkles, rheumatism, hardening of the arteries, high blood pressure, flatulence, cellulite, overweight, acne, premenstrual syndrome, constipation, irritability and low sex drive. It even helps prevent memory loss, proponents say. And if you can't remember that whole list—well, maybe you need some kombucha.

Experts sincerely doubt it.

In his book *Medicinal Mushrooms*, licensed acupuncturist and herbalist Christopher Hobbs, L.Ac., explains that while kombucha is likely to have some health benefits, there are no studies to support these claims.

Kombucha's detractors, skeptical of the craze, say that airborne molds and other contaminants that can form along with kombucha may pose serious health threats. Two cases of severe acidosis—a condition of high acid in the blood and body tissues—have been reported in recent years. Both occurred after people drank kombucha tea, and one woman died.

Although authorities haven't established a direct cause-and-effect relationship between the death and the remedy, they caution that you should talk to a doctor before trying the tea, especially if you're pregnant.

New Pills Slaughter Germs! We Can Live Forever!

Phytochemicals

Just when you thought you had your health bases covered with your morning multivitamin, along come some new nutrients on the block, disturbing your peace of mind as advocates brag loudly about their amazing powers.

This new group of nutrition dynamos, called phytochemicals—literally, chemicals from plants—won't let you live disease-free forever. But they may provide the strongest natural protection against our most feared foes, including cancer, high cholesterol, heart disease, arthritis and diabetes.

Phytochemicals—called phytonutrients or phytomins by some—are proof positive that your mom was right: Vegetables are good for you. Really good for you. Broccoli, cabbage, spinach and most of the veggie and fruit families contain thousands of compounds that help the plants fight off bacteria, insects, viruses, fungi, ultraviolet light and other natural enemies. And when you eat these compounds, you get protection, too.

Eager for profits, marketers have already bottled a few key compounds from vegetables like broccoli, spinach and carrots, and they use the catchy-sounding "phytomin" label to sell them. But while these tablets may end up being good for you, it's still too early to tell. Besides, there are literally thousands of phytomins that come from dozens of vegetables, so if you want optimal phytomin benefits, you're best off eating a large variety of vegetables and fruits. Eat them every day, at least five times a day, experts recommend.

But even though the best packaging is nature's, you'll also find phytochemical supplements at health food stores. Here's what you should know about them.

The Fabulous Flavonoids

We've all heard that an apple a day keeps the doctor away. According to research, you should add onions, broccoli and cranberries to that list, as well as other foods rich in tiny color crystals. Those crystals are the visible evidence of bioflavonoids or flavonoids that give fruits and vegetables their

The Top Ten Phytofoods

Whether or not you decide to supplement your diet with vitamins, minerals or "broccoli-in-a-bottle" pills, you should always be sure to eat foods that are packed with healthy substances, especially what are called phytochemicals or phytomins— protective, disease-fighting compounds found in fruits and vegetables. The following, suggests Elson Haas, M.D., medical director of the Preventive Medical Center of Marin in San Rafael, California, and author of *Staying Healthy with Nutrition*, are the top ten phytofoods to include in your diet.

1. Broccoli
2. Soy
3. Garlic (crushed or sliced to release phytochemicals)
4. Onions
5. Tomatoes
6. Citrus fruits (especially the white pulpy parts)
7. Cabbage
8. Cantaloupe or watermelon
9. Beans
10. Tea (green or black)

lovely yellow, red or blue hues. Flavonoids also pack a powerful protective punch, strengthening capillaries, improving immunity, reducing inflammation and maybe even fighting cancer.

We have the French to thank for much of the revealing research that's been done on these compounds. After studying the diets and lifestyles of the originators of the luxuriously buttery croissant, scientists found an inconsistency more annoying to health-conscious Americans than Pepe LePew is to Bugs Bunny. It seems that even though the French eat lots more butter and lard, have higher cholesterol and smoke just as much as Americans, residents of the United States have a heart disease rate that's 2.5 times higher than that of the French.

The secret behind this French Paradox turns out to be the Gallic penchant for fresh vegetables, fruits and red wine—all of which contain flavonoids. Experts say that these flavonoids prevent the millions of tiny discs in our blood called platelets from sticking together. Sticky platelets are the main cause of blood clots and consequently of heart attacks. So the anti-sticking campaign of flavonoids is a big boon to arterial health.

Testing flavonoids' power to protect our tickers, researchers studied the eating patterns of 805 men ages 65 to 84. They found that those who got the most flavonoids—specifically from tea, onions and apples—were less likely to die from a heart attack than those who consumed less. The more flavonoids the men got, the lower their risk. Those who got the most had the equivalent of four cups of tea, an apple and one-eighth of a cup of onions a day.

These findings were upheld by a larger study that looked at flavonoid intake across seven countries. Investigators found that the more flavonoids people ate, regardless of their culture, the less likely they were to die from heart attacks.

Flavonoids also keep your arteries free and clear, say researchers. Essentially, they just use their antioxidant powers to prevent "bad" LDL cholesterol from oxidizing, and if cholesterol doesn't oxidize, it doesn't adhere to artery walls.

In the wine rack, flavonoids enter the picture in the form of quercetin. This antioxidant, found in all red wine, is as active as the well-known antioxidant vitamin E, and perhaps even more so, says long-time flavonoid researcher Elliot Middleton, Jr., M.D., professor of medicine and pediatrics at the State University of New York at Buffalo.

Flavonoids also activate enzymes that actually neutralize cancer-causing substances, say experts. In particular, the flavonoids found in crciferous vegetables like broccoli and cabbage are so effective that researchers at Fox-Chase Cancer Center in Philadelphia studied the effects of supplements on people with a high risk for colorectal cancer. The study participants took two 500-milligram tablets of dehydrated broccoli three times a day for a year. Although the effects weren't dramatic enough to warrant starting your own broccoli dehydrating business, preliminary results indicate that they did have a protective effect, says Christine Szarka, M.D., medical oncologist at Fox-Chase.

Researchers can foresee a day when people will be using flavonoid supplements to prevent disease, but in the meantime they don't think enough evidence has accumulated. Plus, there are more than 4,000 flavonoids. Researchers still don't know if the ones they've isolated and used in supplements work as well separately as they do when they're combined with the others, says Dr. Middleton.

"Flavonoids affect lots of life processes—the immune system, cancer, atherogenesis (hardening of the arteries) and maybe even aging," says Dr. Middleton. "But they're not mainstream yet, and things have to be mainstream before studies are funded."

Meanwhile, the produce section of your supermarket is well-stocked with flavonoid-rich foods. The best are onions, kale, green beans, broccoli, endive, celery and cranberries. You'll also get a fair amount from tomatoes, sweet red peppers, apples, green and black tea and grape juice.

And, oh, yes, they're also in wine.

The Courageous Carotenoids

If you're into vitamins at all, chances are you've taken beta-carotene. Known as the compound that puts the color in cantaloupe and carrots, beta-carotene—the most abundant carotenoid in foods—has enjoyed immense popularity and remains one of the best-selling supplements.

Scientists have discovered, however, that while beta-carotene is still the king of the carotenoids, there are others that flex a considerable amount of antioxidant muscle. Many deserve credit for scooping up cell-damaging free radicals. In fact, some of the other carotenoids may be even better than beta-carotene when it comes to fighting certain cancers.

Of the more than 600 carotenoids in existence, scientists are investigating lycopene, found primarily in tomatoes, and lutein, found with beta-carotene in vegetables such as spinach and kale. They're also looking at canthaxanthin, which is found in certain mushrooms. Studies so far show some promise of cancer-fighting potential.

In the case of lycopene, there could be an interesting spin on *Attack of the Killer Tomatoes*. Investigators researching the power of the tomato's potent flavonoid have found that tomatocs seem to have cancer-killing abilities. In fact, it's been shown that people in northern Italy who eat seven or more servings of raw tomatoes every week have a 60 percent lower chance of developing colon, rectal and stomach cancer than those who eat only two servings or less. You can find this powerful carotenoid in supplements labeled "tomato extract with lycopene." Dr. Haas notes that taking these supplements may be just as effective as eating tomatoes as long as lycopene is the main active ingredient. Check the label to be sure. If other active ingredients are listed, you may lose the protective effect.

Queen Stays Wrinkle-Free with Royal Jelly!

Royal Jelly

If you were to listen to the advertising, you'd believe that a thick, milky substance known as royal jelly can turn anyone into the highness of the hive, transforming every plain-Jane drone into a luminous, radiant queen bee.

You'd also believe that this substance can reverse aging, lower cholesterol and triglycerides, alleviate rheumatoid arthritis, beat chronic fatigue, help emotional disorders, treat bronchial asthma, stomach ulcers, liver disease and kidney problems and even prevent cancer!

As you've probably guessed, the vast majority of these claims are unsubstantiated. And even those that have some substantiation are pretty shaky. What researchers know for sure is that royal jelly is a good source of B vitamins, especially pantothenic acid. And maybe, just maybe, it helps soothe the joint pain and other symptoms caused by rheumatoid arthritis. But experts warn that we're a long way from knowing that yet.

Straight from the Bee's Mouth

If you're wondering where this majestic jam comes from, the answer is straight from the honeybee's mouth. Or more specifically, its pharyngeal glands, which are found in the throat.

Honeybees feed royal jelly to their queen bee larvae. It's this substance that turns the queen bee into the impressive specimen she is—much bigger than other bees and able to lay several hundred thousand eggs each year.

Although it may sound as if royal jelly must contain some magical ingredient, it's really just a concoction of common nutrients—mostly protein.

Because of its high protein content, some supporters believe that smearing royal jelly on your skin as well as ingesting it can dramatically delay aging. They also think that it provides the skin with the amino acid that forms collagen, the "scaffolding" that holds the skin firmly in place.

But "there's really no evidence that royal jelly works for any of these things," says Dr. Gerson. "It may have some nutrients that are good for your skin. But there are no miracle age-reversers. And you have to be suspicious of anything that says it cures everything."

Aches Away?

Because royal jelly also contains the B vitamin pantothenic acid, many people tout it as a cure for the aching, inflamed joints of arthritis, says Won O. Song, R.D., Ph.D., assistant professor at Michigan State University in East Lansing, who has been studying pantothenic acid for more than ten years.

"Royal jelly is a very good source of pantothenic acid," says Dr. Song, "and people with rheumatoid arthritis have low levels of pantothenic acid in their blood serum. That doesn't mean that you can just give people pantothenic acid or royal jelly and their arthritis will go away, as some people say. It doesn't work that simply."

Because royal jelly also contains inositol, a nutrient that helps keep membranes healthy and may reduce triglycerides, other people claim that it can lower your cholesterol.

Scientists are very skeptical.

"We've found that while inositol can reduce triglycerides, it doesn't reduce blood cholesterol," says Dr. Holub. "Besides, it's very doubtful that there is enough inositol in royal jelly to make any difference."

Not for Everyone

If you're still tempted to try royal jelly, consider some health factors before you do. Although it is nutritious and nonthreatening to most people, for anyone with asthma or allergies, royal jelly can be harmful.

Deaths are rare, but taking royal jelly can be fatal, doctors say. Australian researchers have reported several cases of anaphylactic reactions—allergic responses that restrict breathing—caused by royal jelly. An 11-year-old girl and a 34-year-old woman, both with a history of asthma, died. Dr. Haas notes that he has also seen cases of reactions to royal jelly, although they were mostly mild to moderate in nature.

Researchers speculate that the attacks are triggered by one of the proteins in royal jelly and strongly caution people with a history of asthma against its use.

Spirulina

Fish Food Discovered! Manna from Heaven!

The 1970s sure were an interesting decade. John Travolta strutted his way through *Saturday Night Fever*. We embraced "tube tops." Roller disco became a bona fide craze. And we heard about the emergence of a strange blue-green plankton that some zealous scientists declared "manna from heaven"— literally, divinely supplied spiritual nourishment.

That plankton was spirulina, a type of blue-green algae growing in lakes in Mexico and Africa that had long been used as a dietary staple by the Aztec Indians and some African tribes. Health enthusiasts in the United States embraced it as "the most nutritious food on the planet" during the late 1970s and early 1980s. They believed it could detoxify the blood, cleanse the intestines, increase vitality, improve absorption of other nutrients and help us attain higher intelligence. One researcher even proposed the idea of starting an "algae bank" to squirrel away this ultimate survival food should our nation's economy crash.

Obviously, the Spirulina Savings and Loan never got off the ground. But this once-super seaweed remains very popular, especially among vegetarians, who use it as a source of protein, iron and vitamin B_{12}—nutrients commonly found in animal products. Some studies also hint that it may increase immunity. At the very least, it definitely is good for you.

Brimming with Vitamins and Minerals

Spirulina may have one of the highest nutrient concentrations of any food in the world, concedes Dr. Gerson. "If you're deficient in some nutrients, it'll definitely make you feel better," he says. Other experts agree. "It's a really great nutrient," says Dr. Haas. "We use it at our house!"

Research shows that they're right. Fishy smell notwithstanding, spirulina is a nutritional powerhouse. Besides being 60 to 70 percent protein, spirulina contains large quantities of beta-carotene. And nutritional researchers say it's the richest nonanimal source of vitamin B_{12}, providing more than 0.25 milligram of the nutrient per 100 grams of dried spirulina. That's about 40 times the Daily Value for B_{12}, which is 6 micrograms.

Spirulina is also a good source of iron and gamma-linolenic acid (GLA), an oil that turns into prostaglandins in your body. The benefit of prostaglandins is that they help keep your blood vessels, gastrointestinal tract and blood sugar healthy and stable.

Spiraling Claims

Because spirulina is so nutritious, some researchers believe that it can boost immunity. In one study, Japanese investigators found that mice that were fed spirulina had more antibody-producing cells than those deprived of it. And in a study from India, pregnant rats that were fed spirulina gave birth to more pups in one litter than pregnant rats that didn't eat spirulina.

There has been precious little medical research on spirulina, so whether it does for people what it seems to do for mice and rats is still unknown. "Spirulina, among many other green food sources, including other algae, has nutritional value. But once again, claims for it are exaggerated," adds Dr. Janson. And he notes that there has also been some controversy concerning contamination problems in the production of some algae.

Expressing the same concerns about contamination, researchers at the United Nations Industrial Development Organization sponsored toxicity studies on rats and mice in 1980. They found that spirulina is safe for human consumption.

So far, researchers have concluded that while they know the nutritional benefits of spirulina, they still don't know what benefits it provides above and beyond those of a healthy, well-balanced diet. Most experts don't think it's worth the money. But if you want to try it, you can look for spray-dried spirulina to add to rice and other dishes. Since it's difficult to find the spray-dried form, however, you may want to skip the deep-sea smell and buy spirulina capsules.

Glamorous Grain Reverses Every Known Problem!

Wheat Germ

It's an oldie but a goodie. Wheat germ won't make blind men see or restore mobility to people who use wheelchairs, but it sure is a heart-healthy source of vitamin E.

Wheat germ is the heart of the wheat berry, and like wheat bran, it is removed during the production of white flour. But the wheat germ is where much of the flavor and nutrition are. Crumbly in texture and nutty in flavor, a quarter-cup of the golden stuff packs 40 percent of the Daily Value for vitamin E—a high-scoring antioxidant that "captures" the free radicals that speed up cell aging and has earned many a gold star for preventing heart disease. Although wheat germ is technically a food, most people who sprinkle it on their cereal in the morning are doing it to supplement their diets, not simply to add flavor.

Initial research has suggested that wheat germ may have the power to lower artery-clogging cholesterol as well triglycerides, which are dangerous in high amounts.

People who were included in one study showed a 7.2 percent decline in cholesterol after just 14 weeks of eating raw wheat germ. And their triglycerides dropped 11.3 percent. The study participants consumed about four tablespoons, or a quarter-cup, of wheat germ daily. Some of us may have trouble fitting that much into our diets, but it can be done, and experts suggest sneaking it in by adding it to lean ground beef or sprinkling it on cereal.

"It's a highly nutritious food, but the oils that it contains are very fragile and are readily oxidized," says Dr. Janson. "If someone is going to use it, it needs to be used up quickly to avoid the problem of rancidity."

If you think you'd like to add some lovin' spoonfuls of the golden, nutty stuff to your daily diet, however, no one will discourage you, says Dr. Haas. Just be sure to buy wheat germ in vacuum-packed packages and store it in an airtight jar in the refrigerator or freezer once it's been opened.

13 Herbal Nutrition

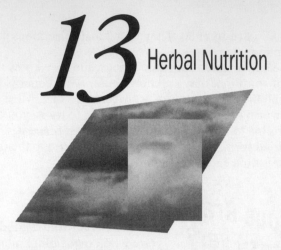

Where Kitchen Meets Pharmacy

Fettucine with pesto sauce. Taco chips with zesty salsa. A bracing after-dinner cappuccino, dusted with cinnamon.

What do these foods have in common, besides the ability to make your mouth water? They all owe their appeal to judicious use of herbs and spices.

It's hard to imagine cooking a delicious meal without at least a sprinkling of herbs and spices. Yet when it comes to healthy eating, these flavorful plants are usually an afterthought: We plan our meals around fish or beef, grains or greens—rarely around basil or garlic.

Herbs and spices are more than just tasty extras, however. A growing body of knowledge—one that marries scientific research with ancient folk wisdom—suggests that these plants may have untapped powers to help prevent heart disease and cancer. And there are some that you can use to treat everyday health problems more safely, gently and sometimes more effectively than you can with anything in your medicine chest.

"Grandmother Medicine" for What Ails You

Generations ago, before the advent of over-the-counter medicines and 24-hour drugstores, herbs were the treatment of choice for everyday health problems from headaches to upset stomachs and from head colds to menstrual cramps. Herbal treatments were shared among friends and families, exchanged by neighbors and taught by one generation to the next. In many parts of the world, herbal remedies are still the chosen way for people who tend to their families' health without the aid of medical doctors.

In modern America, we're more likely to reach for a bottle of pills than a pot of herbal tea when we're under the weather. But herbs haven't disappeared from the therapeutic landscape. Americans are likely to spend over $1.5 billion a year on herbal products.

Most of those dollars are spent in natural food stores, for everything from concentrated herbal essences and capsules to beauty products—those mysterious herbal lotions and potions you may have seen lurking on the shelves but couldn't find a use for.

But the simplest—and surely the most pleasurable—way to unleash the healing power of herbs is the way generations before us did: by using them to lend flavor to their food and brewing flavorful teas. There are many ways to do this. Try a tabbouleh (buckwheat) salad spiked with the crisp flavors of parsley and mint. Add a heavy sprinkling of cinnamon to your fresh-baked rolls or prepare a steaming cup of chamomile tea to help you unwind after a nerve-shattering day. Since most herbs are flavorful, including more herbs in your diet is sure to add spice to your life.

Healing with Herbs

Throughout the ages, herbs have been used to treat just about every conceivable human ailment. The trouble is, unlike prescription or over-the-counter drugs, a plant growing in the woods doesn't come with a label explaining its recommended uses and possible side effects.

This chapter is a guide to some simple ways to add the right herbs to your diet to prevent or treat a variety of health problems. There are in fact hundreds of herbs that have been linked to curing disease and restoring health, and we have included the leading herbal remedies for specific conditions, based upon recommendations of doctors and a review of research. (To find out more about the herbs not included here, see "Resources for Healing" on page 252.)

We've done our best to explain how and why the herbs are believed to work, but keep in mind that while people may have been using herbs for thousands of years, many modern Americans are unfamiliar with their uses and effectiveness. Most of the information we have about herbs is either anecdotal—based on the claims of people who've used them and say they're helpful—or highly scientific, originating in laboratories and reported in science journals. On the following pages you'll find, in alphabetical order, many health conditions—from cancer to yeast infections—that herbs may help prevent or cure.

Cancer Prevention

The idea that herbs can fortify our bodies' defenses against cancer isn't a new one—but even those well-versed in herbal medicine admit that there isn't much scientific evidence to support it. "There's so much we don't know about the role different herbs play in the treatment of cancer," says Daniel Mowrey, Ph.D., director of the American Phytotherapy Research Laboratory in Salt Lake City. "There's a lot more research that needs to be done."

If you would like to include herbs in your personal cancer prevention strategy, it's important to have a realistic sense of what these plants might be able to do and what's better left to conventional medical treatment, cautions Dr. Mowrey. Remember that when it comes to cancer, herbal nutrition is probably more effective as a preventive measure than as a cure.

"I think that once certain severe cancers get going, a complete cure may be beyond the reach of any of our simple herbal remedies," says Dr. Mowrey. "But I believe that the proper herbs, when combined with expert medical supervision, can be used to treat some forms of cancer with success." Dr. Mowrey also thinks it's probable that people can prevent a large number of cancers by including a wide variety of herbs and spices in their diets.

A Stinking Rose to Guard Your Innards

While many different herbs are believed to have cancer-fighting potential, none has been the subject of as much scientific research as garlic. As it turns out, "the stinking rose" comes up smelling sweet in cancer studies.

Epidemiological studies in both China and Italy compared the rates of stomach cancer in people who ate garlic regularly with the cancer rates of others who rarely included garlic in their diets. In both of the studies, the group with the more pungent diet had significantly less stomach cancer.

Garlic also appears to offer some protection against colon cancer. In the Iowa Women's Health Study, which examined the diets and rates of cancer in 41,837 women, women who ate the most garlic—along with other vegetables—had the lowest incidence of colon cancer.

Scientists are only beginning to unlock the secret of garlic's cancer-fighting prowess, but they do have a few theories on the ways in which it might work.

Researchers at Pennsylvania State University in University Park have focused on a compound in garlic called diallyl disulfide (DADS), which has been shown to kill colon, lung and skin cancer cells that were taken from humans and grown in the laboratory.

Of course, killing cancer cells in a test tube is one thing. What scientists still don't know is how this compound might affect cancer cells in the human body. But while DADS still hasn't been studied in humans, researchers have begun to look at its effect on animals, with encouraging results.

In a laboratory experiment, one group of mice that had been injected with human colon cancer cells was treated with DADS, while another group was given plain corn oil. After three weeks, DADS had shrunk the cancer cells by 60 percent, while the tumors in the other mice continued to grow.

Researchers think that DADS works by altering a substance in cancer cells that allows them to grow and multiply. When exposed to DADS, the cells simply stop growing.

Another compound in garlic has been shown to block carcinogens from binding to breast cells in rats, and by checking that process, it helps to prevent tumor or cancer growth in the animals.

When it comes to getting the health benefits of this pungent bulb, the more garlic you eat, the better. In studies in which garlic was associated with a lower risk of cancer, there was a clear dose-response effect. In plain English, the more garlic people ate, the more their cancer risk plummeted.

Green Tea: The Eastern Secret

If you follow health headlines, you probably remember hearing about the benefits of green tea, a cousin of the familiar brew that's popular in Europe and America.

A tempest in a teapot? Hardly. While research is still in the early stages, studies suggest that green tea may be a valuable weapon to add to your anti-cancer arsenal.

Research conducted in China shows that tea drinkers have a significantly lower risk of developing esophageal cancer than people who don't drink tea. The risks are about 50 percent lower for women and 20 percent lower for men. The more green tea people drink, the lower their risk, these studies suggest.

These findings are supported by a mass of animal research that associates drinking green tea with a lower incidence of many types of cancer. In a study at Rutgers University in New Brunswick, New Jersey, mice that were given the equivalent of six cups per day of green tea instead of water were about 40 percent less likely to develop lung cancer than their water-drinking cousins. The mice that took a tea break were also 30 to 60 percent less likely to get stomach cancer and nearly 70 percent less likely to develop esophageal cancer than the water-drinking mice in control groups.

In another study with a different procedure, Chinese researchers who injected laboratory mice with green tea extracts found them much less likely to develop colon cancer than mice that didn't receive the injections.

Another study showed a similar relationship between green tea and skin cancer. Researchers gave one group of mice drinking water that was spiked with GTP, a chemical compound that's plentiful in green tea, while a second group got plain water. After 50 days, the mice were exposed to cancer-causing chemicals. The mice in the GTP group got 40 percent fewer cancerous skin tumors than those that drank plain water.

Green tea has also been shown to reduce the genetic damage caused by aflatoxin B_1, a cancer-causing compound produced by certain molds that is believed to lead to liver cancer.

Of course, a mouse and a human being are two different animals, so the real proof of green tea's effectiveness won't come until it's tested on humans. In the meantime, those concerned about cancer might want to adopt a healthy habit practiced by millions of Chinese.

It's easy to develop a taste for this healthful brew. Green tea bags are available in health food stores and Asian markets. While two to three cups a day is reasonable, up to six may give more health benefits, says Elson Haas, M.D., medical director of the Preventive Medical Center of Marin in San Rafael, California, and author of *Staying Healthy with Nutrition*. Just follow the directions on the package.

Black Tea, Too?

But what if you prefer your tea black rather than green? Black tea—the type most popular in the United States and Europe—hasn't gotten as much scientific attention as the green variety, but some research suggests that it may also offer protection against cancer.

Green tea and black tea come from the same plant, *Camellia sinensis*. The difference is that green tea is made by steaming or drying the leaves, while black tea is fermented, giving it a darker color and stronger flavor.

Most of us know black tea best as orange pekoe, commonly found in Tetley, Lipton and similar tea-bag varieties that you get in restaurants and supermarkets. But whether your tea is green or black, it's rich in a class of chemical compounds called polyphenols, which may have something to do with its cancer-fighting powers. Polyphenols are potent antioxidants, capable of scavenging harmful free radicals to prevent the cellular damage that some experts believe leads to cancer.

Animal studies show that many types of tea—whether green or black, decaf or high-octane—may offer significant protection against skin cancer. Laboratory mice exposed to ultraviolet light and given any type of tea in place of drinking water had 70 to 80 percent fewer tumors than mice that drank only water.

Which type of tea has more cancer-fighting potential isn't yet clear. One study found that green tea was slightly more effective than black tea in preventing lung tumors in animals that had already been exposed to cancer-causing chemicals. But when the animals were given tea before being exposed to these chemicals, both types proved equally effective. In another study, black tea was slightly more effective than green tea in preventing esophageal cancer.

Since the jury's still out on which kind of tea is better for cancer prevention, Dr. Haas says the best advice is to drink the one you like. No one knows yet how much tea it would take to have a protective effect. But since we don't know of any harmful side effects from drinking a normal amount of tea, you might as well enjoy it to your heart's content.

Black tea contains about one-third the caffeine of brewed coffee (35 milligrams or so), and green tea has slightly less than that. Steeping time affects the caffeine content as well—the longer you soak, the stronger the cup. If caffeine is a concern, note that decaffeinated tea contains roughly the same amount of polyphenols as regular, so researchers have reason to believe that it may have the same protective effects.

Turning to Turmeric

When it comes to fending off cancer, some researchers believe the sun-colored spice turmeric is as good as gold. A favorite in Indian cooking, this pungent flavoring gives food a distinctive yellow color when it's added in cooking. Turmeric can be found in most supermarket spice sections and is also an ingredient in commercial curry powder.

A number of studies suggest that including turmeric in your diet may give you an extra edge when it comes to fending off cancer. In studies of laboratory animals exposed to cancer-causing chemicals, researchers supplemented some diets with the compound called curcumin, the active substance in turmeric. (Curcumin is known to have antioxidant and anti-inflammatory properties.) The animals on this supplemented diet were less likely to get colon cancer than those that didn't get turmeric. Other studies have shown that the herb has a similar protective effect against oral and stomach cancer. Some studies even suggest that turmeric can help heal liver damage caused by aflatoxin B_1, a toxic substance produced by certain molds, which is believed to lead to liver cancer.

Just how turmeric protects against cancer isn't entirely clear. But scientists do know that the curcumin it contains has been shown to disarm free radicals, helping to counteract these unstable molecules that are manufactured by the body and cause cellular damage.

This may explain why curcumin seems to offer protection against cancer-causing substances in the environment. A study of 16 smokers found that those who were given turmeric had fewer cancer-causing substances in their urine. Another study found that laboratory animals that were given curcumin in addition to their regular diet were less than half as likely to develop colon cancer as animals that didn't eat the herb.

That said, research on turmeric is very preliminary, and right now experts have more questions than answers about this intriguing herb. In the meantime, fans of Indian cuisine may find themselves with a leg up on cancer prevention.

Other Cancer-Fighters from Your Spice Rack

While research on other potential cancer-fighting herbs is sketchy, some experts believe that many common cooking herbs and spices may offer extra protection against cancer.

Included among these are a number of herbs that you probably have in your spice rack right now, including ginger, oregano and chili powder. All three have been shown to contain effective antioxidants, chemical compounds that protect your cells from damage by rounding up and disarming potentially cancer-causing free radicals. Since free radicals are both ingested and manufactured in the body in response to high-fat diets, smoking and sun exposure, anything that helps prevent the cell damage they cause may also help prevent cancer. Using these spices liberally in cooking will certainly add flavor, and their antioxidant properties might end up reducing your cancer risk.

Another common spice with antioxidant effects is rosemary. In one study, laboratory animals that were fed rosemary extract each day had 47 percent fewer breast tumors than a control group that didn't get the herb. Rosemary's cancer-fighting potential also seems to have something to do with its antioxidant properties.

Two other herbs that might have cancer-fighting potential are dill and caraway. Both contain a compound called d-limonene, which has been shown in animal studies to inhibit the formation of breast tumors. D-limonene seems to increase production of an enzyme called glutathione S-transferase, which disarms cancer-causing chemicals and also has antioxidant properties.

Colds and Flu

Humans have been coping with seasonal hacking and sniffling for as long as anyone can remember. But it wasn't until fairly recently in the course of human history that you've been able to pick up cold relief in the form of decongestants and cough syrups at the corner drugstore. Way back when, our ancestors picked up medicinal plants at nature's pharmacy.

Colds are easier to prevent than they are to cure, so the time to start taking herbals is before you get symptoms, says Dr. Mowrey. Face the sneezing season with herbs that fortify the immune system, and you just might beat that bug before it has a chance to do its dirty work.

Upping Immunity with Echinacea

When it comes to warding off colds, no herb has better word-of-mouth endorsements than echinacea. A plant that's native to North America, echinacea seems to work by pumping up the immune system to help your body keep infections at bay.

Animal studies show that substances in echinacea root stimulate the immune system to produce more of the proteins alpha-interferon, beta-interferon and interleukin-1. These proteins are necessary for the production of immune system cells, the hardworking foot soldiers that defend your body against infection.

Echinacea works best if you start using it as soon as you feel a cold coming on, says Tori Hudson, M.D., a naturopathic physician in Portland, Oregon, who uses herbs in her practice. For mild symptoms, drink two or three cups of echinacea tea a day. If your symptoms are severe, you can drink up to six cups a day.

Building Defenses a Clove at a Time

Garlic is better at preventing colds than at treating them, says Dr. Mowrey, so the best time to use it is before you start sniffling. Just chomp on some raw cloves. Or if raw garlic is a little sharp for your taste, sauté it for a minute or two. That will eliminate some of the bite.

Going with Ginger

Ginger is a traditional cold remedy in Chinese medicine, says Charles Lo, M.D., a physician specializing in preventive medicine in Chicago. "Ginger is considered to have warming properties and is the first choice for cold symptoms like chills, low-grade fever and headache," he says.

Dr. Lo recommends taking ginger at the first sign that a cold is coming on. At different times throughout the day, chew on three or four very thin slices of fresh ginger root, he suggests. You can supplement this daily chew with hot ginger tea, which is especially soothing if you are bothered by nasal congestion.

To brew ginger tea, use a teaspoon of grated fresh ginger per cup of boiling water. Steep for three to ten minutes, or to taste.

Coughs

The next time you buy a package of cough drops, take a look at the label and you'll probably see ingredients like eucalyptus, anise or peppermint. Herbs have long been used to quiet coughing, notes Varro E. Tyler, Ph.D., professor of pharmacognosy at Purdue University School of Pharmacy in West Lafayette, Indiana, in his book *Herbs of Choice*. If your cough is accompanied by congestion or a sore throat, a cup of hot herbal tea may be more soothing than anything you can buy at the drugstore.

You can buy or order peppermint, eucalyptus leaf, aniseed or fennel seed tea at a health food store. Or look for it in supermarkets, which are now carrying more herbal teas. Follow the directions on the package. The herbs stimulate your salivary glands, which makes you swallow more, and the urge to swallow suppresses the urge to cough.

Some herbs for tea are sold loose rather than in tea bags. You'll need one to two teaspoons of the herb per cup of boiling water; try different amounts until you find the strength that tastes best to you.

If you're using the roots of the herb, put some water in a pan, bring it to a boil, add the roots and simmer for about 15 minutes over low heat. When using leaves, bring the water to a boil but remove it from the stove before adding the tea leaves. Then steep it for up to 10 minutes. After steeping, strain the leaves or roots from the tea and enjoy.

Diarrhea

"Blackberry tea is one of the oldest remedies for diarrhea and is generally pretty effective," says Dr. Tyler. Health food stores carry blackberry tea in bags, ready to brew. But read the label before you buy: Some are just blackberry-flavored and don't contain any blackberry leaves. They may taste good, but they won't do a thing for diarrhea.

To make sure you're getting the real thing, you can buy dried blackberry leaves in most health food stores. Use a teaspoon or two of the herb per cup of boiling water and steep for ten minutes. You can drink blackberry tea all day with no ill effects, but it takes about three to six cups a day to help stop diarrhea, according to Dr. Tyler.

Heart Disease Prevention

Every year, some 1.5 million Americans have heart attacks. These people and countless others pop pills to lower their blood pressure or cholesterol, or they cut back on everyday activities because their hearts just can't go the distance. Heart disease is so common in this country that just being an American adult puts you at risk.

When it comes to this ruthless killer, an ounce of prevention is worth a pound of cure. Recognizing this, more and more Americans are taking steps to lower their heart disease risk by exercising and sticking to a low-fat diet.

If you're already on a low-fat diet, you probably think you're doing everything you can to protect yourself from heart disease. But advocates of herbal healing say you're not doing enough unless you're including the right herbs in your diet.

Of course, no herb is a replacement for a heart-healthy lifestyle, including a low-fat diet and regular exercise. But if you're already working out, eating right, having regular checkups and following your doctor's advice, adding a few herbs to your diet may give you a leg up in the race against heart disease.

Guarding Your Heart with Garlic

A decade or two ago, garlic was the herbalist's best-kept secret. Today garlic's benefits are so well known that major pharmaceutical companies are producing and selling garlic capsules. But herbalists feel that to get the full healing potential, you need to eat the real thing—and that means adding some garlic cloves to your menu.

Why the renewed interest in a funny-looking herb that's so odoriferous that it's sometimes called the stinking rose? After all, garlic has been around for as long as anybody has kept track of plants and their uses. Why all the renewed attention?

Chalk it up to a recent spate of scientific studies proving garlic's value in helping to prevent heart disease.

Garlic appears to protect your heart and blood vessels in a number of different ways. You may have already heard that garlic helps lower cholesterol levels. What's more, a study performed at the University of Kansas Medical Center in Kansas City showed that garlic actually helps change the way cholesterol behaves in your bloodstream.

"We're still in the very early stages of understanding how garlic works," says William S. Harris, Ph.D., director of the Metabolism and Vascular Research Laboratory at the Mid America Heart Institute of St. Luke's Hospital in Kansas City, Missouri, who was one of the authors of the study. "It does seem to have a beneficial effect in many areas related to heart disease, including blood pressure and cholesterol and perhaps dissolving clots. It looks promising, and there's no health risk associated with eating garlic that we know of, so there's no reason not to."

The easiest and tastiest way to get garlic's health benefits is to use it generously in cooking. Every day, try to sneak a few cloves into your soups, sauces and stir-fry dishes. Before you know it, garlic will be creeping into your casseroles, marinades and even salad dressings.

Just keep in mind that when it comes to cooking garlic, less is definitely more: Heat is believed to rob the herb of its potency, according to Dr. Mowrey.

"Very lightly fried garlic tastes best, and it's still beneficial as long as it's freshly fried," he says. "If you reheat the leftovers two days later, I doubt you'll get much of a benefit."

If you eat out often, it's easy to get your daily dose of this healthful herb, since flavorful ethnic cuisines like Italian, Chinese and Thai are often seasoned with liberal amounts of garlic.

For those who want the health benefits of garlic but can't stand the odor, deodorized garlic supplements—sold in health food stores and many drugstores—are the best solution.

Heart Protection in the Bag

"What would the world do without tea?" asked nineteenth-century essayist Sydney Smith. For the folks in Smith's native England, life would indeed be different without the daily ritual of afternoon tea. For one thing, if what some Dutch researchers believe is true, they might have a lot more heart disease.

Exactly what is it in tea that could have an effect on heart disease? The answer is flavonoids, a class of compounds found in many different fruits, onions and tea. Not all types of flavonoids protect the heart specifically, but flavonoids in general possess protective antioxidant properties, says Andrew Waterhouse, Ph.D., assistant professor of vitriculture (grape-growing) and enology (wine-making) at the University of California at Los Angeles. The flavonoids most abundant in tea seem to be capable of disarming harmful particles that, if left unchecked, can encourage LDL (low-density lipoprotein, the "bad" cholesterol) to stick to the walls of your arteries. Antioxidant flavonoids halt that process, which means that they can reduce the plaque clogging your arteries and decrease your risk of heart attack.

Dutch researchers saw this effect illustrated in the Zutphen Elderly Study, which kept track of the health and dietary habits of 805 elderly men. At the end of the five-year study, researchers found that tea drinking was associated with a lower risk of heart disease. The men's diets included not only tea but also onions and apples, two other good sources of antioxidant flavonoids. Those who had the most of these foods were half as likely to have a heart attack during the five-year period as men who didn't include these foods in their diets.

Other Herbs for the Heart

While garlic and tea are among the best-researched herbs for heart disease prevention, a few other herbs also show promise.

Eugenol, the active ingredient in cloves, has antioxidant properties. Like garlic and tea, it may reduce the oxidation of LDL so that less of it ends up clogging your arteries. One study suggests that it makes blood less likely to clot, which is good news if you're worried about your heart, since a blood clot in a clogged artery is all it takes to kick off a heart attack.

Research is still sketchy, but a few studies have suggested that ginger may also be of some help in keeping heart disease at bay. Ginger seems to reduce the production of thromboxane, a chemical compound that causes blood vessels to constrict and blood to clot—a potentially lethal combination for people with heart disease. And animal research has suggested that it might have some effect on cholesterol levels if used often enough.

Turmeric, the golden-yellow spice often used in Indian cooking, also contains compounds with antioxidant properties. One of these compounds, curcumin, also appears to inhibit cancer initiation and development.

All in all, the evidence isn't strong enough to suggest that you start loading up on these herbs. But if you already enjoy them and use them in cooking, you may be getting benefits you never realized.

High Blood Pressure

A number of scientific studies suggest another reason that garlic is your heart's friend: Its ability to bring down high blood pressure.

Exactly how much can garlic reduce your blood pressure? It's not as fast-acting as high blood pressure medication, says Dr. Mowrey. But over time, he says, garlic can be almost as effective as lifestyle changes like weight loss, regular exercise and cutting back on salt intake. For people with mild high blood pressure who are already watching their diets and staying active, garlic therapy may be enough to keep blood pressure in the safe range without the help of drugs, says Dr. Mowrey.

High Cholesterol

If cholesterol is a problem for you, you're far from alone: Experts estimate that more than half of Americans have cholesterol levels above 200 mg/dl (milligrams per deciliter), putting them at increased risk for heart disease.

In addition to a eating a low-fat diet and getting regular exercise, adding the right herbs to your diet can also have a beneficial effect on cholesterol levels. Here's how.

Garlic Does It Again

You've traded butter for olive oil, hamburgers for fish and doughnuts for bagels. You're eating less fat and more fiber. You're even exercising. And while your cholesterol numbers have dropped, you're still in that risky range above 200.

You may think you've tried everything, but you haven't—until you've tried garlic.

Studies on the cholesterol-lowering power of garlic abound. While some studies find it to be more effective than others, the benefits are usually provable—studies show that, on average, garlic therapy lowers total cholesterol by about 12 percent. That may not sound like much, but for those with high levels, it can take a huge bite out of their risk of having a heart attack.

For every 1 percent reduction in total cholesterol, you cut your risk of heart disease by 2 percent. So if your total cholesterol is 240 mg/dl and you bring it down to 216 (a decrease of 24 points, or 10 percent), your risk plummets 20 percent.

Garlic also seems to be helpful in lowering triglycerides, another type of fat in the blood. Elevated triglyceride levels are strongly associated with heart disease.

"On a percentage basis, garlic may be even more effective in lowering triglycerides than in lowering total cholesterol," says Dr. Tyler. "Some people will be able to reduce their levels by about 15 percent."

Best of all, garlic doesn't seem to lower HDL (high-density lipoprotein) cholesterol, the "good" type that actually protects you from heart disease. So while it whittles away the harmful blood fats, it seems to leave the beneficial HDL right where it was.

"I believe garlic is the best proven herbal treatment for high cholesterol," says Dr. Tyler.

Research suggests that garlic also helps prevent the oxidation of "bad" LDL cholesterol. Oxidation is a chemical process that makes LDL more likely to attach to the walls of your arteries in the form of plaque.

Researchers at the University of Kansas Lipid Laboratory gave ten people garlic powder supplements for two weeks, then examined samples of their blood. They found that LDL cholesterol in the blood was much more resistant to oxidation after those two weeks of steady garlic consumption.

In animal studies at Penn State, researchers have found that garlic affects the body's ability to *produce* cholesterol. The studies showed that liver cells of rats treated with garlic produced less LDL and fewer triglycerides compared to livers of mice that didn't get garlic. And the less cholesterol that's produced in the liver, the less there is floating around in the blood and clogging up the arteries.

But if you do decide to try garlic for cholesterol control, be patient: In one study, it took about four months for garlic to have a noticeable effect on cholesterol.

The Japanese Advantage

When it comes to managing cholesterol, Americans have a lot to learn from the Japanese: In general, the serum cholesterol levels of Japanese are low by Western standards. Experts attribute the difference mostly to the super-healthy Japanese diet, which is heavy on fish, rice and vegetables and light on red meat, junk food and other fatty fare.

But some experts believe it's not just what the Japanese eat that gives them an advantage over cholesterol, it's also what they drink. A study of 1,306 Japanese men found that those who drank lots of green tea had lower levels of total cholesterol than those who drank it rarely or never.

If you'd like to try green tea to see if it lowers your cholesterol levels, it might take quite a bit of tea to produce an effect: The men in the study with the lowest levels drank nine or more cups per day. And since green tea is made from the same plant as black tea, it's quite possible that regular tea could have the same cholesterol-lowering effect.

Indigestion

Deep inside the twists and turns of your digestive system, there's ample room for discomfort—ranging from excess gas to indigestion and heartburn. But herbalists have some healing drinks that could relieve whatever ails you.

A Minty Solution

One of the most popular herbal remedies for indigestion is peppermint, which is especially helpful if you have problems with excess gas. The plant's leaves contain an oil that's been shown to relax the lower esophageal sphincter, which can help you release gas. Peppermint also stimulates the flow of bile, a fluid produced by the pancreas that plays an important role in digestion.

If you're prone to indigestion, a cup of peppermint tea is a pleasant and therapeutic after-dinner ritual, says Dr. Mowrey. Peppermint tea, either loose or in tea bags, is widely available in health food stores and most supermarkets. To brew it, follow the instructions on the package.

Sweet Relief with Bitters

Bitter herbs such as dandelion also work for common digestive disturbances like heartburn and excess gas, says Dr. Mowrey. Dandelion root stimulates the production of digestive enzymes all along the digestive tract, from mouth to stomach to small intestine, he explains. This property makes it an excellent after-dinner tonic for those prone to indigestion.

A cup of dandelion tea after dinner is a great way to give your digestion a boost, although the bitter taste may be hard to take, says Dr. Mowrey. To prepare the tea, use two teaspoons of dried dandelion root per cup of boiling water and simmer for ten minutes. An alternative to tea would be dandelion root capsules. Dr. Mowrey suggests one or two capsules after meals.

A Stimulating Proposition

If you're an underachiever in the digestion department, two other herbs to try are ginger and cayenne pepper, says Dr. Mowrey.

"These herbs stimulate the musculature of the entire gastrointestinal system," he explains. "They improve mobility so that nutrients are carried into the blood faster and assimilation is improved." If you often feel sluggish after a meal or are prone to constipation, spiking a meal with ginger or cayenne can help get things going, Dr. Mowrey concludes. "I like to include both of those in my diet a lot," he says.

Good Gastro with Garlic

"Garlic improves the digestion of many foods it's combined with," says Dr. Mowrey. "It improves the digestion and utilization of fatty things in particular, which might be why foods like sausage often contain garlic."

If a special occasion calls for a meal that's a little richer than your stomach is used to, you might try adding garlic to a few of the dishes as you're cooking, he says. Your stomach may thank you later.

Or if you have gallbladder problems, you "can really benefit from a lot of garlic in your diet," says Dr. Mowrey.

Toning Up with Turmeric

Another helpful herb for poor digestion is turmeric. This herb stimulates and tones the liver and gallbladder and stimulates the production of bile, according to Dr. Mowrey. "Proper bile secretion is absolutely critical to good digestion and to good cleansing of the blood," he says.

Chamomile for IBD

Another popular herbal remedy for digestive disturbances is chamomile. Researchers have traced its beneficial effect to chamazulene, a chemical compound in chamomile known to have anti-inflammatory properties.

For this reason, chamomile tea is often used to soothe inflammatory bowel disease (IBD), which can have many uncomfortable symptoms, including abdominal pain, bleeding and diarrhea. (It takes a doctor's diagnosis to determine if you have IBD or another intestinal problem.) While the tea contains only minute quantities of chamomile's antispasmodic and anti-inflammatory components, herbalists believe that drinking it regularly has a cumulative effect. Chamomile tea is also rich in a number of flavonoids, a class of phytochemicals that are believed to have beneficial effects.

To prepare chamomile tea, pour a cup of boiling water over a heaping tablespoon of chamomile flower heads or a chamomile tea bag and let the mixture steep in a covered teapot for 10 to 15 minutes. Drink the tea between meals, three or four times a day, for stomach or intestinal discomfort.

Insomnia

The herb valerian is a well-known traditional remedy for insomnia. A mild tranquilizer, valerian has been used for centuries to treat sleeplessness, nervousness and anxiety and is the primary ingredient in a number of herbal sleep aids. Scientists still haven't pinpointed exactly which substances in valerian have sedative properties, but a cup or two of valerian tea at bedtime is considered safe and has no known side effects, says Dr. Tyler.

The only problem: Valerian tea tastes bad—really bad. "I would describe it as a bitter, dirty taste," says Dr. Hudson. Unless that appeals to you, this is one case where a newfangled herbal product—a capsule or tincture (a liquid concentrate usually containing alcohol as a base)—is in order. "A teaspoon of the tincture or one to two capsules before bedtime is usually enough," says Dr. Hudson. "Just follow the directions on the package."

Menstrual Cramps

Menstrual cramps are a fact of life for many women, and a week of suffering every month is a lot! If you're one of the many women who dread cramps, you owe it to yourself to find a safe, gentle treatment that works.

To ease menstrual cramps, try a soothing cup of chamomile tea, says Dr. Hudson. Chamomile's antispasmodic activity makes it a natural choice for easing the back and abdominal pain that many women face each month. It also tastes good, she says. And it's easy to find—looseleaf or in bags— at many supermarkets and nearly all health food stores. Drink the tea throughout the day whenever cramps bother you, she suggests.

Nausea

To put your stomach on the road to recovery, ginger is the Cadillac of herbal remedies, according to Dr. Mowrey.

"In my experience, ginger is effective against nausea no matter what the cause," he says. "It's also very safe. In fact, there are no side effects at all except for a little aftertaste."

A number of studies have shown that ginger is particularly effective for treating motion sickness. In one study conducted by Dr. Mowrey, college students who were prone to motion sickness volunteered to be strapped into a rotating chair and spun around until their stomachs churned. All of the students were given a capsule to swallow, but they weren't told whether it was dimenhydrinate (Dramamine), powdered ginger root or a completely inactive placebo. Of the three groups, the students who got the ginger felt better most quickly.

Ginger seems to counteract motion sickness by absorbing stomach acids and interrupting nausea signals sent from the stomach to the brain, according to Dr. Mowrey. If your mother gave you ginger ale for your upset tummy, her instincts were right on target. Ginger ale really does contain enough ginger compounds to be effective, at least in very mild cases, according to Dr. Mowrey.

In fact, if you're only slightly queasy, either ginger ale or ginger tea can be quite effective, he says. "What form you take it in depends upon the severity of the condition." If you're not very susceptible to motion sickness but just get mildly queasy, he recommends ginger ale or a tea made by steeping slices of ginger root in boiling water. For more serious symptoms,

Dr. Mowrey recommends encapsulated ginger root, available at most health food stores. "Just take it as needed every couple of hours," he says. "If you get really seasick, you may need up to a dozen or so capsules a day."

Premenstrual Syndrome (PMS)

"Women were coping with premenstrual syndrome long before Midol was invented," says Dr. Hudson. In the absence of drugstore remedies like Midol for PMS, women turned to nature for relief.

One of the most common premenstrual complaints among Dr. Hudson's patients is water retention, a condition she treats successfully with herbs.

"Either parsley or dandelion leaf tea is effective for water retention," she says. "Even better, mix them. I'd advise drinking at least three cups a day, but you can drink as much as you want. Parsley is also rich in minerals, which is a nice bonus."

Even more bothersome than water retention are the tension and anxiety that many women feel when they're premenstrual, and this is another symptom that can be relieved with herbs, according to Dr. Hudson.

"Probably the best-tasting tea for anxiety is lemon balm," she says. "You can ask for it in just about any health food store, and it's got a very nice taste. Just follow the directions on the box and drink it as needed throughout the day."

Ulcers

An herb that seems to have potential for ulcer prevention is cinnamon. Japanese researchers found that small doses of Chinese cinnamon helped prevent alcohol-induced ulcers in laboratory animals. Cinnamon seems to increase the blood flow to the stomach lining, which may help keep the cells healthy and free of injury. While the effect of cinnamon on ulcers still hasn't been studied in humans, Dr. Haas says it can't hurt to include a little more of it in your diet.

Other research suggests that hotshot herbs like chili peppers may be just the ticket for keeping ulcers at bay. That's right—the spice that fires up a five-alarm chili won't burn a hole in your stomach. In fact, it may actually prevent one.

When researchers looked at Indian and Malaysian residents of Singapore, whose traditional diets include lots of chili, they came up with a surprising revelation. The chili eaters were less prone to ulcers than Chinese residents, who rarely use the fiery spice.

Chili peppers owe their zesty flavor to a chemical compound called capsaicin, which has been shown to protect the stomach lining from damage caused by too much alcohol or by anti-inflammatory drugs like aspirin. Robust herbs such as hot pepper, cayenne and paprika all contain capsaicin. "The healing effect of capsaicin may be due to its ability to increase circulation," says Dr. Haas. "That explains the feeling of warmth."

Of course, if you're prone to ulcers, it's important to follow your doctor's dietary advice. It's also important to listen to your body. "If chili peppers and cayenne give you discomfort, don't eat them!" says Dr. Haas.

Another herb that you may not have considered for ulcer healing is licorice root. This super-sweet, woody herb has been used for centuries to flavor food and drinks. Today it's more commonly thought of as the chewy black whips found in the candy aisle, although those are most likely flavored with anise.

Licorice contains glycyrrhizin, a compound shown to possess notable anti-inflammatory properties. Dr. Mowrey recommends whole licorice root (rather than the candied version) not only for ulcers but for other inflammatory stomach troubles as well. "Whole-herb licorice, in powder or root form, can be very effective for soothing irritated stomach tissue," he says.

Twiglike sections of licorice root, found in health food stores, can be chewed, and the syrupy juice can be swallowed. Capsules are also available, and Dr. Mowrey recommends up to six a day for mild stomach complaints. Bulk licorice root powder is the strongest approach, he says. Dr. Mowrey suggests up to a tablespoon of the sweet stuff per day mixed with juice or water. "In my opinion, licorice is one of the top five healing herbs in the world," he notes.

Urinary Tract Infections (UTIs)

To nip infections in the bud, Dr. Hudson recommends homemade cranberry tea. Try making it part of your daily routine as a preventive, especially if you've had UTIs before. "Two or three cups, spaced throughout the day, should have a preventive effect," she says.

To brew one cup of cranberry tea, fill a standard-size tea ball with dried cranberries, then pop the tea ball in a small pot of boiling water. Let the tea steep for 20 minutes on low heat—just hot enough so that it simmers, says Dr. Hudson.

Yeast Infections

The wonders of garlic may never cease.

Now add this: Including more garlic in your diet may be helpful in warding off recurrent yeast infections, according to Dr. Hudson.

Scientists at Boston University Medical Center found that when garlic went head-to-head with a variety of common infection-causing bacteria, the fragrant bulb came out a winner every time. Scientists think garlic owes its

Resources for Healing

Books

The Complete Book of Natural and Medicinal Cures
The Editors of *Prevention* Magazine
   Health Books
Rodale Press

The Healing Herbs
Michael Castleman
Rodale Press

Herbs of Choice
Varro E. Tyler, Ph.D.
Haworth Press

Herbs for the Home: A Definitive Source-book to Growing and Using Herbs
Jekka McVicar
Studio Books

bacteria-slaying powers to allicin, the same compound that's responsible for its characteristic odor.

But garlic's effectiveness goes beyond killing bacteria. "Garlic does things antibiotics can't do," Dr. Hudson says. "It doesn't just kill bacteria; it's also antiviral and antifungal, which makes it terrific for any type of infection."

If you want to keep yeast infections away, make a point of eating at least a clove of fresh garlic every day, suggests Dr. Hudson.

"Raw or very lightly cooked garlic is best," she says. "If you don't want to smell it or taste it that much, you can get the same effect with prepared garlic capsules. I would suggest taking one capsule in the morning and another one in the evening."

Part

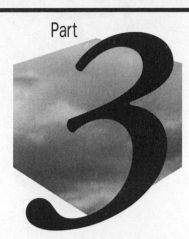

The New Nutrition for Healing

14 Arthritis

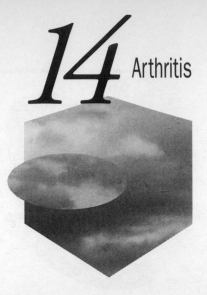

Quench the Fire in Your Joints

In 1960, actor James Coburn played a knife-hurling cowboy in the classic western *The Magnificent Seven*. But by 1980, the rawhide-tough Coburn couldn't grasp a knife or even get out of bed due to the crippling effects of rheumatoid arthritis.

When conventional medical treatments failed, Coburn turned to alternative measures for relief from arthritis pain. Finally, he resorted to radically altering his diet.

Coburn fasted. Then, through his own trial and error and medical blood tests, he discovered that he had an allergic reaction, in the form of arthritis flare-ups, to more than half of the foods he was tested for.

"It was a gradual process," he says. "Today, I live a relatively pain-free life and I continue to carefully watch my diet."

Pain Relievers—Or Fishy Promises?

Like Coburn, many Americans are digging into alternative diets to unlock their prisons of pain. For some, conventional medical approaches have been unsuccessful. Others are looking for a natural, drug-free system for coping with the pain and inconvenience of arthritis.

The range of diets that claim to ease arthritis is vast, from eating more fish to cutting out tomatoes, potatoes and other vegetables from the plant family called nightshades, and from near-vegetarian, peasant-style cuisine to fasting.

These eating systems have strong advocates among practitioners of alternative nutrition, such as California nutrition researcher Joseph Scala, Ph.D., and New Jersey fasting authority Joel Fuhrman, M.D., and equally strong detractors among conservative arthritis experts.

But while the experts debate, the joint-searing pain, stiffness and swelling experienced by the 37 million Americans with arthritis motivates many to look for some kind of relief. Complicating their search is the fact that there are actually more than 100 forms of this debilitating disease, which can inflame joints as well as muscles, tendons and even the skin and internal organs.

Among the most common types is osteoarthritis, a problem that often accompanies aging when the cartilage "cushion" between the bones in a joint breaks down. Another common form is rheumatoid arthritis (RA), in which the body's immune system attacks joint membranes, causing pain and even deformities. The onset of RA can occur at any age: It's not associated with aging, as osteoarthritis is.

Yet another kind of arthritis is gout, in which an excess of uric acid (a substance that the body usually eliminates in urine) irritates joint linings, most often in the big toe.

Different Views of Foods

Just how strong is the link between arthritis pain and what you eat?

"We've known that gout can be helped by weight reduction if the individual is overweight and by reducing sources of uric acid in the diet. And that being overweight can make osteoarthritis worse, particularly in the weight-bearing joints," says Doyt L. Conn, M.D., senior vice-president for medical affairs at the Arthritis Foundation in Atlanta. "And we think that substances in certain foods could make RA worse for some patients."

But beyond that, arthritis experts differ sharply over the effectiveness of diet for controlling achy arthritis.

Some arthritis researchers now say that roughly one-quarter of those with RA report responding to dietary changes and that people with other forms of arthritis could benefit, too. Advocates of new nutritional therapies are the most optimistic, saying that nearly 70 percent of patients could improve if they changed their diets.

Other experts target "problem foods" rather than overall diet. "I suspect that there are just a few people who experience flare-ups of arthritis after eating certain foods, and it's pretty clear to them and to their physicians," says Dr. Conn. "By eliminating the problem food, those people may do better. But if there were a sizable number of people with arthritis for whom diet was really making a difference, we would know that already."

Gunning for Gout

It's a long way from your mouth to your toes. But if your big toe is throbbing with painful gout, the culprit is usually something you ate.

"There has long been a well-described connection between gout and diet," says Christopher Wise, M.D., associate professor of internal medicine at Virginia Commonwealth University Medical College of Virginia in Richmond.

A gout attack occurs when crystals of uric acid, a natural substance that is normally excreted, find their way into a joint. Uric acid is a waste product, and if the kidneys can't remove it all, crystals start to form. Like sugar settling in the bottom of a cup of tea, the crystals settle to the body's extremities—the hands and feet.

Certain foods are very high in the purines that break down into uric acid, Dr. Wise says. These foods include sardines, mussels, anchovies, liver, cheese and red meat. And worst for gout is alcohol. Although not high in purines, it has an adverse effect on the kidneys' ability to excrete uric acid.

Meanwhile, researchers are uncovering some tantalizing links between food and arthritis. At Vanderbilt University School of Medicine in Nashville, Tennessee, researchers have seen a possible link with food allergies or sensitivities in some people who have pain from RA. In Belgium, fish oils have been shown to reduce joint pain in people with RA, and they may reduce the need for some medication. In Norway, a two-year study of a low-fat, vegetarian diet found that it helped substantially to soothe RA.

What can *you* do? If you think you have arthritis, says Dr. Conn, see a doctor first for appropriate treatment, which could vary depending on the type of arthritis. "Even if you follow a specific diet," he says, "you shouldn't delay looking into established treatments." But beyond those treatments, there's more you can do to help yourself find relief. One place to begin is with fasting.

Fasting for Fast Relief

You don't have to be a prophet to profit from fasting, say nutrition experts. The practice of abstaining from food for a few days or even a few weeks has proven effective for some people in easing the pain of RA.

"I use fasting, allowing only water for seven to ten days usually, to help many people with arthritis," says Dr. Fuhrman, a nutritional medicine specialist, director of the Amwell Health Center in Belle Mead, New Jersey, and author of *Fasting—and Eating—for Health*. "Sometimes the body needs a rest from food altogether."

The culprits that are responsible for joint pain, swelling and stiffness are often partially digested animal proteins that "leak" through weak intestinal membranes into the bloodstream, according to Dr. Fuhrman. In his view, the body's immune system identifies these big protein molecules as foreign invaders. In response, antibodies attach themselves to these invaders and form immune complexes. These complexes cause trouble in large numbers, inflaming joints such as the fingers, toes, wrists, knees and ankles.

"Fasting may work by cleaning these proteins out of the bloodstream," says Dr. Fuhrman. Fasting also seems to change the dynamic state of the body by altering intestinal flora, the "good" bacteria that help us digest food. As a result, we absorb food better after fasting, says Dr. Fuhrman.

Don't Fast Alone

In Dr. Fuhrman's view, fasting is "more powerful than the strongest and most toxic drugs at reducing inflammation." Mainstream medical researchers don't go that far, yet in four studies, people with RA did see improvement after fasting.

But don't try this without talking to your doctor. Dr. Fuhrman says a doctor should be consulted before anyone gives up food, even for a few days. And many people should not consider it at all, including those who have damaged livers or kidneys, are pregnant or nursing or take medication regularly for a medical condition. Your doctor won't want you to fast if you have anemia, Type I (insulin-dependent) diabetes, cancer, epilepsy, an eating disorder, AIDS or tuberculosis, says Dr. Fuhrman. And for those with a rare enzyme defect called MCAD (medium-chain acyl-CoA dehydrogenase) deficiency, fasting is strictly forbidden: They can lapse into a coma if they go without food for several days.

Is fasting alone the key to soothing the pain of RA? No, says Dr. Fuhrman. After all, human beings need to eat. "A fast prepares your body for the next step: a change of diet," he says. "Without a new way of eating, your arthritis symptoms will return as soon as you go back to your previous diet."

Eliminate the Ache

In addition to fasting, many of Dr. Fuhrman's patients also try an elimination diet. The goal is to hunt down and eliminate foods that spark painful flare-ups.

How do you play the elimination game?

Whether or not you've fasted beforehand, Dr. Fuhrman suggests you begin by adopting a restricted vegetarian diet with no dairy foods, fish, wheat, citrus or caffeine—all foods that may cause flare-ups. You can eat all the green and yellow vegetables, wheat-free whole grains and noncitrus fruits you want. But be sure to check with your doctor before eliminating food groups, just to make sure you don't shortchange yourself on some nutrients.

"If your arthritis quiets down, in a few months you can try adding

Sleuthing Clues for the Diet Detective

Become a mealtime Sherlock Holmes to unmask potential ache-making foods that could make arthritis-wracked joints throb, suggests nutritional medicine specialist Joel Fuhrman, M.D., director of the Amwell Health Center in Belle Mead, New Jersey.

"For people who do not want to fast or don't have the time for a fast, an elimination diet is a good way to find troublemaking foods all by itself," says Dr. Fuhrman. How? Try this system.

Start with reaction-free fare. If you eat a limited diet to begin with, says Dr. Fuhrman, it will be easier to determine which foods jar your joints. He recommends eliminating foods such as citrus fruits (including tomatoes), wheat, dairy products, eggs and all meats for at least four weeks.

When planning a restricted diet, consider which foods might be suspects. Among the leading culprits are corn, wheat, bacon, pork, oranges, milk, oats, rye, eggs, beef and coffee. In fact, these foods are the ones most likely to cause discomfort for people with rheumatoid arthritis, according to researchers at Epson General Hospital in Surrey, England.

Test your reactions. After following the restricted diet for a month or more, Dr. Fuhrman suggests that you try eating one of your food suspects and note whether or not the fire in your joints flames up. Then, after returning to your limited menu for a few days, eat the food again and note whether pain returns. To be certain you've either caught the culprit or found a friend, repeat the routine once more: Eliminate the food for a few days, then eat it and note your reaction. Only then, if you experience a return of symptoms, should you eliminate the food entirely from your diet, Dr. Fuhrman advises.

Banish with care. Take note: Any elimination diet requires a doctor's supervision. Consult your doctor or a nutritionist before removing any large food groups—such as all dairy products, all protein sources like meat or fish or most fruits or vegetables from your diet—to help you replace important nutrients. For example, cutting out all dairy products on a long-term basis could rob your body of bone-building calcium.

Allow room for cheating. Often, after a two-month recess, you can sometimes eat a forbidden food every now and then without an adverse reaction, says David Edelberg, M.D., director of the American Holistic Health Center in Chicago. So if ice cream is your off-limits delight, sample it like caviar—have a scoop on rare special occasions.

---

citrus or other potentially irritating foods to see if you get inflammation or not," he says. Add one potentially irritating food at a time, then wait several days to see if there's an effect before adding others.

Common irritants reported by arthritis sufferers in one Vanderbilt

University study included pork, beef, citrus, sugar, food additives and dairy products as the worst offenders.

"If there's a negative reaction, the food is eliminated from the diet," says Dr. Fuhrman. "This approach helps 70 percent of the people I see with RA, and 40 to 60 percent might have total relief. Milder cases respond really well. And advanced cases show significant improvement."

The improvements that people reported include more hand strength, less tenderness in their joints and more flexibility. And some people were impressed that they developed the ability to move without being halted by pain.

Dr. Fuhrman recalls one 62-year-old woman with RA who could finally close her hand into a fist after ten years of pain so severe that she couldn't close her fingers over her palm—a simple movement necessary for grasping everything from a fork to a comb to a car's steering wheel.

The Norwegian Experience

A two-year study of fasting and restricted vegetarian meals at Norway's University of Oslo showed that this kind of eating can dramatically reduce arthritis symptoms such as tender, stiff joints.

After a seven- to ten-day fast during which they ate only broths and juices made from vegetables, 27 women and men who had RA were put on medically supervised vegetarian diets for one year. For the first three and a half months of the diet, milk, meat, eggs and any foods that contained gluten (such as bread or pasta) were forbidden. These foods

A New Way in Norway

When 27 Norwegians with rheumatoid arthritis agreed to give low-fat, vegetarian fare a test drive for one year, researchers at the University of Oslo found that the entire group reported less pain and fewer swollen, tender joints. After two years, more than half the members of the group still reported significant improvement.

What were they eating? Their diets were restricted to some fruits and grains, vegetables and beans. Some participants added dairy products and gluten-containing grain products, such as whole-wheat bread, as well. They were permitted to continue having these foods as long as their arthritis didn't flare up.

Restricted foods at the beginning of the study included dairy products, meat, fish, citrus fruits, refined sugar, salt, strong spices, preservatives, tea, coffee and alcoholic beverages.

Such a small study is far from conclusive, yet findings like this have led arthritis researchers—and some doctors who treat arthritis—to look at diet as a contributor to arthritis pain.

"I encourage people to minimize high-fat foods, cut out animal foods and focus on whole, natural foods," says Joel Fuhrman, M.D., a nutritional medicine specialist and director of the Amwell Health Center in Belle Mead, New Jersey. "It helps."

were slowly reintroduced over the rest of the year to check for reactions. Coffee, alcohol, citrus fruits and even fish were also eliminated. Another 26 patients stayed at a convalescent home for a month but continued to eat a nonvegetarian diet.

After one month, the vegetarian dieters had fewer tender and swollen joints, less morning stiffness and pain and greater grip strength. Two years later, more than half of the vegetarians were still enjoying those benefits. Meanwhile, the other arthritis patients who never went vegetarian were experiencing worse symptoms by the end of the first year.

Retiring the Fat

Performing liposuction on your refrigerator may be the best thing for your joints. That's the opinion of Charles Lucas, M.D., director of the Division of Preventive and Nutritional Medicine at William Beaumont Hospital in Birmingham, Michigan.

In the 1980s, Dr. Lucas and Lawrence Power, M.D., of Wayne State University in Detroit, reported that when people stop eating high-fat foods like cheese, butter, whole milk, red meat, cakes and pastries, as well as anything that's fried, their RA improves in many cases.

"The medical community didn't exactly embrace our findings," Dr. Lucas says. In those days, the connections between food and arthritis were treated with skepticism by mainstream doctors.

The low-fat approach works by switching off the power supply to joint pain, according to Dr. Lucas. "The body needs fat to produce prostaglandins—substances that fuel inflammation," he says. "Take away the fuel, and you take away the inflammation." If you load your plate with fruit, vegetables, fish and beans, you automatically reduce production of inflammatory prostaglandins.

Other medical researchers agree with Dr. Lucas that a lean, meat-free diet rich in fruits and vegetables may bring relief. And they also agree that prostaglandins are among the chemicals responsible for the pain and swelling of RA. But when the University of Oslo team tried to pinpoint a connection between dietary fat and the chemical changes that produce pain-provoking prostaglandins, they came up empty-handed.

Going for Fish

Greenlanders. Folks from the North Atlantic's windswept Faeroe Islands. Villagers in coastal Japan. What links them together? All belong to an exclusive "club" whose members feast on fish-rich diets—and they're all people who don't get much arthritis.

James Scala, Ph.D., a nutrition researcher from Lafayette, California, and author of *The Arthritis Relief Diet*, says that Americans can reap the same pain-reducing benefits if they just look to the sea for sustenance. The secret, he says, is to use breakfast, lunch and dinner to balance between two kinds of prostaglandins in your body—the beneficial, pain-reducing kind and the joint-torturing, pain-producing kind.

Your body will make more of the "good-guy" prostaglandins that keep joints feeling oiled, smooth and pain-free if you eat more fish, says Dr. Scala. But not just any fish.

Cold-water denizens of the deep—like salmon, mackerel, tuna and herring—are best. Why? They're richest in omega-3 fatty acids, the chemical building blocks that your body uses to produce the beneficial prostaglandins. A study at Albany Medical College in New York adds support for a diet rich in fish oils. When people with RA took 130 milligrams of omega-3 fatty acids daily in capsule form, they found that tender joints and morning stiffness lessened. They also had less pain.

You need a minimum of one gram of omega-3's a day—about the amount in a 3½-ounce serving of canned salmon—to produce enough of these pain-easing substances to relieve arthritis, Dr. Scala says. But three to four grams is even better, he adds. Although it's best to get this from fish (see "Pain Tamers from the Deep"), some experts say that supplements can also be helpful.

Adding Fiber, Subtracting Animal Fats

But eating more fish isn't the whole story.

Add at least nine servings of fruit and vegetables and plenty of pasta and whole-grain breads and cereals to your plate every day, Dr. Scala suggests. This not only gives you the edge on overall good nutrition but also provides 25 to 35 grams of fiber a day. Fiber, he says, may escort inflammation-causing substances out of the body.

For extra nutritional insurance, Dr. Scala suggests taking a multi-vitamin/mineral supplement. To find a supplement that doesn't exceed the Daily Value (DV) of any nutrients, check the labels.

At the same time, Dr. Scala recommends that you steer clear of the animal fats found in meat and full-fat dairy products like whole milk, cheese and ice cream, since animal fats prompt your body to make the bad-guy prostaglandins.

If you follow Dr. Scala's recommendations, he claims that "in two to three weeks, you'll feel a lot better. In three months, you'll forget how bad you once felt. Stick with this diet for life, and you'll never know how badly deformed your joints could have become."

Dr. Dong and the Faucet Effect

According to an ancient Chinese proverb, "Sickness enters through the mouth, and catastrophe comes out of the mouth."

This age-old saying led Collin H. Dong, M.D., a family practice physician in San Francisco, to delve into his Chinese cultural heritage for a food plan to conquer arthritis.

So crippled with arthritis that he was confined to a wheelchair, Dr. Dong was told by his doctors to "live with it!" Instead, he abandoned the traditional American diet, laden with caffeine, red meat, dairy products and preservatives, and switched to classic Chinese peasant cuisine—mostly fish, vegetables and rice. In a matter of weeks, Dr. Dong's pain diminished so much that he could play golf.

Ecstatic, he outlined his discovery as co-author of *New Hope for the Arthritic* and author of *The Arthritic's Cookbook*. In his view, the Western idea of a "balanced diet" just plain isn't—with dairy products, processed sweets, alcohol and animal fat causing the most harm. He also advocates an elimination diet, saying that different foods aggravate arthritis in different people.

"I call it the faucet effect," says Dr. Dong. "You turn off the food tap that is harming you and turn on the food tap that will benefit you."

First published in the mid-1970s, his books flew in the face of conventional medical wisdom about arthritis. But later, a study of 26 people with RA found that some "responded excellently" to the Dong diet.

Saying No to Nightshades

Maybe summertime doesn't seem complete without potato salad. And spaghetti isn't the same without tomato sauce. But if you've got arthritis,

The Do's and Don'ts of Dr. Dong's Diet

It's what you choose to eat that counts most, according to Collin H. Dong, M.D., a family practice physician in San Francisco, co-author of *New Hope for the Arthritic* and author of *The Arthritic's Cookbook*.

Dr. Dong says some foods are okay once in a while, such as on special occasions. These include chicken breast, wine for cooking, a small amount of bourbon or vodka and a small amount of hot spices and pasta.

Dr. Dong also has a list of other foods that you can eat as often as you want. The "acceptables" include:

- All seafood
- Vegetables
- Vegetable oils
- Margarine (look for types without milk solids added)
- Egg whites
- Honey
- Sugar
- Nuts
- Sunflower seeds
- Soybeans
- Rice
- Bread with no additives
- Tea
- Coffee
- Plain soda water
- Parsley
- Onions
- Garlic
- Bay leaf
- Salt
- Flour
- Chicken broth

Dr. Dong recommends avoiding some foods, since he says they can aggravate arthritis. Stay away from:

- All meat, including meat broths
- All fruits
- Tomatoes
- Dairy products such as milk, cheese and yogurt
- Egg yolks
- Vinegar
- Peppers and all hot spices
- Chocolate
- Dry-roasted nuts
- Alcoholic beverages and soft drinks
- All additives and preservatives, particularly monosodium glutamate

---

you might want to give up that salad, that sauce and everything else that contains potatoes, tomatoes and a number of other veggies that are close relatives.

Calling off a love affair with potatoes and tomatoes, as well as the rest of the botanical family called nightshades, could stop the pain and disfigurement of arthritis, according to Norman F. Childers, Ph.D., courtesy professor in the horticulture sciences department at the University of Florida in Gainesville and author of *Arthritis: Diet to Stop It*.

Dr. Childers' no-nightshades diet forbids all nightshade foods—including eggplant, potatoes, tomatoes and peppers, such as red and garden bell types, paprika, pimiento, cayenne and chili. (Black pepper doesn't

Shady Hideaways of Nightshades

If you're testing a nightshade-free diet to deliver a knockout punch to arthritis, it's easy enough to identify the offenders that are fresh from the garden. But it gets trickier when you try to eliminate the nightshades that may be hidden in processed and packaged foods. To do that, you have to read ingredient labels, warns Norman F. Childers, Ph.D., courtesy professor in the horticulture sciences department at the University of Florida in Gainesville and author of *Arthritis: Diet to Stop It.*

When you're reading the fine print on ingredient labels, watch out for hidden nightshades such as potato flour, cayenne pepper, tomato sauce and chopped red or green pepper. (Black pepper is okay, since it isn't in the nightshade family.) You'll often find these ingredients in foods such as biscuits, fish cakes, sausage, tortilla chips, meatballs and meat loaf, soups, horseradish, meat pies, relishes, sauces, seasoned salts, tacos and stuffed salad olives.

come from the nightshade family, so it's allowed.) Tobacco, on the other hand, is a nightshade, so Dr. Childers tells smokers to kick the habit.

How could vegetables hurt your joints? Dr. Childers believes that people with a sensitivity to nightshades are slowly being poisoned by minuscule amounts of a chemical called solanine, which is dangerous in large quantities and is found in tiny concentrations in nightshades.

Nutrition experts disagree with Dr. Childers' claims about solanine, but the diet, Dr. Childers says, has helped at least 546 people with arthritis who tried it and wrote to him. The diet seems to work fastest for people with early stages of the disease.

After a year of debilitating arthritis, Pat Claudio, a fourth-grade teacher from Burke, Virginia, quit eating nightshades and says her pain literally disappeared in six weeks. "If I eat the tiniest bit of a nightshade vegetable now, I'm crippled with arthritis for a week or two," she says.

15 Cancer

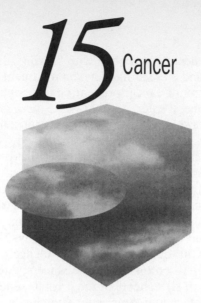

Recipes for Protection

Sweet, juicy peaches. Fresh spinach spiced with garlic and a glisten of olive oil. Tart, sun-bronzed apples. Fragrant whole-wheat bread.

The menu for a romantic *al fresco* lunch? Yes—and much more.

An increasing body of research has been suggesting what nutritionists, cancer experts and natural healers have suspected all along: Fruits, vegetables and whole grains can play powerful roles in preventing cancer, the second leading killer of men and women in the United States.

Switch on your television or radio or browse at the newsstand, and you'll hear plenty about cancer-preventing foods and diets. The one place you may not hear much at all about them is at your doctor's office.

"The American medical system is still oriented toward fixing cancer, not preventing it," says Daniel W. Nixon, M.D., associate director of the Division of Cancer Prevention and Control at the Hollings Cancer Center of the Medical University of South Carolina in Charleston and author of *The Cancer Recovery Eating Plan*. "Soon your doctor's office will become a prevention center as well as a treatment center. But for now, the focus is still on treating cancer—even though it can be expensive and painful and often doesn't really work."

Nutritional Links

The history of healing is replete with "curing" diets, like the South African grape cure and the German Gerson treatment. Doctors like Susan Mayne, Ph.D., director of cancer prevention and control research at the Yale University Cancer Center, say that while these and many other early practices are now considered potentially dangerous, the link between special diets and cancer prevention is well-established.

"We've found in large population studies that people who eat more fruits and vegetables have a lower risk of cancer," says Dr. Mayne. "We know that fruits and vegetables contain antioxidants and other substances that in laboratory studies block or suppress cancer growth."

While no diet can cure cancer, what you put on your plate can have a far-ranging impact on whether or not it occurs, says Dr. Nixon. More and more research bears this out. Consider the evidence:

• Half of the nation's colon and rectal cancers, one-fourth of all breast cancers and one out of six cancers of the prostate, endometrium and gallbladder might be prevented if Americans switched to diets low in fat and high in fruits, vegetables and whole grains, says Dileep G. Bal, M.D., chief of the cancer control branch of the California Department of Health Services in Sacramento.

Researchers at the University of North Carolina found that women who helped themselves to more than three servings of fruit a day cut their risk for developing precancerous colon lesions by nearly 60 percent.

• At China's Jiangsu Institute of Cancer Research, scientists examining the diets of 564 smokers and nonsmokers found that even heavy smokers who ate fruit every day cut their risk of lung cancer by 60 percent. Those who ate green vegetables daily reduced their risk by nearly 70 percent.

Of course, kicking the cigarette habit is the best way to prevent lung cancer. But positive changes in diet are especially important for anyone who breathes secondhand smoke—at home, in the car pool or at work.

• When University of Toronto researchers followed the eating habits of 56,837 Canadian women, they found that those who consumed the most fruits and vegetables rich in vitamins A and C lowered their breast cancer risk by 30 percent.

• The typical American diet—one that's high in fat, bereft of fiber, high in calories and skimpy on fruits, vegetables and whole grains—is thought to play a contributing role in about one in three cancer cases in the United States. Some experts put the number even higher, saying that as many as 60 percent of cancers in women and 40 percent in men may be linked to nutrition.

"Our eating habits are the major preventable cause of cancer," says Dr. Bal. "But people don't want to think it's as simple as eating a lot of fruit and vegetables and whole grains, reducing fat in the diet and exercising every day. They are more inclined to blame something like fast-food restaurants or even genetics."

The Powers of "Pharmafoods"

In recent years scientists have begun exploring a host of powerful compounds with tongue-twisting names like sulforaphane, phytosterols and isoflavones. If "drugs" like these came in a bottle, you'd certainly need a prescription. But nature is generous with her favors; these and similar compounds are plentiful at every produce stand and supermarket—and, says Dr. Bal, they appear to be one of your best hopes for winning the cancer war.

Experts have discovered that many fruits and vegetables, sometimes called nutriceuticals or pharmafoods, contain a variety of cancer-preventing compounds. Some you already know about. Antioxidant vitamins such as beta-carotene and vitamin C, occurring naturally in food, help protect cells from free radicals—unstable, high-energy molecules that can damage healthy cells and set the stage for disease, including cancer. The following are some other powerful substances found in food.

Flavonoids. Present in almost all fruits and vegetables, this class of compounds is able to keep potential carcinogens out of cells, where they do their damage.

Indoles and isothiocyanates. These compounds are responsible for the biting taste of broccoli, cauliflower and other cruciferous vegetables and also help keep harmful substances out of cells.

Isoflavones. Found in soybeans and soybean products like tofu, isoflavones provide multiple benefits. They act like antioxidants and also help block tumors from getting started.

Organosulfur compounds. Found in garlic and onions, these appear to play a powerful role in helping to block the formation of tumors.

Monoterpenes. Occurring in citrus fruits, monoterpenes help protect cells by interfering with the harmful action of carcinogens.

Even some well-known nutrients like folate and calcium now appear to have larger cancer-fighting roles than researchers previously thought. "There is compelling evidence from both animal and human studies that suggests that folate may prove to be an effective nutrient in our fight against colon cancer," says Joel B. Mason, M.D., assistant professor of medicine and nutrition at Tufts University School of Medicine in Boston. Calcium, he adds, plays a protective role by disarming the toxins that can lead to colon cancer.

Food to Favor

Regardless of the protective power of individual nutrients, a diet that's high in fruits, vegetables and whole grains provides what scientists call synergy—protective powers that may be greater than the sum of the individual parts. "We don't know exactly which nutrients are most important for people," says Dr. Mayne. "I suspect it's a combination."

The National Cancer Institute (NCI) and the American Cancer Society (ACS) have formulated simple dietary guidelines that if followed by more people could save literally thousands of lives a year. Perhaps it's not surprising that these modern guidelines really aren't very different from the basic, good-health diets that people have traditionally followed for thousands of years.

"No one fruit or vegetable will prevent cancer," says Carolyn Clifford, Ph.D., chief of the diet and cancer branch of the NCI and co-author of the institute's diet guidelines. "What we do know is that a low-fat, high-fiber diet containing fruits and vegetables is associated with less cancer. We don't yet know all the reasons why. But as a plan, it seems to work."

In a nutshell, here's what experts advise.

Pile your plate. Eat at least five servings of different fruits and vegetables every day. A serving is a half-cup of cut vegetables or fruit, a cup of raw salad greens, one-quarter cup of dried fruit or a hand-size piece of fresh fruit.

This is one area in which most of us can use improvement. According to the Centers for Disease Control and Prevention in Atlanta, only one in four women and one in five men eat five or more helpings of produce a day. Most of us manage about three.

With today's busy schedules, it's sometimes difficult to eat the way you'd like. It's easy to boost your fruit and vegetable quotient with a glass of 100 percent pure juice or a piece of fruit at breakfast. Or simply pick up a lunchtime salad or take an extra helping of vegetables at dinner.

"There's more to fruit and vegetables than science ever realized," says Dr. Clifford. "This is such an active area of research right now that I sometimes make the analogy to the 1940s and 1950s, when all the essential vitamins were being discovered and named. Now we're looking into the potential of preventing chronic diseases like cancer."

Eat by the colors. Try eating fruits and vegetables of at least three different colors daily. Each color means you're getting a different type of protective nutrient. Be sure to include cruciferous vegetables like broccoli, cabbage, cauliflower and bok choy. Get plenty of citrus fruit and dark green, leafy vegetables as well.

"No one food item can provide all of the essential nutrients," notes Dr. Clifford. "So you need a variety. Green, leafy vegetables are good sources of B vitamins and carotenoids. Yellow and orange vegetables are also good sources of carotenoids and other important compounds."

Focus on fiber. One of the easiest—and most important—ways to keep yourself healthy is to eat foods that have an abundance of dietary fiber. High-fiber diets have been linked to a lower risk of both colon and breast cancer.

"Fiber is important," says Charles B. Simone, M.D., founder and director of the Simone Protective Cancer Center in Lawrenceville, New Jersey, and a former NCI researcher. "It acts like a sticky substance, pulling fats and carcinogens and sugars out of the body with it. It also speeds the movement of food through the intestines, giving the bacteria there less time to produce carcinogens."

Although cancer experts advise raising fiber intake to about 30 grams a day, most of us eat less than 13 grams a day. To make up the difference, enjoy five servings of fruits and vegetables a day, along with four or more servings of whole grains. It sounds like a lot, but consider that one slice of bread or a half-cup of pasta each counts as one serving.

Cut back on fat. Most Americans get at least 34 percent of their daily calories from fat, which experts say is way too high. Research suggests that reducing your daily fat intake to 30 percent or less of total calories could substantially lower your risk of colon, breast, prostate, rectal and endometrial cancer. "Fat is carcinogenic," says Dr. Nixon. "It works several ways, including promoting the growth of cancer cells."

Studies have shown, for example, that diets high in fat and calories are associated with a higher risk of rectal cancer, especially in men. In addition, a major analysis of data from 59 countries showed that those who eat more animal fat and meat have higher risks of oral and esophageal cancer, while those who eat more fruit and cabbage have lower risks.

There are many ways to eat lean. Select the leanest cuts of meat or choose fish or skinless chicken, suggests Dr. Bal. Forgo gravies and sauces. Don't go overboard with creamy, high-fat desserts—select fresh fruit instead. Go light on salad dressings, and use low-fat or nonfat types. You could even try topping a salad with naturally fat-free salsa. Switch from whole-fat milk, yogurt and cheese to low-fat and nonfat varieties.

Curb the calories. Being overweight or taking in more calories than you burn each day may contribute to cancers of the colon, breast, prostate, endometrium, kidney, cervix and thyroid. One of the most dramatic anti-cancer steps you can take is to restrict calories and maintain a lean body weight, according to the NCI.

When you take in extra calories without increasing exercise, experts say, the cargo that accumulates in the form of body fat may increase cancer risk. "Fatty tissues may promote cancer, especially the hormone-related types such as breast and prostate cancer," says Dr. Bal.

Go easy on party fare. Foods that have been barbecued, smoked or pickled have been linked with some cancers of the stomach and esophagus. "When foods are overheated by frying or grilling, cancer-causing chemicals form," explains Sidney Weinhouse, Ph.D., professor emeritus of biochemistry at the cancer center of Jefferson Medical College of Thomas Jefferson University in Philadelphia and co-author of the ACS dietary guidelines. Pickled substances, he says, tend to be high in salt, which may encourage stomach cancer. "Foods prepared that way taste good, but they aren't good for you."

Be a moderate drinker. Heavy drinking has been shown to weaken the immune system, which can give cancer cells the "breathing space" they need to get a head start. Excessive drinking has been linked to some cancers of the rectum, mouth and esophagus, and even moderate drinking has been linked to an increased risk of breast cancer. When drinking is combined with cigarette smoking, there's a higher risk of lung cancer as well.

On-Target Diets

Prevention is always the best medicine, and there's abundant evidence that a healthful diet can help reduce the risk of many different cancers. Even if you've already had cancer, eating the right foods can help your body mount a helpful defense, says Daniel W. Nixon, M.D., associate director of the Division of Cancer Prevention and Control at the Hollings Cancer Center of the Medical University of South Carolina in Charleston and author of *The Cancer Recovery Eating Plan*.

The diet you choose depends in part on which type of cancer is involved. Here are some of Dr. Nixon's specific nutrition plans.

Breast cancer. Drop fat consumption to 20 percent of daily calories. Increase fiber intake to 25 grams a day or more. Eat plenty of fruits and vegetables.

The advantage of this diet is that it's fairly low in calories, which may shut off food energy to growing tumors. At the same time, it lowers levels of fatty acids and estrogen that might stimulate tumor growth.

Prostate cancer. When the cancer has been successfully treated, Dr. Nixon rec-ommends following the National Cancer Institute's basic nutrition plan, which emphasizes cutting back on fat and increasing the amount of fruit and vegetables and whole grains in the diet. Men with more advanced disease should reduce fat to 20 percent or less of total calories and also try to get more fruits and vegetables in their diets.

Colon cancer. Increase fiber intake to 30 to 35 grams a day. Eat plenty of fruits and vegetables. Decrease fat to 20 percent of total calories. Emphasize high-calcium foods like spinach, salmon (eat the small bones) or skim milk and fill up on garlic, onions, leeks and other members of the allium family. Calcium and the sulfur compounds in garlic may have protective effects against colon cancer, Dr. Nixon explains.

Skin or lung cancer. Eat 11 or more servings of fruit and vegetables a day and lower fat intake to 25 percent or less of daily calories.

Skin, lung and other "squamous" cancers are often linked to poor nutrition in which essential nutrients—particularly those found in fruits and vegetables—are missing from the diet.

Cook for Protection

The kitchen, as we've seen, can be a powerful protection center. All you need is a plan—a special way of eating to help prevent cancer from taking hold.

Some diets emphasize low fat intake as the key to warding off cancer. Others push for more produce. Still others emphasize the healing power of individual foods, like soy. A few are intended especially for people who have had cancer and traditional treatments, like chemotherapy, and who want extra nutritional protection against a relapse.

In the following pages we'll discuss a few of the more popular anti-cancer diets. It's important to remember, however, that virtually every good eating plan shares at least two key points: Eat less fat and more fiber and eat the widest possible variety of fruits, vegetables and whole grains.

"I'm a strong advocate of diet for getting nutrients," says Dr. Mayne. "Foods are extraordinarily complex. They contain all sorts of compounds we really know nothing about. It's not right to equate an orange with the amount of vitamin C in a vitamin pill. There's so much more there—so much that we need."

Macrobiotics

"Disease is imbalance." So says Michio Kushi, international spokesman for the macrobiotic movement, founder of the Kushi Institute in Becket, Massachusetts, and co-author of *The Cancer Prevention Diet*. "It all boils down to too much protein, too much sugar and not enough carbohydrates."

Cancer, as macrobiotic proponents like Kushi see it, is the result of excess and extremes—too much food or too much of the wrong foods overwhelming the body's natural, healthy balance. They say that macrobiotics—a diet philosophy that stresses grains and vegetables, with a minimum of meat and no sugar—can restore equilibrium.

In the macrobiotic view, cancerous tumors are literally waste dumps created by the body to store an overload of toxins. The cancer process begins with food: If your diet is unbalanced or you're just eating too much, the body cannot discharge all of the by-products of digestion. Mucus and fat deposits accumulate under the skin, in the kidneys, lungs and breasts, on reproductive organs and even within the heart and liver. Blood cells become less healthy, and without the ability to cleanse itself, the body resorts to storing toxins and the sickly blood cells as tumors.

Medical researchers don't agree with this theory of cancer's origins. Yet followers say that a diet focused on whole grains and vegetables and supplemented with soups, beans and sea vegetables helps prevent the disease. Meat and dairy products should be eaten sparingly, if at all. Seafood is included in small amounts. Sugar and alcoholic beverages are ruled out. Fruit should be seasonal—and local.

"To eat," notes Kushi, "is to take in the whole environment: sunlight, soil, water and air."

A naturally balanced diet, Kushi says, changes with the seasons and includes long-cooking foods in winter and raw salads and lightly cooked dishes in summer. It also conforms to climate: Folks living in temperate zones, says Kushi, lose natural immunity to local diseases if they eat tropical foods like pineapple, bananas, grapefruit and avocados. Local eating also means that people living close to the equator should steer clear of dairy products, for example, because such foods aren't natural to that area.

An Anti-cancer Balance

In the world of macrobiotics, dietary balance goes beyond eating healthful, locally grown foods. Foods also reflect yin and yang, in Kushi's view—that is, each kind of food reflects the universal forces of contraction and expansion, outwardness and inwardness.

• Yin foods grow in hot climates. Sour, bitter, sweet, hot or aromatic, they include fruits, sugar, spices and dairy products.

In the macrobiotic view, cancers in more hollow, expanded organs—including the breast, the outer regions of the brain, the esophagus, mouth, skin and stomach—are usually considered yin and can often be traced to an overabundance of yin foods.

• Yang foods come from cold climates. Dry, salty or pungent, they include eggs, meat, poultry, salty cheeses and fish.

Cancers that appear in deeper, lower, compact organs of the body—such as the bones, brain (inner regions), colon, ovary, pancreas, prostate and rectum—are said to be the result of too many yang foods.

• Cancers thought to be caused by an excess of both yin and yang include skin cancer (malignant melanoma) and tumors of the bladder, kidney, liver, lung, spleen, lower stomach, tongue and uterus.

To avoid extremes, macrobiotics stresses foods poised between yin and yang, such as vegetables, grains and beans. Building a diet on these "balanced foods," says Kushi, promotes health and decreases cancer risk.

While no one has studied the cancer-preventive impact of a macrobiotic diet in particular, research along more conventional lines indicates that some elements of this eating plan may have scientific merit. Soy, for example, is often incorporated into a macrobiotic diet. Soybeans and soy-based foods like tofu, tempeh and soy milk contain a phytochemical known as genistcin, a weak plant estrogen that has proved in test-tube studies to block the growth of breast cancer cells and precancerous cells in the prostate. Evidence is accumulating that the rates of breast cancer and prostate cancer are considerably lower in cultures that include soy dishes in their diets.

Banned from the Macro Table

A macrobiotic diet is helpful not only due to the foods it includes but also because of those it excludes. For example, meat plays only a small role at the macrobiotic table, and that may be a good thing. When researchers at New York University Medical Center in New York City examined the diets of 14,291 local women, they found that those who ate the most meat had an 87 percent greater risk of breast cancer than those who ate the least.

At the University of Florence in Italy, researchers discovered a link between a person's taste for refined sugar—as measured by the amount of sugar spooned into coffee—and colon cancer. Cancer risks rose 40 percent in those who added one spoonful, 50 percent in those adding two and 80 percent in those who added three or more spoonfuls. Researchers speculate that sugar may play an influential role in colon cancer growth. As for a macrobiotic diet, since it's free of refined sugar, the cancer risk is likely to be much lower.

The same goes for meats and other sources of saturated fats: Take away the fats, and cancer rates go down. In a University of Toronto study of 1,014 Canadian women, for example, those who reported consuming the most saturated fat and eggs and getting the least dietary fiber had the highest rates of ovarian cancer.

Not for Patients

It's important to note, however, that eating a macrobiotic diet during conventional cancer treatment can be dangerous, warns Dr. Mayne. "One key sign of cancer is weight loss," she says. "Many macrobiotic diets are very low in fat and therefore very low in calories. For a cancer patient who's losing weight, restricting calories may not be a good idea."

In addition, without careful monitoring, macrobiotic diets may be deficient in vitamin B_{12}, an essential nutrient found in meat, poultry and other animal foods, and vitamin D, which is important for the body's growth and development. If you're following a completely vegetarian macrobiotic diet—one containing no animal products—be sure to ask your doctor about supplementation.

Cancer patients who adopt any macrobiotic program should be sure they're getting adequate supplies of both of these important nutrients. They should also be under the care of a physician to ensure that they're getting adequate amounts of calories and protein.

Low-Fat Anti-cancer Diets

When it comes to fat, is lower always better? While cancer researchers debate how much fat we can safely eat, some argue that we should be getting considerably less than the amount recommended by the NCI.

"I personally try to get just 20 to 25 percent of my calories from fat," says Dr. Mayne. "While the government recommends 30 percent or less, there's a large debate about whether that's low enough. My personal feeling is, the lower the better, within reason. In parts of China, people eating a diet that provides 12 percent of calories from fat are very healthy and have low rates of chronic disease."

When Dr. Simone counsels men and women at his New Jersey cancer center, his message is "lower is better." Less fat, he maintains, means less cancer risk.

"Really rigorous research shows that protection against cancer begins when fat is in the 20 percent range," says Dr. Simone, who outlines his low-fat, high-fiber eating plan in his book *Cancer and Nutrition: A Ten-Point Plan to Reduce Your Risk of Getting Cancer*. "People who think they're protected by eating 30 percent of calories from fat are misleading themselves."

Studies suggest that there's a strong link between a high-fat, low-fiber diet and breast and colon cancer, and there's also some evidence that dietary fat is linked to prostate cancer. But not all researchers agree about the interpretation of the evidence.

For instance, population studies suggest that women who eat more fat have more breast cancer. Yet a major Harvard University study of 89,494 nurses found no difference in cancer rates between women who got more than 49 percent of their daily calories from fat and those who consumed less than 29 percent of calories from fat. Critics argue, however, that the Harvard study didn't go low enough—that cancer prevention doesn't occur until the percentage of fat in the diet falls to much lower levels, say, below 20 percent of total calories.

"I have no doubt that fat causes cancer," says Dr. Simone. "Eating less is important for two reasons—it helps control your weight, and it gets carcinogens out of your diet."

Estimating the Risk

It's easy to talk about daily percentages of fat as though the numbers were as obvious as speed signs on the highway. In fact, you have to do a little figuring to know whether or not your fat intake is in a healthy range. Here's how to do it.

1. When buying food, check the label for the amount of fat (in grams) per serving.
2. Multiply the number of grams of fat by 9—the number of calories in each gram. If the label lists two grams of fat per serving, for example, that means you're getting 18 calories from fat.
3. To determine the percentage of calories from fat, divide the number of fat calories by the total number of calories in a serving. If fat accounts for 20 percent or less of the total calories, Dr. Simone says, it's a "safe" food.

Here's a real-life example. You pluck a pint of frozen yogurt from the freezer case and read the label. Each serving has 140 calories. It also has four grams of fat. Multiply the grams of fat by 9 and you get 36 fat calories. To get the fat percentage, divide 36 by 140. You'll see that the amount of fat in each serving is about 25 percent of total calories—not bad, but a bit too high, in Dr. Simone's estimation.

Not every food in the supermarket has a label, of course. Trust your instincts. "Fruits, vegetables, grains and cereals are low in fat. Fish, as well as turkey and chicken without skin, generally derives 20 to 30 percent of calories from fat," Dr. Simone says. "Everything else is off-limits. That includes pork, beef, lamb, veal, dairy products (except for skim or nonfat products), diet margarines and cooking oils."

Back to Basics

Watermelon on a hot summer's night. Peppers and onions in pasta primavera. Extra helpings of vegetables—from broccoli and beets to summer squash.

Pat Boehle, director of volunteers and bereavement at the Comprehensive Home Health and Hospice in Brisbane, California, and mother of three, adopted this dairy- and red-meat-free eating plan for one good reason: to improve the odds that breast cancer won't return.

After a malignant tumor was removed from her right breast in 1991, Boehle was treated with chemotherapy and radiation. At the same time, she took control of her own health. She stopped eating ice cream, hamburgers and butter and switched to a diet high in fiber, low in fat and high in fruits and vegetables. So far she's cancer-free.

The hardest part? Feeding a family. "I try to follow a low-fat diet,"

Boehle says. "But I'm married, with three sons!"

Her motivation?

"I can remember sitting at the doctor's office," Boehle recalls. "I told him, 'My husband and I just redid our kitchen. I created a big sink. I want to be able to bathe my grandchildren.' I don't have any yet."

Her new eating strategy was recommended by her doctor, Robert Kradjian, M.D., a San Francisco breast cancer specialist and author of *Save Yourself from Breast Cancer*. Among American women, the lifetime risk of developing breast cancer is one in eight, Dr. Kradjian notes. In Asia and Africa, where women routinely follow a low-fat diet, the risk can be between 12 and 25 times lower.

Nutrition, according to Dr. Kradjian, is the only "logical and safe" way to prevent breast cancer.

Putting It All Together

Although some people are perfectly comfortable eating a diet that's extremely low in fat, most of us are more likely to steer a middle course. Even so, there are ways to make a good diet even better.

If you choose to indulge in small amounts of fat, for example—say, a little oil to splash on your tomato salad—make it olive oil, Dr. Simone advises. A monounsaturated fat, olive oil is thought to be healthier than the polyunsaturated kinds like corn oil.

"Research shows that polyunsaturated fats can promote cancer because free radicals attack them," Dr. Simone says. "The more polyunsaturated fats you have in your body, the higher your risk of cancer-causing damage to your cells."

Obviously, there's more to cancer protection than cutting back on dietary fat. Dr. Simone's nutritional plan also calls for maintaining a healthy weight, consuming fewer calories, getting 25 to 30 grams of dietary fiber a day, eating foods high in antioxidants, B vitamins and calcium, limiting al-

Meals to Blitz Breast Cancer

You don't have to be a gourmet chef to enjoy good food that's also good for you. In his book *Save Yourself from Breast Cancer*, San Francisco breast cancer specialist Robert Kradjian, M.D., gives examples of the kinds of meals that should be part of a protective diet. Breakfast in particular is important; it's essential to start the day with foods that are low in fat and filling and also provide plenty of cancer-fighting nutrients, such as beta-carotene.

Breakfast Oatmeal made with vanilla and water and topped with sliced peaches, apples, dates or bananas

1 or 2 slices whole-grain toast with fruit preserves or jam

Cantaloupe

Lunch Low-fat vegetable soup

Tomato-cucumber salad with vinegar or nonfat dressing

Tuna sandwich made with 2 slices whole-grain bread, 1 to 2 ounces water-packed tuna, nonfat mayonnaise, lettuce, tomato and sprouts

Apple, peach or other fresh fruit

Dinner Mixed green salad dressed with vinegar

Bean enchiladas made with corn tortillas and topped with salsa

Spanish rice

Lemon pudding made without egg yolks

---

cohol to one drink a week or less and eliminating barbecued, smoked and pickled foods.

Beyond diet, he advocates lifestyle changes such as giving up cigarettes, getting regular exercise and avoiding cancer threats like unnecessary x-rays and prolonged sun exposure. At the same time, you should have regular checkups, so if cancer does occur, you can catch it early.

"Cancers take 15 or more years to become evident," Dr. Simone says. "Changing your eating habits and lifestyle could slow the progression of any existing cancers dramatically. It's worth doing."

Going Even Lower

To decrease breast cancer risk, it's not enough for a woman to lower her intake of fat to 30 percent, the amount recommended by the NCI, says Robert Kradjian, M.D., a San Francisco breast cancer specialist and author of *Save Yourself from Breast Cancer*. He recommends that women begin by reducing dietary fat to 15 to 20 percent of daily calories. The eventual goal, he says, is to get that number down to 10 percent.

That's radical, according to some experts, but Dr. Kradjian bases his recommendation on population studies in rural countries that have low breast cancer rates and correspondingly low intakes of dietary fat. Some rural Chinese women, for example, derive just 6 percent of their daily calories from fat. They also have some of the world's lowest breast cancer rates.

While researchers continue to debate the role of dietary fat in breast cancer, Dr. Kradjian says he's convinced the link is powerful. At the same time he recommends a diet based on rice, potatoes, corn, beans, whole grains and pasta—and yes, lots of fruits and vegetables, which naturally contain cancer-inhibiting fiber, nutrients and protective food chemicals known as phytochemicals. Alcohol and tobacco should be avoided because of their known links to cancer, Dr. Kradjian says.

Eating Your Fill

Don't call Dr. Kradjian's meal guidelines a diet. They're not just short-term changes, he emphasizes, but a lifetime plan. The reason it works is that the foods taste good and are sufficiently healthful that you can eat as much as you like. In summary, here's what he recommends.

• Base your diet on foods that grow from the ground, such as rice, potatoes, corn, beans, whole grains and pasta made from wheat.

• Reduce total dietary fat to no more than 20 percent of total calories. Eventually, try to drop the number to 10 percent of calories.

• Eat a lot of cancer-fighting fresh fruits and vegetables. Of special importance, of course, are the pharmafoods, including soybeans, chick-peas, lentils, cruciferous vegetables, dark green, leafy vegetables and fresh fruits.

• Build up to 30 to 35 grams of fiber daily. Since most of us eat about half that amount or less, a gradual increase will ensure digestive comfort.

• Avoid dairy products—even nonfat milk. Dairy products contain what Dr. Kradjian considers to be excessively high amounts of animal protein— protein that he believes may lead to higher cancer rates. Low-fat or nonfat soy cheese, rice milk and soy milk make good substitutes.

You can get plenty of calcium from spinach, collards and other plant foods, says Dr. Kradjian: "After all, that's where the cow gets her calcium." However, once you cut back on dairy foods, it may take some careful planning to get the recommended daily amount. Green vegetables like broccoli and kale and soy products like tofu contain helpful amounts of calcium. If you're considering a supplement, check with your physician.

• Minimize or avoid alcohol. Water is the "ideal beverage," so drink lots of it with every meal and in between as well, suggests Dr. Kradjian.

• Avoid oils. If you must have a splash on your salad, make it olive oil—it's high in monounsaturated fat and has the least cancer-enhancing effect. Steer clear of polyunsaturated fats like corn, safflower, soybean, peanut, cottonseed, sunflower and sesame-seed oils, Dr. Kradjian says, because laboratory studies show that such vegetable oils are potent breast cancer promoters.

• Take a daily vitamin supplement containing vitamins C and E and beta-carotene.

• Go ahead and enjoy small amounts of nuts and seeds. Despite their high fat content, they're good sources of vitamin E and beneficial oils.

Essentially, this meal plan is very similar to ones practiced by our hunter-gatherer ancestors, says Dr. Kradjian. The benefits of such a plan make sense. After all, our bodies evolved on low-fat, plant-based nutrition. Modern diets have changed in a hurry; our bodies, however, have not.

"Not one in a hundred doctors accepts my viewpoint," Dr. Kradjian acknowledges. "But women who radically change their diets do better."

The Powers of Soy

Why do the Japanese have less prostate and lung cancer and also dramatically lower rates of fatal breast and prostate cancer than Americans? The secret may be soybeans.

"There is a theory, gathered from population studies in Japan and other Asian countries, that lower rates of some cancers may be due not just to a low-fat, high-fiber diet but also to soy," says Dr. Clifford. "Researchers are finding phytochemicals in soy that have anti-carcinogenic properties."

While Americans are familiar with soy as a milk substitute in baby formulas, other soy products like miso (a savory condiment), soy flour, tempeh (a meatlike patty) and tofu have been staples of Asian cuisine for thousands of years. In fact, Asians use soy in many of the same ways that Americans use meat.

In Asia, people eat about two to three ounces of soy a day, while Americans get about one-tenth that amount, if any. It's our loss. Many researchers, like Kenneth Setchell, Ph.D., of Children's Hospital Medical Center in Cincinnati, believe that soy can help prevent some cancers by blocking the harmful effects of estrogen, a hormone that's vital for a woman's reproductive health but can also spur production of cancerous cells.

Soy to the Rescue

Soybeans and soy products, notes Dr. Setchell, are major sources of genistein, which in laboratory studies has been shown to block animal estrogens and suppress the growth of tumor cells.

Soy may also reduce breast cancer risk by lengthening the menstrual cycle. Early in every cycle comes a burst of estrogen, so longer cycles would mean, over a lifetime, fewer estrogen surges. The menstrual cycles of Asian women are two to three days longer than those of Western women, which researchers speculate may partially explain the lower cancer rates.

Soy isn't for women only, of course. The same estrogen compounds that benefit women may help men stave off or at least survive cancer of the prostate, a gland that produces fluid for carrying sperm. As with other foods that contain phytochemicals, soybeans contain compounds that help block the action of cancer-causing enzymes and can help squelch tumor growth.

"All available evidence thus far suggests the idea that soy may be beneficial in preventing breast cancer and some other cancers," Dr. Setchell says.

What Are You Waiting For?

You don't have to wait for the final research results before slipping a little soy into your own diet. "Two to three ounces of soy protein a day will give you all you need," says Earl Mindell, Ph.D., professor of nutritional science at Pacific Western University in Los Angeles and author of *Earl Mindell's Soy Miracle*. "It's really not much at all. But it could be the next nutritional revolution."

Crumble tofu into chili. Broil marinated tempeh until brown. Substitute soy milk for regular milk in recipes, on cereal or in coffee.

Soy is excellent cuisine, but Dr. Mindell offers these cautions to keep in mind if you want to start eating more soy foods.

• Soy is no substitute for healthy eating. In other words, you can't munch doughnuts and fast-food hamburgers all week, then try to "recover" with a serving of soy. "I recommend a diet that gets 20 percent or less of its calories from fat," says Dr. Mindell. "You can't eat soy and expect it to overcome a high-fat, low-fiber diet."

• Soy products can be very high in fat. Three ounces of firm tofu, for example, contains seven grams of fat; in other words, more than half of its calories come from fat. "But remember, the fat is unsaturated, so it doesn't pose the dangers that saturated animal fats do," notes Dr. Mindell. It's also possible to buy low-fat soy products.

Tofu Temptation

A mild, cheeselike cake made from soy milk, tofu is high in protein and a variety of cancer-fighting compounds. It's also a very versatile ingredient. Tofu soaks up flavors from whatever it's cooked with, making it a great meat substitute in dishes such as chili, enchiladas and casseroles. It can also serve as a stand-in for cream cheese or ricotta cheese in a chocolate "cheesecake."

Depending on the brand and variety, a three-ounce piece of tofu has between 50 and 118 calories and up to 150 milligrams of calcium—the same amount as in a half-cup of milk. In general, the firmer varieties are higher in protein, fat and calcium.

There are two main types of tofu. Which you use depends on the recipe.

• Firm tofu holds its shape well during cooking and is recommended for recipes such as soups and stews. It can also be marinated, baked or grilled or crumbled into dishes such as salads and lasagna.

• Soft tofu is used when a soft, smooth texture is important, as in cream sauces, thick soups and puddings.

Nutrition for Recovery

If you have cancer or have recovered from it and want to do everything you can to stay in remission, what you eat can be a strong ally. Eating for recovery means more than just getting extra calories, says Dr. Nixon, whose book outlines a dietary recovery strategy. The point is to eat fewer of the foods that promote cancer and more of those that can prevent or even help reverse it.

"There's more and more data that fat and fiber can change what's happening with existing cancers," he says. "There's more and more evidence that fruit and vegetables play a strong role in preventing cancer. The major point is to do as much as you can to fight the disease."

The foods they eat can be particularly potent for people with those types of cancer that appear to have the strongest dietary links, like breast and colon cancer.

Lowering fat intake to 20 or 25 percent of total calories can help shut off a tumor's energy supply, says Dr. Nixon. Fruits and vegetables—like apricots, broccoli, carrots, spinach and sweet potatoes—are vital for their many cancer-fighting abilities. That's why Dr. Nixon recommends that you gradually change your diet until you're including as many as 11 servings of fruits and vegetables a day.

"If fruits and vegetables protect against cancer, it is reasonable to think that they support recovery as well," he notes. "While you're undergoing medical treatment, good nutrition is a bonus."

In Dr. Nixon's view, you don't have to give up good taste to have a great diet. You can enjoy fat-free chocolate pudding or angel food cake as an occasional snack. Try broiled tuna as a main course. If you find it hard to do without red meat, you can eat lower-fat cuts like top round and sirloin. And sweet pineapple and juicy strawberries are excellent dessert options.

"There are so many ways to tailor your diet and make it enjoyable," he says. "You can follow a healthy, cancer-preventive food plan and eat very well at the same time. That's what my wife and I do. We enjoy the heck out of our food."

16 Chronic Fatigue Syndrome

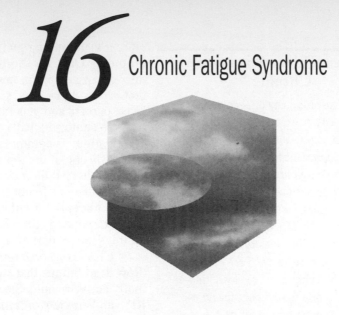

Eating to Build Energy

After Pat Hopkins was stricken with chronic fatigue syndrome, there wasn't much left that she could do.

"I could sit in a recliner and do some crosswork stitching," recalls Hopkins, of Bonner Springs, Kansas. "But that was only on good days.

"On bad days—which was every day during the first year—I couldn't even get out of bed. I might have an hour or two where I could sit up," she says.

Hopkins, now in her early sixties, recalls that her problems began in the early 1970s, years before doctors started diagnosing the syndrome. It wasn't until 1988, after batteries of tests and several misdiagnoses, that Hopkins was diagnosed correctly.

Today, she still has "good energy" for only about three hours a day. But she keeps herself going by following some simple rules: "I'm thankful for what I have. I get plenty of rest. And I'm careful about what I eat."

What's in a Name?

It's been called the yuppie flu and was thought to be caused by the Epstein-Barr virus (which causes mononucleosis) or possibly to be related to postpolio syndrome. It's been misdiagnosed countless times by countless health professionals. Even worse, it's been dismissed as "all in the head."

When Fatigue Becomes Chronic

The vast majority of people who feel fatigued are experiencing nothing more than a bout of tiredness due to a hectic lifestyle. But for the handful of people who have chronic fatigue syndrome (CFS), fatigue can persist for months or years, whittling away at their professional, social and family lives.

What are the clues that your fatigue may be caused by CFS? For one thing, CFS is characterized by a kind of fatigue that starts suddenly, for no explainable reason, and drags on for at least six months. If you have CFS and not just regular tiredness, sleep is no help. In fact, all the sleep in the world won't make it go away. It's generally accompanied by a host of other symptoms, including:

- Headache
- Low-grade fever
- Swollen lymph nodes
- Sore throat
- Depression
- Lack of ability to concentrate
- Some loss of mental quickness or fuzzy thinking
- Muscle and joint aches and pains
- Allergies
- Digestive problems
- Weight loss
- Rashes

If you have a number of these symptoms along with oppressive fatigue, experts recommend that you see your doctor.

It's chronic fatigue syndrome, or CFS, for short—a cornucopia of symptoms and signs that brings its victims' social lives, careers and general activities to a sputtering halt.

Fatigue is common. Nationwide, It's one of the top reasons that people visit their doctors. But CFS is vastly different from just feeling under the weather, burned out or depressed, although these feelings are all part of it.

CFS is out-of-the-blue, drop-dead fatigue that strikes normally active people. Sleeping like Rip van Winkle won't make it go away. It can drag on for months or years. The effects are so devastating that those with CFS often contemplate taking their own lives. Although many people with CFS recover on their own in a year or two, some never return to their old selves.

People with CFS also endure a whole lot more than just being tired. The balls and chains of this disease include short-term memory loss, diminished concentration, sore throat, painful lymph nodes, muscle pain (myalgia), headache, low-grade fever, muscle weakness and soreness and difficulty sleeping.

How many people have it? The answer to that question is almost as much of a mystery as the disease itself. Reports from the Centers for Disease Control and Prevention (CDC) in Atlanta have put the prevalence of CFS at between four and ten cases per 100,000 Americans over the age of

18. But those figures include only people who have been officially diagnosed by physicians according to the more stringent 1988 CDC criteria. Using other methods of counting, doctors believe that a more realistic number is between one and two million sufferers in the United States, according to Paul Cheney, M.D., a CFS specialist and director of the Cheney Clinic in Charlotte, North Carolina.

We do know that while it seems that white women have this burdensome disease more often than members of any other group, the syndrome may be undercounted among African-Americans, who tend to seek care for CFS less often. The incidence of CFS among African-Americans may actually be higher than among Caucasians, according to Dr. Cheney. It's also known that CFS generally strikes its victims around the age of 30 and most frequently sticks with them for a decidedly unlucky 7½ years.

Causes, Coping and Cure-Alls

As with arthritis, cancer and all the other mysterious diseases under the sun, you'll hear plenty of self-proclaimed authorities say that they've got a theory for CFS—and a cure. But none of the theories or the cures is proven.

That's not to say that reputable researchers don't have their educated theories. They do.

One of the most popular theories is that a virus triggers CFS and that somewhere along the line, the immune system goes haywire and starts attacking the body's healthy tissues. This is much like the progression that doctors see in people with rheumatoid arthritis, the inflammatory joint disease that can result in lifelong deterioration of bone and tissue.

Now scientists have added an interesting twist to that theory. It seems that people with CFS have a defect in an enzyme called carnitine acyltransferase, which is as serious as it sounds. Carnitine acyltransferase is the taxi service that transports fats into our cells and disposes of toxins, the waste products of cell operation. If the taxi doesn't run right, the cells don't get enough fuel, and their garbage disposal system goes on strike.

"A defect like this makes it a lot harder for people to create energy, and when they do, they build up toxins that they cannot remove," explains Dr. Cheney. "The more you push emotionally, physically or mentally, the more energy you make and the more toxins you build up. Then you crash."

What causes the carnitine acyltransferase defect? While no one can say for sure, researchers suspect free radical foul play. Free radicals are highly charged molecules in our bodies that wreak havoc on our healthy cells, damage body tissue and ultimately cause disease and aging. We create free radicals just by breathing, but we dramatically accelerate their production when we stress our bodies or increase our activity level.

"This theory makes sense when you look at people who commonly get this disease," says Dr. Cheney. "They are people who tend to be under tremendous stress and who push themselves."

Although there is no single cure for CFS, medical professionals armed with a knowledge of how this disease works biologically have been able to manipulate people's diets and lifestyles to make them feel more energetic and alive, if not shorten the disease process. Although these techniques are largely unproven, there is both clinical and anecdotal evidence that they can work.

"I treat CFS as if it's a pile of straws that has broken the camel's back," says Michael T. Murray, N.D., a naturopathic physician in Seattle and author of *Chronic Fatigue Syndrome: Getting Well Naturally*. "I try to eliminate as many straws as I can. Then I strengthen the camel."

The following are diet strategies recommended by a number of experts who practice alternative or complementary medicine. Even if you're receiving conventional medical treatment for CFS, these experts say that there are important alternative nutrition strategies that may help lighten your load.

No Artificial Ingredients

If your first stop in the morning is the local doughnut shop for a Danish-and-java breakfast and your last stop of the day is a fast-food drive-through window for a burger-and-fries dinner, you're just piling more straws on your already broken back.

Our modern diet of artificially colored, artificially flavored, processed and refined foods hurts our bodies on many levels, say alternative nutrition experts. This is especially true for people with CFS, whose immune systems are already compromised.

Some of the chemicals that are pumped into these foods, such as pesticides and preservatives, are potentially toxic to your system, says Allan Magaziner, D.O., director of the Magaziner Medical Center in Cherry Hill, New Jersey, who has been treating people with CFS for more than ten years. In addition, he says, the processed foods can rob you of essential nutrients.

"Processed foods are loaded with sugar, which may give you a very short burst of energy but in the long run suppresses white blood cell activity and depletes essential vitamins and minerals," says Dr. Magaziner. "You end up using the vital nutrients like B vitamins and chromium that you've gotten from healthy foods to metabolize all the sugar in your diet."

Not surprisingly, the diet that many doctors recommend for people with CFS is the same as what nutritionists have been recommending for years: Eat lots of vegetables, beans and rice, with very little red meat, fat, sugar and caffeine.

The Yeast-Free Diet

One early theory held that chronic fatigue was actually caused by chronic candidiasis, or a severe overgrowth of yeast in the body. Yeast is an organism that typically lives peacefully in the body's mucous membranes. But under certain conditions—sometimes related to taking antibiotics, birth control pills or steroids—the yeast can proliferate and crowd out the body's friendly bacteria.

Since women are more prone to yeast infections, some researchers believed that this "yeast connection" explained why women were overwhelmingly more likely to get CFS.

Although yeast overgrowth may not be the cause of CFS, experts agree that rising levels of candida yeast are a definite problem for people with CFS because yeast can weaken the immune system. And this yeast overload can make people with CFS feel even worse, say experts.

To fight yeast, some practitioners suggest following a special diet designed to exclude foods that may encourage yeast growth. Some clinical studies have found low-yeast diets to be of benefit in the treatment of CFS. Certain practitioners and their patients swear by them, especially for people who are exceptionally sensitive to yeast-containing foods.

If yeast is a problem for you, experts recommend clearing your cupboards of foods that either contain yeast or promote yeast growth. Top offenders include foods that need yeast to rise, such as breads, rolls, cakes and pizza crust; fermented foods, such as beer, wine, soy sauce and vinegar; and foods that contain mold or fungi, such as cheese and mushrooms.

You should also shake your sugar habit, say alternative healers. And that's not just the granular white stuff that you spoon into your coffee. It includes anything containing sucrose, glucose, fructose (fruit sugar), corn sweeteners, honey and maple syrup. Sugar not only robs your body of important nutrients, it also encourages yeast growth, according to doctors.

Playing Musical Foods

Some practitioners believe that the aches, tiredness and other symptoms that go with CFS are the result of the body's allergic reaction to some common foods.

You may be allergic to wheat, for instance. So while you think you're eating well by noshing on whole-wheat products, you're really filling up on food that your body will reject, making you feel worse.

At least that's the theory. But it's controversial. Although a few folks with CFS may have bona fide food allergies, most people with CFS really have food sensitivities, says Dr. Cheney.

"We've found that people with CFS become sensitive to almost anything they eat," he says. "That's because they have leaky guts," he observes—which is not quite as disgusting as the phrase implies. It simply means that they have trouble digesting protein, so bits of undigested proteins get into the small bowel and leak out, wreaking havoc on the body for a few days.

Fixing this is pretty simple, says Dr. Cheney. "Choose your proteins wisely, so digestion is easier. Flaky white fish is obviously a better choice than steak."

If you try this and still have trouble, you may have an actual food allergy, says Dr. Cheney. Some practitioners suggest trying an intricate food rotation plan, in which you rotate possibly allergenic foods in and out of your diet and monitor your reactions, or an elimination diet that requires you to replace foods you commonly eat with those you rarely eat.

Approach such diets with caution, warn experts. Studies have found them to be nutritionally incomplete, so you may run low on vitamins and minerals—and consequently on energy—when you're rotating out or eliminating nutrient-rich foods.

A more commonsense approach that most doctors recommend is to simply pay attention to how you feel after you eat. If you feel bad, try to figure out which food caused the reaction and eliminate it.

The Usual Allergy Suspects

If you do suspect that "something you ate" has made you feel worse, you probably won't need Sherlock Holmes to find the culprit. Those knowledgeable about CFS can round up the usual suspects pretty quickly.

One top offender is alcohol, which has the obvious drawback of being a big-time depressant. Others include sugar, fat and dairy products. And you're likely to give your body a boost if you avoid other tough-to-digest items such as fried foods and red meat, say experts.

Although sugar and fat are pretty well known nutrient robbers and energy sappers, the dairy dilemma often surprises a generation brought up on milk as the provider of strong bones and healthy teeth. While it may still give a killer smile to those who can stomach it, it means bloating, gas and diarrhea for those who are lactose-intolerant, meaning that they can't digest milk sugar. (For the full story on lactose intolerance and what to do about it, see "When Milk's No Natural" on page 312) The thing to remember is that all of the intestinal problems may be even worse for those with CFS.

Doctors report that people with CFS seem to do worse when they overload on dairy foods, simply because they are tough to digest. Digestion requires a lot of energy, and that's something people with CFS don't have.

"Most of us become lactose-intolerant as we grow older," says Peter Manu, M.D., director of the Medical Services Department of Psychiatry at

Long Island Jewish Medical Center in Glen Oaks, New York, and associate professor of medicine and psychiatry at Albert Einstein College of Medicine of Yeshiva University in the Bronx. Dr. Manu simply recommends cutting out dairy. "We eat too much cheese and drink too much milk," he says. "They are highly indigestible foods."

Building Strength with Supplements

Everyone knows that vitamins and minerals are an integral part of a good diet. The right nutrients keep our immunity strong and our bodies running at peak efficiency. It only makes sense then that people with CFS need at least the Daily Value (DV) of essential vitamins and minerals, and probably much, much more, say experts.

That's why doctors say that nutritional supplements are as important to the diets of people with CFS as fruits, vegetables and grains. The following are the key nutrients that experts recommend you include in your daily regimen.

Muscling Up with Magnesium

When a group of British researchers found that people with CFS had below-normal levels of magnesium within cells and that the same people felt better when they received supplementation, some thought magnesium was going to be the great glistening hope for those with CFS. Without question, it's an important mineral for energy production at the cellular level.

Today researchers concede that getting more of this mineral may not work for everyone, but many still stand by the scientific and anecdotal evidence supporting magnesium supplementation.

"Whether we give it orally or by injection, we see people with CFS gain energy when we supplement them with magnesium," says Dr. Magaziner.

Magnesium works not necessarily because people with CFS are magnesium-deficient, explains Dr. Cheney, but because they have enzyme deficiencies that impair their cells' ability to convert food into energy. Magnesium supplementation seems to stimulate production of such enzymes, so cells generate more energy.

Experts who recommend supplements often specify a daily dose of about 500 milligrams, which is 25 percent above the DV that's recommended for health maintenance. They recommend chelated magnesium, either magnesium glycinate or magnesium asparate, which are rapidly absorbed by the gastrointestinal tract. If you have kidney or heart problems, you should check with your doctor before taking supplemental magnesium.

You can also up your dietary intake of this energy-boosting mineral by including more peanuts, bananas and wheat germ in your diet.

Because magnesium increases your body's need for calcium, you should take calcium supplements as well, say experts, who generally recommend taking twice the amount of calcium as of magnesium.

Ante-ing Up with Antioxidants

But what about the theory that CFS is the result of free radical damage to cell membranes? If that theory is true, it only makes sense that you'd want to take antioxidants that bond with the free radicals and slow the destruction that they can cause. It's a way to help preserve the cell membranes so that they can do their job by letting in the nutrients that make energy.

Antioxidants, which include vitamin C, vitamin E, beta-carotene and selenium, are important members of your body's vice squad—sucking up free radicals and helping deactivate them before they can do their dirty deeds.

As important as antioxidants are, however, researchers are finding that they're not lone heroes and are best used in combination with natural compounds called bioflavonoids.

"We're finding that the people we treat actually get worse if we give them only vitamins and minerals," says Dr. Cheney. "That's because antioxidants themselves can sometimes become free radicals, so we need compounds to buffer the free radicals once the antioxidant has scavenged them, and those are bioflavonoids, such as proanthocyanidin."

"By using a combination of antioxidants, bioflavonoids and chelated minerals, we have been able to reduce people's free radical levels within five weeks," he observes. "Although reducing free radicals doesn't make you feel better per se, people do notice that they have more endurance, so they can push further before crashing."

Experts recommend that people with CFS take the following antioxidants daily: 1,000 to 3,000 milligrams of vitamin C, 25,000 international units of beta-carotene, 400 to 800 international units of vitamin E and 50 micrograms of selenium. These recommendations are higher than DV levels. For some people, this much vitamin C can cause diarrhea. And you should talk to your doctor before taking more than 600 international units of vitamin E.

They also recommend that you include more antioxidant-rich foods in your diet. Citrus fruits, tomatoes and red bell peppers are great sources of vitamin C. Include wheat germ, almonds and some vegetable oils in your diet to get your vitamin E. Carrots, broccoli and sweet potatoes will provide beta-carotene, while canned tuna is a convenient source of selenium.

Beating Fatigue with the Bs

Anyone who's experienced chronic fatigue knows that the mental depression and stress it causes can be even more crippling than the physical fatigue itself.

When it comes to lightening that mental load, experts agree, the *B* in B-complex vitamins stands for "boost."

"The B vitamins are important for people with CFS because they're key vitamins for brain and central nervous system function, and they're involved in energy production," says Dr. Magaziner. They also help support the adrenal glands, which are important players in the body's reactions to stress, he says.

"When you're stressed or fatigued, your body uses more B vitamins," adds Dr. Manu. "Making matters worse, people with this condition also tend to suffer from malnutrition because they're not eating as much as they should, and they're eating the wrong things, like sugary, processed, refined foods that actually rob the body of B vitamins."

Because B vitamins are so important, vitamin B_{12} is actually used as a drug by some doctors, who inject massive doses of the nutrient into the muscles. This technique works to improve energy levels in about 30 percent of people with CFS, reports David S. Bell, M.D., a clinical instructor at Harvard Medical School and co-author of *Curing Fatigue: A Step-by-Step Plan to Uncover and Eliminate the Causes of Chronic Fatigue*.

You can also get B-complex vitamins in most multivitamin/mineral supplements, say the experts. Dr. Cheney recommends that people with CFS get at least 50 milligrams each of thiamin, pantothenic acid and vitamin B_6, along with 400 micrograms of vitamin B_{12}.

To get more vitamin B_{12} in your diet, reach for foods such as tuna, nonfat yogurt, fish, chicken and low-fat cheese, which are rich in this vital nutrient.

Charging Up with Coenzyme Q_{10}

Ask someone if he's had his dose of coenzyme Q_{10} today and he'll probably give you a look usually reserved for alien life forms. But even though it sounds like something from *The X-Files*, coenzyme Q_{10} (coQ_{10}) is a common nutrient that may be just what you need for fatigue, say experts.

CoQ_{10} is one of those nutrients, like vitamin K, that our bodies make for themselves, although we also eat it in foods like soybeans, vegetable oils and meats. It's similar in structure to a vitamin, and it has super antioxidant powers like vitamins C and E and beta-carotene. These qualities alone make it a good supplement for those with CFS.

But there's more. This supernutrient acts like a spark plug for your body, reacting with other enzymes so your cells can convert protein, carbohydrates and fats into energy.

"People with CFS frequently say they feel better with coQ_{10} supplementation," says Dr. Magaziner.

Does that mean they're deficient in coQ_{10}? Not necessarily, says Dr. Cheney. "More likely, they're low in the enzymes that defend against free radicals produced in our bodies' energy factories, the mitochondria," he explains. Such a deficiency may be counteracted by coQ_{10}, Dr. Cheney says.

"We recommend using sublingual coenzyme Q_{10} lozenges instead of tablets; otherwise the liver uses it all," adds Dr. Cheney. He recommends supplementing with about 200 milligrams of the nutrient daily. Lozenges are difficult to find, but you can ask your pharmacist about ordering them for you. Some pharmacies may also be able to make lozenges using coQ_{10} powder, a process known as compounding. But you'll need to discuss this with your doctor, because a prescription is required.

More Iron for Your Fire

When we think of iron, we think of power and force, à la "Iron" Mike Tyson, which is why women with CFS should also think of iron, according to Dr. Murray.

Iron deficiency can be an underlying cause of fatigue problems among women in their childbearing years. "It can also really exacerbate an existing problem with fatigue," says Dr. Murray.

"I love it when someone has an iron-deficient blood sample, because it means they'll be easier to treat," says Dr. Murray. He recommends that people with iron deficiencies take two 500-milligram capsules of hydrolyzed (liquid) liver extract a day. "It provides the best iron without the fat and cholesterol," he says. You can also add iron to your diet by eating Cream of Wheat cereal, tofu and quinoa, a grain that can be cooked like rice.

17 Diabetes

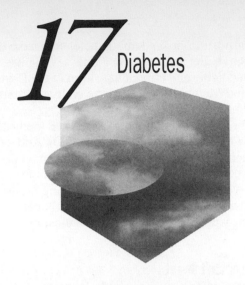

Big Benefits from Small Changes

Once in a while, Barbara Parks plucks a tiny Tootsie Roll from her secretary's candy jar, indulging her abiding love for chocolate.

These days it's a special treat, because Parks, a Minneapolis working mother with two children, has completely revamped her diet since learning she has diabetes.

Out went potato chips, sugar-saturated desserts and oversize portions at meals. In came fiber-rich fruits and vegetables, low-fat pretzels and granola bars. When Parks gives in to her sweet tooth and enjoys a Tootsie Roll or a piece of chocolate cake, she compensates by not eating something else that day.

Because of her diligence, she hasn't needed medication at all for her diabetes. "My doctor gave me some time to see if food and exercise could control it. I'm lucky: They did. Now I feel much better. I've lost 32 pounds. And I exercise five or six days a week on my stationary bike," she says.

Little adjustments—for great rewards. If you are one of the approximately 16 million Americans with diabetes or if your doctor says you're at risk for developing it, food can be your most powerful ally. In fact, by controlling blood sugar levels with diet, you can prevent a host of diabetes-related health problems, from fatigue and weakness to heart disease, blindness and kidney failure.

So powerful is the role of diet that up to two-thirds of people with

Type II, or non-insulin-dependent, diabetes (the most common type) can manage it through diet and exercise alone, says James Anderson, M.D., professor of medicine and clinical nutrition in the Division of Endocrinology and Metabolism at the University of Kentucky College of Medicine in Lexington.

"Even for people with diabetes who need medication, diet still matters for controlling blood sugar and blood fats," Dr. Anderson adds.

How effective is diet? In a study at the University of California, Los Angeles, 652 people with Type II diabetes ate a low-fat, high-carbohydrate diet for three weeks. Most also added a walking program. Afterward, 71 percent of those taking oral medications and 39 percent of those using insulin injections were able to stop using medication.

When Sugar Isn't Sweet

As many people know, or quickly learn when they develop diabetes, controlling this condition hinges on controlling blood sugar, or glucose.

People with diabetes have no trouble making glucose, which comes from complex carbohydrates like pasta and bread and from simple carbohydrates like sugars. Their problem is getting glucose into cells where it's needed. The reason is that they lack a chemical "key," called insulin, that essentially unlocks cells to let glucose in.

When insulin is in short supply or isn't working efficiently, glucose accumulates in the bloodstream and relatively little finds its way into cells.

In people who have the more severe form of diabetes, called Type I, or insulin-dependent, specialized cells in the pancreas that make insulin are largely inoperable. This condition requires treatment with synthetic insulin.

Type II diabetes is far more common and generally less severe. About nine out of ten people with diabetes have Type II, which typically strikes after age 40.

With Type II diabetes, the pancreas produces some insulin, but not quite enough. Some people will feel quite ill, but more often the effects are subtle. You may feel tired and hungry—a result of your cells not getting enough glucose. You may be very thirsty and have to urinate often, sometimes three or four times a night. Over time you may begin to lose weight as your body draws on fat reserves to make up for the missing glucose.

Even in those who don't know they have diabetes, however, damage is being done. "The long-term complications with diabetes are life-threatening," says Aaron Vinik, M.D., Ph.D., director of the Diabetes Research Institute in Norfolk, Virginia. Impotence. Heart attacks. Strokes. Kidney damage. Blindness. Nerve damage. Without treatment, the consequences can be dire.

Can you relieve or even reverse this condition? In most cases, experts say, the answer is yes. Here's how.

Healing Yourself with Food

"Nutrition therapy is absolutely the cornerstone of diabetes control," says Marion Franz, R.D., director of nutrition at the International Diabetes Center in Minneapolis. "To be honest, it's also the most challenging aspect of living with diabetes. After all, food is with us all the time."

The link between diabetes and diet has been suspected for a very long time—although the "solutions" weren't always the best. As early as 1500 B.C., health-conscious Middle Easterners wondered if a diet of fruit, wheat and sweet beer could dry up the excessive urination caused by diabetes. In the eighteenth century, experts advocated a protein-only plan. As recently as 1900, near-starvation was generally the treatment of choice.

Today, nobody's recommending beer, wall-to-wall protein or an empty plate for good health. But proper nutrition is still considered the key for controlling diabetes. The approach you choose, however, depends on your particular circumstances. The best eating plan is one that's tailored to your total health, not just your diabetes, says Abhimanyu Garg, M.D., associate professor of internal medicine at the Center for Human Nutrition at the University of Texas Southwestern Medical Center in Dallas.

"It's an individual decision, based on taste and food preferences and also on what a person's doctor perceives as the goals for that person, such as weight control or lowering the risk of heart disease, along with controlling blood sugar," says Dr. Garg.

Custom Cuisine

If everyone with diabetes were the same, it would be easy to create a one-size-fits-all eating plan. But there's a huge variation, not just in how people react to the condition itself but also in lifestyle factors that affect how they handle it.

Eight of ten people with diabetes are overweight—but two of ten are not. Four of ten could have high levels of LDL (low-density lipoprotein) cholesterol, the "bad" kind of blood fat that raises your risk of heart disease and stroke—but six of ten may not.

For one person, giving up or cutting back on sweets might be as easy as a shrug and a "no thanks" at dessert time. For someone else, a strictly controlled diet might feel like a prison sentence.

Since everyone is different, experts have devised a number of scientifically proven meal plans. Each of these plans can help get blood sugar under control. You and your doctor or dietitian will want to choose a plan that takes a number of different factors into account: whether you also have high cholesterol, for example, or whether you need to lose a few pounds. Or you might choose one diet over another simply because you'll enjoy it more.

If you have diabetes, you should consult a doctor or nutritionist about a food plan that's right for you. For virtually everyone, however, one of the diets that follow—or a combination of elements taken from each one—will help keep blood sugar under control.

The American Diabetes Association Diet

More a set of flexible guidelines than a rigid diet, the American Diabetes Association (ADA) plan stresses getting an abundance of fiber and carbohydrates and also recommends cutting back on saturated fat. And unlike the ADA's older recommendation to eliminate sugar, this new approach allows for the occasional sweet treat and offers new choices for controlling the amount of carbohydrates and fat you consume. The plan can be adjusted to help you lose weight or maintain a healthy weight and lower cholesterol and triglycerides as well.

Experts have long recognized that giving up favorite foods can be one of the most troublesome aspects of controlling diabetes. In fact, when doctors advised complete abstinence from birthday cake, sweet sodas, snack foods and so on, more often than not people cheated and ate them anyway. As it turns out, there's nothing inherently bad about sugary foods if they're eaten in moderation and as part of a sensible eating plan.

The guidelines also let you adjust the amounts of fat, carbohydrates and protein you eat, and as long as you keep your blood sugar, weight and cholesterol under control, how you apportion these different elements is to a certain extent up to you. For most people, following the guidelines will readily control high cholesterol levels and reduce excess pounds while controlling blood sugar, says Christine Beebe, R.D., vice-president of the ADA and diabetes program director at St. James Hospital and Health Center in Chicago Heights, Illinois.

Beef up with carbs. According to the ADA guidelines, carbohydrates should make up the bulk of your diet. The actual amount will vary from person to person. For some people, carbohydrates will make up 40 percent of the diet; for others they'll be as high as 70 percent. You'll need to work with a doctor or nutritionist to find the amount that's exactly right for you.

Cut back on protein. In people with diabetes, too much protein, particularly animal protein, may be harmful to the kidneys. (Plant proteins appear to be less harmful.) The ADA plan recommends getting between 10 and 20 percent of daily calories from protein.

Slice off the fats. For the population at large and for people with diabetes, experts generally advise getting 30 percent or less of total calories from fat. More specifically, try to limit saturated fats to 10 percent or less of total calories, with the rest coming from polyunsaturated and monounsaturated fats such as olive oil.

Enjoy a snack—sometimes. Dessert lovers rejoiced when the ADA reported that some sugar, at least for most people with diabetes, is perfectly fine. This was quite a breakthrough, because for years it was thought that a candy bar, a piece of cake or a bowl of ice cream could have dangerous re-

Easy on the Sweets

The alternative diet for people with diabetes has traditionally focused on the importance of avoiding sweets. Now the guidelines from doctors in the American Diabetes Association (ADA) permit people to enjoy small amounts of sweets. But that doesn't mean that the old sweet-free diet is out the window; going overboard can still cause problems.

"If I had pie and cake every day I'd be obese—and I'd miss the nutrition found in fruits, vegetables and other carbohydrates," says Davida Kruger, R.N., senior vice-president of the ADA.

Every time you have a sweet, you need to subtract another carbohydrate (or even two or three) from your diet in order to keep blood sugar levels stable. Here's how it works.

Check your treat for carbohydrates. For every 30 grams of carbohydrates listed on the label, you need to remove one carbohydrate serving from somewhere else in your diet.

For example, one serving of vanilla ice cream may contain 30 grams of carbohydrates. In terms of carbs alone, that means giving up a large apple or one-third cup of rice, for example, or a small potato or four or five crackers.

Check the fat. For every five grams of fat in the sweet treat, you'll have to remove one fat serving from elsewhere in your daily diet. How can you cut out that teaspoon of fat? By eliminating a teaspoon of oil, mayonnaise or peanut butter.

Consider the consequences. Even though a small piece of cake may be "equal" to a piece of whole-wheat bread and a teaspoon of margarine in terms of carbohydrates, it doesn't have the same power to fill you up, and it may have much more fat. So you have to swap carefully in order to fill up without filling out. "You have to look at the pluses and minuses," according to Kruger.

---

sults for someone with diabetes. Experts now know that all carbohydrates, not just sugar, raise blood sugar levels and that careful eating will keep them under control.

"Sugar is no longer off-limits," says Beebe. "Of course, you can't pig out on cake. What we're saying is, sweets are carbohydrates, and people with diabetes need to pay attention to all the carbs they eat. That's the big message."

Plan ahead. Since as far as your body is concerned, all carbohydrates are created equal, sometimes having one food means going without something else later on. The goal is to keep your blood sugar levels as steady as possible, no matter what you eat.

Don't forget fiber. Experts advise getting 20 to 35 grams of fiber a day, which is two to three times the amount most of us currently get. There are a number of ways to load up each day. Having three to five daily servings of vegetables is a good start (a serving is a half-cup of cooked vegetables or one cup of raw veggies). Add two to four servings of fruit (a serving is one piece or one cup of fresh fruit). In addition, you'll need one to two servings of whole grains daily.

The advantage of the ADA's plan is that it's supremely flexible. "We adjust the plan to meet people's needs," says Franz. "Maybe someone just needs to lose a few pounds and would eat less fat. Or maybe their weight is fine but their blood cholesterol or triglycerides—kinds of blood fats—are high, and they may experiment with a diet that's higher in monounsaturated fat for that. Or blood sugar control may be your only issue. We can help by raising or lowering calories and carbohydrate and fat levels."

Critics of the plan argue, however, that it may be too flexible—that many people with diabetes should be getting tougher rules and restrictions than the ADA delivers. It's really up to you and your doctor. You may be one of those who need a very specific diet. "Many people with diabetes are overweight and have high blood lipids and high blood pressure," says Dr. Vinik. "You need some rules."

The High-Carbohydrate, High-Fiber Diet

Developed at the University of Kentucky, this plan stresses whole grains, beans, fresh fruit and vegetables and is often recommended for those who need to lose weight and lower cholesterol. Fiber-rich foods are at the heart of this diet, which was pioneered by Dr. Anderson, author of *Dr. Anderson's High-Fiber Fitness Plan.*

"I believe fiber—particularly the soluble fiber found in large amounts in beans, oat bran and some fruits—has a dampening effect on absorption of sugars into the bloodstream," says Dr. Anderson. "You don't get a rush of glucose. That way, if your body still makes some insulin, that insulin will work better because it can handle smaller amounts of glucose."

This diet calls for 25 to 40 grams of fiber a day. Just as important, he says, the plan lowers fat to 20 to 25 percent of daily calories and protein to 15 to 20 percent—in both cases, about a third less than most of us consume daily.

"Fat sort of dissolves insulin receptors," explains Dr. Anderson. "Cutting it makes your cells more sensitive to insulin again. And I personally believe that animal protein is detrimental to the kidneys, which can fail in people with diabetes. Why wait for kidney failure to cut your protein intake? I think it's helpful to reduce the protein sooner and avoid kidney damage."

Joining the Bean Counters

High-fiber breakfast cereals, lunchtime salads with low-fat dressings, broiled fish and generous amounts of produce are the stars of this plan. And so are beans. Just ask Norman Atkins of Lexington, Kentucky, who has been following this diet for more than three years. He eats beans at lunch and dinner.

"The diet really helps me," says Atkins, who is in his early seventies. "Before, I had such blurry vision I couldn't keep the car on the road. I had to stop driving. Now I drive everywhere, and I walk two miles every day. I feel great—and I don't take diabetes medication anymore."

Becoming drug-free is a hallmark of this diet, says Dr. Anderson. By his own count, normal-weight people with Type II diabetes can cut their insulin needs in half—or even down to zero—on this plan. Cholesterol readings drop 30 percent, and blood pressure goes down 10 percent. People with Type I diabetes have been able to reduce their insulin use by 10 to 35 percent, he says.

The Mediterranean Plan

Based on the traditionally healthy diets of Italy, France and other Mediterranean countries, this diet differs from our own in that most of the fat calories are derived from plant-based monounsaturated fats such as olive and canola oils. Unlike the saturated fats that come from animals, monounsaturated fats seem to reduce LDL cholesterol. And some studies suggest that monounsaturated fats may help reduce blood pressure and blood sugar as well.

For thousands of years, people living in Mediterranean countries have enjoyed diets rich in fruits, vegetables, whole grains, olive oil and small amounts of protein, says David Robbins, M.D., director of research in atherosclerosis and diabetes at Medlantic Research Institute and professor of medicine at George Washington University, both in Washington, D.C.

"People who eat this way traditionally have less diabetes and heart disease," says Dr. Robbins. "Of course, they exercise regularly, too."

Now scientists here have been able to confirm what researchers witnessed overseas. In a study conducted at the University of Texas Center for Human Nutrition, people who were given a diet quite high in monounsaturated fats—that is, a diet similar to those enjoyed in the Mediterranean region—did better at controlling blood sugar levels, LDL cholesterol and triglycerides than did people on a high-carbohydrate diet.

For this diet to work, however, it's essential to cut back on saturated fats and get more of the heart-healthy monounsaturated kind, says Dr. Garg, who led the study. The diet he recommends gets less than 15 percent of calories from animal fats and polyunsaturated vegetable fats and 20 to 25 percent from monounsaturated fats, found in olive oil, canola oil, nuts and avocados.

"I think we can recommend this higher monounsaturated fat diet as a lifetime diet for many people with diabetes," Dr. Garg says. "The fat level is closer to what Americans already eat—they would just have to switch the

Mediterranean Flavor

Beef sizzled in olive oil. A snack of almonds. Sugar cookies. Muffins made with canola oil.

Even before researchers in Texas, Minnesota and California concluded that a Mediterranean diet could lower blood sugar and cholesterol in people with Type II diabetes, volunteers in the study were sure of one thing.

"They loved it!" says Pat Schaaf, R.D., research dietitian and certified diabetes educator at the General Clinical Research Center of Stanford University Hospital in California, who helped plan the menus for the study.

Not intended for weight loss, the diet was designed to keep the volunteers' weight constant throughout the study, so total daily calories were calculated specifically for each participant. The diet gets 40 percent of calories from carbohydrates, 15 percent from protein and 45 percent from fat—including 25 percent monounsaturated fats like olive or canola oil, avocados and nuts. The moderate fat content makes this menu satisfying to eat, but if you try this plan, remember that you need to carefully measure all of the ingredients to keep total calories, carbohydrates, protein and fat in check. "This nutrient distribution isn't a license to eat as much fat as you desire," notes Schaaf. Here's a sample of the foods from one day's research menu.

Breakfast ⅔ cup grapefruit sections with 1 teaspoon sugar
Medium oat bran muffin with 1 ounce peanut butter
½ cup skim milk
Black coffee or tea if desired

Lunch Sandwich made with 2 ounces beef fillet (sautéed in ½ tablespoon olive oil), 2 slices wheat bread, lettuce and ½ tablespoon mayonnaise
Carrot sticks
Medium sugar cookie

Dinner 2 ounces chicken breast served over ⅔ cup spaghetti and topped with olive oil gravy*
½ cup broccoli
Salad made with lettuce and tomato, with ½ tablespoon olive oil and vinegar to taste
½ cup canned peaches

*To make olive oil gravy: In a medium nonstick skillet, whisk 1 tablespoon whole-wheat flour into 1 tablespoon olive oil over medium heat, then thin with ¼ cup water and simmer gently.

kinds of oils they use and choose more monounsaturated-fat foods over foods high in saturated fat, like meats and cheese."

He recommends it particularly for people whose diabetes is not well-controlled on a high-carbohydrate diet. "If LDL cholesterol and triglycerides are remaining high, then this program may help," he says.

It's worth noting that this diet is perhaps most unlike the traditional American diet in its sparing use of protein. "Meat and fish become a seasoning, sprinkled in smaller amounts on top of pasta or vegetable dishes," says Dr. Robbins. "I prefer keeping total fat to 20 to 30 percent of calories, with most as polyunsaturated or monounsaturated fat."

One word of caution: A gram of fat has about twice as many calories as a gram of carbohydrates. "People with diabetes have to watch their calories, no matter what the source," adds Dr. Garg. "Obesity makes this disease worse."

An "Eating Smart, Eating Easy" Plan

Some people with diabetes do best with a highly structured, day-by-day eating plan. But for others, "one or two small changes might be all a person needs in order to have big success controlling diabetes," says Susan Thom, R.D., a nutritionist and certified diabetes educator who owns a consulting company, Nutri-flex, in Cleveland.

Indeed, this is often the secret of success, nutritionists say. Small changes can help control blood sugar and lower the risk of heart disease and other diabetes-related complications later on. "One woman who came to me was drinking six cans of sugary cola a day," Thom says. "She said it would be easy to switch to diet soft drinks and she did, cutting out almost 1,000 calories per day. She lost weight, and her blood sugar dropped to normal in two weeks."

Whittle your weight. If you're overweight, dropping even a few pounds can dramatically improve your blood sugar control, says Dr. Robbins. As a result, you'll feel more energetic, and diabetes-related complications like blurry vision, tingling fingers and a too-frequent urge to urinate may become things of the past.

"Most research suggests that losing just 10 percent of your weight can help," Beebe says. "That means if you weigh 200 pounds, you don't have to get down to 140. You could get down to 180 and see improvements."

What's more, the benefits are almost immediate. "The impact comes within two days to six weeks of beginning a weight-loss plan," says Dr. Robbins. "Blood sugar levels improve. Cholesterol and triglyceride levels do, too. Consuming less calories seems to make the cells of your body more sensitive to insulin."

If you are at high risk for diabetes, weight loss is your best prevention plan, he says. "Staying close to your ideal, healthy weight, through diet and exercise, is the most effective way to avoid diabetes.

Trimming a little flab may save you a little money as well. In a study at the University of Kentucky College of Medicine, researchers found that people with diabetes who lost—and kept off—about 20 pounds spent $440 less a year on diabetes medicines and supplies.

Cut back on saturated fats. "High-fat diets make people more insulin-resistant," says Dr. Anderson. "They also tend to make you overweight. And eating too much saturated fat can raise your chances for heart disease, which

Taking Charge with Exercise

If stumbling to the coffee pot at dawn and reaching for the potato chips at night is your idea of staying in shape, you're missing out on a powerful weapon against diabetes: burning calories.

"People with diabetes spend so much time talking about food that they often forget about the other facet of diet—the energy they're expending," says David Robbins, M.D., director of research in atherosclerosis and diabetes at Medlantic Research Institute and professor of medicine at George Washington University, both in Washington, D.C. "If you have diabetes, exercise improves blood sugar levels." At the same time, your body's cells become more sensitive to insulin almost immediately.

Any exercise is good. At a minimum, say experts at the Joslin Diabetes Center in Boston, you should aim for 20 to 40 minutes of continuous activity at least three or four times a week. Brisk walking, dancing, stair climbing and team sports like soccer and basketball are all great for diabetes control.

How important is regular exercise? In one study, Swedish researchers put 41 men with Type II diabetes on a weight-reduction and exercise program. After six years, half no longer had symptoms of diabetes.

In the same study, 181 men with borderline diabetes went on a weight-control and exercise program. Five years later, three-quarters of them had normal blood sugar levels.

is already a problem for people with diabetes." Here are some ways to reduce saturated fat in your diet.

• Sauté foods in water or low-salt broth instead of using oil or butter. Use enough liquid to keep the foods from sticking to the pan, and add more liquid as necessary. Or you can use a nonstick pan lightly misted with nonstick cooking spray.

• Substitute plain, nonfat yogurt in recipes that call for sour cream.

• Swap low-fat or skim milk for whole milk.

• In recipes that don't require cooking, replace sour cream with a look-alike consisting of equal parts of low-fat yogurt and low-fat cottage cheese beaten until smooth.

• Replace each whole egg in recipes with two egg whites plus a tablespoon of vegetable oil. Or use egg substitutes.

• Eat more fish or skinless chicken and less red meat. When you do decide to have meat, choose the leaner cuts, and make sure you eat less than six ounces per day.

Work on your timing. If you eat large meals close together or let yourself go without eating for so long that your body is running on empty, you're creating fluctuations in blood sugar that may be difficult for your body to handle.

"If you can allow four to five hours between breakfast and lunch and put five to six hours between lunch and dinner on a regular basis, that can make a big improvement in blood sugar levels," says Franz.

Stay in balance. To help keep blood sugar levels constant, you should shoot for an "ideal" balance of protein, carbohydrates and fats with every meal. Generally, this translates into having three or four carbohydrate servings per meal plus a little bit of meat at lunch and dinner, according to Franz. Good carbohydrate choices include:

- A cup of skim or low-fat milk or plain, low-fat yogurt.
- Three-quarters of a cup of dry, unsweetened cereal.
- One-third cup of rice.
- A half-cup of cooked pasta.
- One-half of a medium banana.
- 12 to 15 grapes or cherries.
- One medium apple, peach or pear.
- One-third to a half-cup of fruit juice.

Keep up with fiber. Dietary fiber is one of the most important ingredients in any diabetes control plan. "Putting more fiber in your diet by switching from refined to less refined fruits, vegetables and grains helps improve blood sugar control and can lower cholesterol levels," says Dr. Anderson.

Fiber is found in all fresh fruits and vegetables. Instead of orange juice, have a whole orange. Snack on baby carrots and broccoli florets. Have a baked potato and eat the skin. Other high-fiber foods include brown rice and whole-wheat breads, he says.

Beans, oat bran and fresh fruit like apples and pears are especially rich in soluble fiber, the kind that makes the most positive impact on blood sugar and cholesterol levels. "But Mother Nature provides some soluble fiber in most foods, so you'll be getting some no matter what you eat," Dr. Anderson notes.

Make changes slowly. People who suddenly start eating more fiber often experience cramping, gas and other uncomfortable digestive problems, says Belinda M. Smith, R.D., research dietitian for the Metabolic Research Group at the Veterans Affairs Medical Center in Lexington, Kentucky. That's why experts advise moving gradually to a fiber-filled diet.

Here's Smith's plan for an easy transition.

- This week, have a high-fiber cereal for breakfast three or four days.
- Next week, start adding additional fiber by having some fresh fruit instead of drinking juice, for example.
- The following week, add still more fiber by substituting beans for ground beef or by having an extra serving of vegetables.

"Make one change and see how it goes before making another," she suggests. "We've had people go hog-wild on oat bran muffins, for example, and really feel discomfort. Slower is better."

Stay afloat. Fiber absorbs tremendous amounts of fluid, so when you increase your fiber intake, be sure to drink more water as well. Experts advise drinking at least six to eight full glasses (eight ounces each) of water a day.

Fast Fiber

Even if you're grabbing breakfast, lunch and dinner on the run, you can still have a high-carbohydrate, high-fiber diet.

The following one-day plan is recommended by James Anderson, M.D., professor of medicine and clinical nutrition in the Division of Endocrinology and Metabolism at the University of Kentucky College of Medicine in Lexington. Intended for occasional on-the-go eating, this menu provides 1,800 calories and 32 grams of fiber.

Breakfast Whole-wheat bagel with 1 ounce light cream cheese
Banana
½ pint skim milk
Black coffee

Snack ½ cup raw cauliflower and broccoli from salad bar

Lunch Fast-food, low-fat, light taco
Serving of pinto beans and cheese
Peach
Water

Snack Oat bran muffin

Dinner Fast-food grilled chicken sandwich with 1 packet reduced-calorie salad dressing
Small serving of fast-food chili
Unsweetened iced tea

Snack 1 packet instant oatmeal, made with water, topped with small box raisins.

An added benefit of drinking water is that it keeps you feeling full, which also helps keep weight under control, says Davida Kruger, R.N., senior vice-president of the ADA. While sugar-free liquids like diet soda, coffee or tea can be counted toward your daily water quotient, milk, fruit juice and sugary drinks cannot. "They count as carbohydrates that will raise your blood sugar," says Thom.

Drink cautiously. Most experts agree that a moderate intake of alcohol—one or two drinks a day—usually won't cause problems. For people taking insulin or oral diabetes medications, however, caution is advised.

"The danger is that you may think you're feeling the effects of a drink or two when actually your blood sugar is getting dangerously low," Beebe says. "We recommend having the drink with a meal or a snack to counteract the blood sugar–lowering effect of the alcohol."

Consult the experts. At first, switching to a diabetes diet can feel like trying to learn a new mathematical formula. To make the transition, experts say, it's extremely helpful to consult a nutritionist or certified diabetes educator. Or contact your local hospital or the ADA at 1-800-DIABETES for free diabetes information, including nutrition facts.

18 Digestive Problems

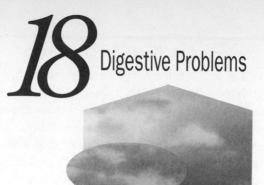

Ease Them with Food

In the Balkans, constipated folks swallowed molasses for relief.

In Wales, mothers cured their children's diarrhea with milk warmed with a poker fresh from the fire.

In England, munching a raw potato is still touted for cooling heartburn.

From burdock root for gallbladder woes to cinnamon for irregularity, food has long been the choice all over the world for relieving digestive problems.

It's different in America today: We go to the drugstore instead, and we spend over $1 billion a year on over-the-counter laxatives, antacids and anti-diarrhea medicines. Yet experts say more than half of us would be better off reaching into the pantry first.

"It's easier to take a pill than to alter your eating habits," notes Steven R. Peikin, M.D., professor of medicine and head of the Division of Gastroenterology at the University of Medicine and Dentistry of New Jersey, Robert Wood Johnson Medical School at Camden. "But so often, food is a better alternative than medicine for digestive problems."

Happily, there are many food alternatives for digestive trouble, so you're likely to find one tailor-made to ease your gut reactions. In this chapter, for instance, you'll find a healing new eating plan for inflammatory bowel disease (IBD), an age-old vegetarian solution to constipation, a

The "Get-Regular" Bran

Wheat bran. For people bothered by constipation, this mildly nutty-tasting outer layer of the wheat grain is proof that good things come in small packages—in this case, in tiny flakes.

"Wheat bran is the first food we recommend for constipation," says Arnold Wald, M.D., professor of medicine and associate chief of the Division of Gastroenterology and Hepatology at the University of Pittsburgh Medical Center. "It's almost entirely insoluble fiber, which bulks up the stool, drawing in water to make it softer. The bowels actually don't have to work as hard to move a big, soft stool."

Flaky or finely powdered, yellowish to russet brown, wheat bran is low in calories and high in fiber. Two tablespoons weigh in with 15 calories and three grams of mostly insoluble fiber, the kind that helps ease elimination.

Wheat *bran* shouldn't be confused with wheat *germ*. Wheat bran is the outer covering of the wheat grain, while wheat germ is the grain's inner core, or embryo. Both have their strengths. Wheat bran is lower in calories and higher in fiber, while wheat germ is nutrient-packed: It's full of folate, a B vitamin vital for producing red blood cells, and vitamin E, which has powerful protectant qualities.

Here's how to get more wheat bran in your diet.

Sprinkle it liberally. Add two to three tablespoons of wheat bran or 100% All-Bran cereal to low-fiber foods like yogurt, applesauce and cornflakes. Mix some into casseroles, meat loaf and homemade breads and muffins, suggests Jennifer K. Nelson, R.D., clinical dietetics project manager in the Division of Endocrinology, Metabolism and Internal Medicine at the Mayo Clinic and Foundation in Rochester, Minnesota. "The key thing is to use wheat bran," she says. "Eating small amounts of bran or other whole grains throughout the day, along with lots of water, can ease constipation."

Choose whole grains. "Make sure your bread and your breakfast cereal contain whole wheat if you're concerned about constipation," says Dr. Wald. "It's the easiest and cheapest way to get bran in your diet." Whole-grain cereals include bran cereals, shredded wheat, Wheatena and Ralston.

When buying bread, look for more than the word *wheat* on the front label—scan the ingredients list and make sure whole wheat is listed first, which means that there's plenty in the loaf.

Bring your own. For an easy, portable snack, carry unprocessed bran, available in the grains section of most health food stores, mixed with a bran cereal in a plastic container, suggests Nelson. "Sprinkle it on salads, have a little snack of yogurt dusted with the cereal or just eat the cereal out of the container," she says. "It's convenient."

doctor-tested strategy that calms irritable bowel syndrome (IBS) and a hospital-endorsed comfort plan for diarrhea, to name just a few.

Getting Regular—Naturally

Smooth, efficient regularity. It's one of the first benefits that people who adopt a vegetarian lifestyle enjoy—and one that you may have noticed without realizing the cause after a vegetarian-style dinner like meatless chili or a vegetable stir-fry over brown rice.

The reason? Things "go" better with fiber, an important, indigestible substance found in the walls of plant cells. And there's fiber galore in the fruits, vegetables, beans and whole grains that are at the center of a meatless eating program.

"Fiber bulks up the stool. It has water-holding properties," says Louis N. Aurisicchio, M.D., a gastroenterologist in private practice in Carmel, New York. "As a result, the stool becomes smoother and passes more easily."

While the American Dietetic Association recommends that we eat 20 to 35 grams of fiber a day, most of us shortchange ourselves, getting less than half that amount. But vegetarians get more than the recommended daily fiber quotient, eating two to three times as much fiber as meat-eaters.

As a result, they're less bothered by constipation. And, says Dr. Peikin, less constipation means more comfort—plus a lower risk of diverticulosis and diverticulitis. Fiber is also recommended if you have IBS with constipation.

A Twinkie or a Strawberry?

The truth is, you don't have to give up meat entirely to benefit from the fiber advantage that vegetarians enjoy. But you do have to eat more like a vegetarian, choosing produce and grains that are as close to "natural" as possible. Unrefined grains that undergo little or no processing contain more fiber.

"A hundred years ago, people went to the grocery store and got bushel baskets of food, like fresh fruit and vegetables," says Dr. Peikin. "Now we come out with Twinkies and potato chips and white bread and other highly refined foods. There's no bulk there, no fiber to maintain gastrointestinal health. Any highly processed, highly refined food will be constipating."

Experts say that insoluble fiber—the kind found in highest concentrations in wheat bran, whole grains and vegetables like cauliflower, green beans and potatoes (with the skin)—is best for beating irregularity. Soluble fiber is the other type of food fiber—the kind that helps lower cholesterol levels—and can be found in beans, peas and some fruits and vegetables.

More Power in Prunes

Nutritionists love to sing the praises of constipation-fighting dried fruit: It's sweet, virtually fat-free, portable and loaded with fiber.

Five dried pear halves weigh in with more than 11 grams of fiber, three dried figs have 5 grams, and a half-cup of raisins has 4 grams. "Look for packages of dried fruit as a convenient way to carry fruit," says Jennifer K. Nelson, R.D., clinical dietetics project manager in the Division of Endocrinology, Metabolism and Internal Medicine at the Mayo Clinic and Foundation in Rochester, Minnesota.

But fabulous fiber can't explain the mysterious laxative power of prunes. A mere handful of these dark, sweet nuggets (1½ ounces, or about five prunes) does have three grams of fiber, but that's not all, according to Stephen B. Hanauer, M.D., professor of medicine and clinical pharmacology at the University of Chicago Medical Center and co-author of *Inflammatory Bowel Disease: A Guide for Patients and Their Families*.

The magic extra in prunes? "It's phenolphthalein," says Dr. Hanauer. "Small amounts in prunes stimulate the intestines to move. It's the same thing used in some laxatives, like Feenamint and Correctol."

Nature has conveniently packed both types into most of the fiber-rich foods you'll find in the grocery store. It's a happy coincidence—in fact, having the two together is a benefit.

"If people simply look for high-fiber foods, they don't really have to worry about whether the fiber is soluble or insoluble," says Henry D. Janowitz, M.D., clinical professor emeritus of medicine and consultant in gastroenterology at Mount Sinai School of Medicine in New York City. "Just getting more fiber into your diet is what's helpful."

A study of elderly patients at a Virginia nursing home found that most cut their laxative use in half after just four weeks on a high-fiber regimen combined with more fluids, exercise and scheduled time on the toilet. "If it works in older people, it should work even better in younger people," says Dr. Janowitz. That's because most younger people have better muscle tone and higher activity levels and are less dependent on laxatives.

Fitting Fiber In

Switching to a meat-free, high-fiber diet can be as simple as ordering the beans and rice at your local Mexican eatery or substituting spinach for ground beef in your favorite lasagna recipe. Here are more fiber-packed, vegetarian-style suggestions from doctors and nutritionists.

Go meatless. Meatless entrées and side dishes that spotlight fresh vegetables, whole grains and fresh fruit can really boost your fiber intake, says

Filling Up on Fiber

You can help prevent constipation by making high-fiber diet choices at breakfast, lunch and dinner, says Steven R. Peikin, M.D., professor of medicine and head of the Division of Gastroenterology at the University of Medicine and Dentistry of New Jersey, Robert Wood Johnson Medical School at Camden. Five servings of fruit or vegetables a day, plus six servings of whole-grain breads, cereals or legumes will give you the 20 to 35 grams of fiber recommended by doctors and dietitians. A typical serving could be one apple or a half-cup of whole-wheat pasta. Here are some great sources of fiber in order of fiber content.

Food	Portion	Fiber (g.)
General Mills Fiber One cereal	½ cup	13.0
Health Valley Fruit & Fitness cereal	¾ cup	11.0
Kellogg's All-Bran cereal	⅓ cup	10.0
Nabisco 100% Bran cereal	½ cup	10.0
Chick-peas	½ cup	7.0
Kidney beans	½ cup	6.9
Lima beans	½ cup	6.8
Refried beans, canned	½ cup	6.7
Black beans	½ cup	6.1
Post Raisin Bran cereal	⅔ cup	6.0
Whole-wheat spaghetti	1 cup	5.4
Lentils	½ cup	5.2
Succotash	½ cup	5.2
Guava	1	4.9
Navy beans	½ cup	4.9
Barley	½ cup	4.4
Pear	1	4.3
Blackberries	½ cup	3.6
Brussels sprouts	½ cup	3.4
Raspberries	½ cup	3.0
Baked potato (with skin)	1 medium	2.2
Broccoli	½ cup	2.0
Spinach	½ cup	2.0

Dr. Peikin. Start by experimenting with meatless lunches or dinners once or twice a week, then add more meat-free days to up your "roughage quotient."

"I think you can acquire a taste for vegetables, beans and whole-grain breads," Dr. Peikin says. "You would be amazed at how many nights you can go without meat and not miss it. Besides being dense in calories and usually high in fat, meat has no fiber—and it tends to be constipating."

Don't be a big cheese. Cheese has no fiber and is high in fat—two rea-

Meeting Emission Standards

You know the old ditty: Beans, beans, they're good for your heart. The more you eat, the more you ... well, the more you pass gas.

By nature, we human beings are gas producers, manufacturing one to three pints daily and releasing it as often as 23 times every 24 hours. It's perfectly normal, yet even the words for gas evoke embarrassment and even discomfort.

But beans may not be the only cause of that unwanted, uh, natural gas. You can often take steps to reduce your gas production and relieve uncomfortable bloating by paying attention to your eating style and food choices, according to Jennifer K. Nelson, R.D., clinical dietetics project manager in the Division of Endocrinology, Metabolism and Internal Medicine at the Mayo Clinic and Foundation in Rochester, Minnesota. Here's how.

Eat less of the gas makers. Many starchy and fiber-rich foods cause gas, as do some natural sugars. Reactions may vary from person to person, according to the National Institutes of Health (NIH) in Washington, D.C. Try minimizing gas by eating smaller quantities of these gas-producing prime suspects.

• Corn, potatoes, noodles and wheat products, which produce gas as they're broken down in the large intestine.

• Soluble fiber, found in oat bran, beans, peas and most fruits. (In contrast, insoluble fibers like wheat bran produce almost no gas.)

• Raffinose, a natural sugar found in large quantities in beans and to a lesser extent in cabbage, brussels sprouts, broccoli and asparagus.

• Lactose, a milk sugar that many people can't digest. African-Americans, Native Americans and Asian-Americans are more likely than others to have trouble digesting lactose.

• Fructose, another natural sugar, which is found in onions, artichokes, pears and wheat and used as a sweetener in soft drinks.

---

sons to enjoy it in moderation if you're concerned about constipation or other health problems like overweight or heart disease, notes Dr. Aurisicchio.

Make fiber an all-day thing. Increase the fiber content of breakfast, lunch and dinner by remembering a few simple rules, says Jennifer K. Nelson, R.D., clinical dietetics project manager in the Division of Endocrinology, Metabolism and Internal Medicine at the Mayo Clinic and Foundation in Rochester, Minnesota. Here's how.

• Aim for at least two servings of whole-grain products at each meal. At breakfast, this could be whole-grain cereal (oatmeal or a high-fiber cold cereal) and a piece of whole-wheat toast, a double portion of cereal (about 1½ cups) or two slices of whole-wheat toast. At lunch and dinner, the choices include whole-grain bread and side dishes like brown rice, barley or whole-wheat pasta.

- Sorbitol, a fruit sugar found in fruits such as apples, pears, peaches and prunes. Sorbitol is also used as an artificial sweetener in sugar-free candies and chewing gums.
- High-fat foods, including fried foods, rich pastries and rich sauces and gravies.

Make low-wind choices. Black-eyed peas, chick-peas and lima beans cause less gas than green beans, pintos or small white beans. Soybeans and black and pink beans are the biggest gas producers.

Rinse away the gas factor. Cut flatulence in half by soaking dried beans for four to five hours before cooking, then discard the water. Add fresh water, cook for a half-hour, then discard that water. If the beans need more cooking time, add fresh water and continue cooking. This helps remove indigestible sugars that cause gas in your gut.

Slow down. If you eat fast, drink fast or even talk fast, you may be swallowing excess air that's bound to resurface with a loud "U-u-u-rp!" says Henry D. Janowitz, M.D., clinical professor emeritus of medicine and consultant in gastroenterology at Mount Sinai School of Medicine in New York City. A mellower pace could banish some belches.

Begin with Beano. Love beans, hate the gas? Sprinkle three to ten drops of Beano, which is available at health food stores and some supermarkets, on your serving. Beano supplies the enzyme that our bodies lack for digesting raffinose, the sugar in beans and many other vegetables, according to the NIH. But it doesn't reduce the gas caused by fiber or lactose.

Swallow some charcoal. Activated charcoal tablets may reduce intestinal gas if you take two to four just before eating and again one hour after meals, according to the NIH.

- Be a fruit fan. Fruit's great with cereal, refreshing at lunch and elegant in a fresh fruit cup for dessert. "The take-home message is, have fruit at each meal," says Nelson. "Try to eat it with the skin on—like a fresh pear or peach—for more fiber." Most berries are also good fiber choices.
- Add vegetables. Have one or two helpings of vegetables with lunch and dinner. Try carrot sticks with a sandwich, a side salad (with low-fat dressing) at a fast-food restaurant or even quick-cooking precut frozen veggies at dinner.

Tote a snack. Pack high-fiber crackers in a sandwich bag and tuck it into your purse or briefcase. That way you'll always have an instant, high-fiber alternative to the typically low-fiber offerings in the office snack machine, suggests Nelson. "Some crackers even come individually wrapped, which makes it very convenient," she notes.

Garnish with the good stuff. For eye appeal and an extra dose of fiber, sprinkle a quarter-cup of raisins over cereal or rice for an extra two grams of fiber. Add wheat germ, with four grams of fiber per quarter-cup, to baked goods or hot cereal. Dust grain dishes with wheat bran—there's an extra three grams of fiber in every two tablespoons.

Build up slowly. Increase your fiber intake gradually to avoid the uncomfortable gas, bloating and even diarrhea that can accompany a rapid change to a fiber-rich regimen. "Add fiber slowly and give yourself time to adjust," says Dr. Aurisicchio. "Go from 10 grams a day to 15, then to 20 and so on until you reach 25 to 30 grams per day. Add a serving or two of a high-fiber food and make sure you're comfortable before adding more." (Some doctors recommend getting as much as 35 grams of fiber a day.)

The Rest of the Regularity Regimen

A strategic diet to relieve constipation can be more effective at keeping you regular than over-the-counter medications, says Dr. Peikin. Beyond fiber, focus also on getting plenty of water or other liquids like juices, soups and skim milk. It also helps if you limit your intake of caffeine and alcohol.

Such a plan works best for mild to moderate constipation, which doctors say you have if you have fewer than three bowel movements per week or if you have difficulty or pain while passing a stool. If you suffer more serious and persistent constipation or are over 40 and have sudden, severe constipation, see your doctor. The cause could be an obstructing growth, impacted fecal matter or the side effect of some medications such as those commonly prescribed to control high blood pressure or depression, says Dr. Aurisicchio.Otherwise, add these steps to your regularity program.

Try psyllium. If you find you cannot eat enough fiber or are ready to reach for a laxative, try psyllium, suggests Roger Gebhard, M.D., professor of medicine at the University of Minnesota in Minneapolis and staff physician at the Minneapolis Veterans Administration Hospital. "For many people, psyllium is the simplest way," Dr. Gebhard says. "Look for products like Metamucil that say they contain psyllium, and follow the instructions on the package."

Quaff, quaff, quaff. It's important to drink plenty of water or other liquids such as juice and soup when embarking on a high-fiber diet. Fiber absorbs liquid in the intestine to form a soft, bulky stool. How much is enough? The Mayo Clinic suggests eight to ten eight-ounce glasses a day.

A Comfort Plan for Diarrhea

Perhaps it was the potato salad that sat too long in the afternoon sun. Or maybe you changed the baby's diaper and forgot to wash your hands.

Whatever the reason, when you've got diarrhea, it feels more like diarrhea's got you. You're running to the bathroom over and over again, cramped with stomach pains, able to think of nothing except reaching the toilet in time.

Well, if you often find yourself in this scenario, here's one small comfort—you are not alone. The National Institutes of Health (NIH) in Bethesda, Maryland, estimates that Americans endure 99 million bouts of the runs every year, caused by everything from drinking tainted water to eating improperly handled food. And if you're a parent or a child-care worker who sometimes forgets to wash up after swaddling your young charge in a clean diaper, you're offering a first-class invitation to diarrhea.

If you add a slew of other factors, including travel abroad, stress, lactose intolerance, antibiotics, long-distance running, antacids and artificial sweeteners such as sorbitol, the number of cases soars past the 100 million mark.

Is it serious? Most often it's not, says Dr. Peikin, but you should see your doctor if diarrhea persists for more than a week, is bloody or is accompanied by a fever or feelings of dehydration. Serious causes that need treatment range from IBS and thyroid problems to a malfunctioning pancreas.

For short-term diarrhea that's caused by the flu or other bug, Dr. Peikin says the main thing is to stay comfortable and drink plenty of soothing liquids until it's over.

"Clear soups, Jell-O and other bland, liquid-based foods are best," he says. "They soothe your stomach and keep you from being dehydrated at the same time."

Coping When You're Out of Commission

A typical run-in with the runs that lasts just a day or two doesn't merit a trip to the doctor's office. Chances are it's a viral or bacterial infection, and the volumes of watery stool you're seeing are the result of toxins given off by the bug invading your bowels. The toxins stick to the walls of the intestine, making cells there secrete massive amounts of fluid.

When you're temporarily grounded, doctors suggest the following tips to help your body weather the thunderstorm in your gut.

Consider clear liquids. The Mayo Clinic suggests a clear liquid diet for sudden, short-term diarrhea. The benefits? This simple plan allows your bowels to rest while replacing the fluids that your body loses to diarrhea.

"Dehydration is the major concern when you're waiting for the end of a bout of diarrhea," says Nelson. "Most of us can go without solid food for a day or two, but you could dehydrate quickly without fluids. This is especially important for older people and young children. Dry eyes, a dry

(continued on page 314)

When Milk's No Natural

They flash 1,000-watt smiles from the pages of glossy fashion magazines: famous athletes and celebrities, each sporting a milk mustache. The commercial message? Drink up—milk's rich in bone-building calcium.

But hold that glass of moo for a moment. If you're one of the 50 million American women and men who are lactose-intolerant, milk's no celebrity. For members of this very large club, downing an ice cream cone or even a frosty glass of skim milk brings on bloating and gas—and maybe diarrhea.

What's going on? If you are lactose-intolerant, your body doesn't make enough lactase, the digestive enzyme that splits big molecules of milk sugar, or lactose, into smaller sugar molecules that your body uses for energy.

"You wind up with unabsorbed sugar in your colon," says Louis N. Aurisicchio, M.D., a gastroenterologist in private practice in Carmel, New York. "This leads to the cramps, gas and bloating."

Lactose intolerance is so common—affecting as many as three out of four African-Americans and nine out of ten Asian-Americans—that doctors actually say that adults who can digest milk are the unusual folks. Most are of Northern European descent.

"No mammal was intended to drink milk past the weaning years," says Jack A. DiPalma, M.D., associate professor of medicine and director of the Division of Gastroenterology at the University of South Alabama College of Medicine in Mobile. "Lactase levels start dropping soon after birth. In some people, the levels drop quickly. In others, it takes longer. In some people, levels never drop low enough to cause a problem."

Leaving Lactose Behind

You may be lactose-intolerant if downing one or two glasses of milk on an empty stomach tends to cause trouble. If the uncomfortable, telltale symptoms arrive within 30 minutes to two hours, the cause is probably dairy products, says Dr. Aurisicchio. But see a doctor to be certain.

"If you're going to make a lifetime change in your diet, it's important to be sure that you have definitely been diagnosed with lactose intolerance," says Dr. DiPalma. "Other digestive problems like irritable bowel syndrome can mimic lactose intolerance."

Fortunately, people with lactose intolerance can still enjoy many dairy products—even a cool glass of milk—and get sufficient calcium by making a few dietary adjustments. Here's how.

Drink just one glass. Most people who are lactose-intolerant can probably digest the 12 grams of lactose found in a single glass of skim or low-fat milk, says Dr. Aurisicchio. Whole milk's got slightly less lactose, but it has more calories due to its higher fat content.

"I suggest, especially to women age 25 or older, who need plenty of calcium in their diets, trying one glass of low-fat or skim milk or an ounce or two of low-fat cheese," he says. "Unless you are highly lactose-intolerant, your body should be able to digest it."

Team dairy with meals. Sip your milk or munch your cheese at breakfast, lunch or dinner to increase lactose digestion. "When you eat dairy products as part of a meal, digestion takes longer, and your body actually has more time to break down the lactose. With more time, whatever lactase you do possess has a better chance to process some of the sugars," says Dr. Aurisicchio.

Go for active cultures. The bacterial cultures that convert milk into yogurt produce an enzyme that breaks down up to 40 percent of the lactose in yogurt. Buy brands that say "live cultures" or "active cultures" on the label, since these can help you digest more of the lactose in the yogurt, says Dr. DiPalma.

Note: Frozen yogurt may lack the enzyme advantage, says Dr. Aurisicchio.

Say cheese. If you're lactose-intolerant, choose hard, aged cheeses rather than softer kinds. Thanks to a process that removes most lactose-rich milk solids, cheeses such as Swiss, Cheddar and Jarlsberg contain less lactose than soft cheeses like mozzarella, notes Dr. Aurisicchio. Reduced-lactose cheese is available in some supermarkets.

Give your lactose a boost. Milk treated with lactase is available two ways—70 percent and 100 percent lactose-reduced. Both kinds cost more and taste sweeter than regular milk, but you can get a wide selection, including whole, low-fat and skim, as well as calcium-fortified and even chocolate varieties.

Improve upon nature. Lactase enzyme supplements, taken just before meal-time, digest milk sugars for you, says Dr. DiPalma. They're handy if you're eating out or are sharing a meal with others who are not lactose-intolerant.

"If I eat a big bowl of ice cream, I get a bellyache, but if I take a supplement first, there's no pain," he says. "I've found that you may need to use a fair amount more than the label says. If it calls for taking two or three pills, you may need as many as six to eight. Through trial and error, you will discover how many are best for you."

Supplements are available under a number of brand names. Of three major brands tested in a 1993 study at Baylor College of Medicine in Houston, Lactrase outperformed Lactaid and Dairy Ease in relieving symptoms.

Put drops in your moo juice. You can purchase liquid lactase drops that convert regular milk right in the carton. Put five drops in a quart of milk, and up to 70 percent of the lactose disappears in 24 hours. To convert more milk sugar, add more drops or wait up to 72 hours.

Sip soy or rice. Soy milk and rice milk, both available in health food stores, are lactose-free. If you like milk for your coffee or need it for your cereal, consider these alternatives.

tongue or a higher temperature could be signs of dehydration."

You can avoid it with plenty of clear liquids such as broth, fruit drinks and juices, carbonated beverages, lemonade and weak tea as well as ice pops and gelatin desserts.

One word of caution: Because this diet is not nutritionally complete, you should follow it for only a day or two before adding more solid foods.

Add a sports drink. Consider a sports drink to offset the loss of electrolytes—minerals and salts vital for the normal functioning of your body's cells. "Diarrhea is not just water. It's also lost electrolytes such as sodium and potassium," Dr. Peikin says. "What helps is something that also has sugar in it, which helps keep the salt in your body."

Don't drink the coffee. Limit your intake of alcohol and caffeinated drinks like coffee, cola and strong tea. These may not only irritate your bowel but can also act as a diuretic and increase urinary fluid loss, Nelson notes.

Rein in the roughage. Bran, whole grains, beans, fruits and vegetables with seeds or skin and other fiber-rich foods may actually aggravate sudden-onset diarrhea. For the same reason, you should try to avoid nuts, seeds, dried fruit like raisins and prunes and raw fruits and vegetables, suggests Nelson. For some people, bananas or applesauce may be helpful. They contain pectin, a gel-like compound that can help firm up loose stools.

Keep it tepid. Some people find that piping hot and very cold foods may bring on more bowel movements, so keep your food and liquids lukewarm or at room temperature to avoid yet another trip to the bathroom, suggests Nelson.

Keep it simple. If you're hungry, stick with light, low-fiber foods like white rice or white toast, suggests Nelson. And keep the menu bland and oil-free: Greasy, fried or spicy dishes may irritate sensitive intestines that are already under siege. Tender meat, fish or poultry, refined cereals like puffed rice, cornflakes and Cream of Wheat, and well-cooked fruits and vegetables without seeds or skin are also good choices.

Say "no, thanks" to milk. Avoid milk and dairy products during—and for a few days after—a bout of diarrhea, suggests Dr. Peikin. "Even people who are not lactose-intolerant could temporarily have trouble digesting lactose (milk sugar) when they have diarrhea," he says. "And that could make the diarrhea worse."

Tiny, fingerlike projections in your small intestine produce the enzyme that digests lactose. But diarrhea can damage them. "They will repair themselves, but it could take a week or so," says Dr. Peikin.

Calming Irritable Bowel Syndrome

Renee Ozier was enjoying lunch with her husband at his Dallas office when suddenly "it hit me out of the blue—cramping, pain and a whooshing

Cooling That Acid-Backwash Burn

A double helping of lasagna. Chocolate chip cheesecake. Espresso with a lemon twist. What a feast—and what a classic recipe for heartburn.

"What people eat and when they eat it are among the causes of heartburn," says Henry D. Janowitz, M.D., clinical professor emeritus of medicine and consultant in gastroenterology at Mount Sinai School of Medicine in New York City. "Often a change in habits can prevent it."

Heartburn is really just a teaspoon or two of stomach juices backwashing out of the tummy and into the esophagus—the tube that carries food from your mouth to your stomach. Laced with harsh hydrochloric acid, the juices burn the tender lining of the esophagus. Over time, acid reflux, as it's also known, can carve deep ulcers. In rare cases, the irritation leads to a precancerous condition called Barrett's syndrome.

Even if you use an antacid, adjusting your eating habits is still an important part of the heartburn control equation. Here's how the experts suggest putting those strategies into practice.

Lose weight. Carrying extra pounds around your middle acts just like tight pants or a girdle, creating pressure that can help propel acid upward, says Dr. Janowitz.

Baby your esophagus. Citrus and tomato juices, alcohol, carbonated drinks and coffee—both caffeinated and decaf—may irritate the esophagus. So can extremely hot, cold or spicy foods, says Dr. Janowitz. Steer clear.

Keep the pressure on. For reasons experts don't entirely understand, fatty and fried foods as well as chocolate and peppermint act to relax the opening to the stomach—and that opens the door for acid reflux.

"Also, something like chocolate, which contains caffeine, could stimulate acid production," says Dr. Janowitz. "So you'd be setting the stage two ways for heartburn by eating chocolate. I advise patients to avoid these foods."

Report to the mess hall on time. Eating meals on a regular schedule is helpful because it prevents a buildup of irritating stomach acids, says Dr. Janowitz. "The size of the meal is important," he adds. "Having a skimpy breakfast and a skimpy lunch, followed by a huge dinner, increases pressure in your stomach, which stimulates acid production."

Be an upright citizen. After dinner, don't lie down for at least three hours. "The goal is to give your stomach time to empty before lying down to sleep," says Dr. Janowitz. And when you do go to bed, you can help keep reflux in its place if you elevate the head of your bed on six-inch blocks or sleep on a specially designed wedge.

---

sound like Niagara Falls in my stomach."

She raced home, reaching the bathroom just in time. Irritable bowel syndrome (IBS) had struck again.

"The attacks of diarrhea and pain would last for two or three hours and really wear me out," says Renee, 33, a former actress and mother of four. "The attacks were happening three times a week. I even had one in the airport in London. I would just pray 'Please, God, get me through this.' "

She got through it. Following a doctor-designed diet, she now avoids trigger foods like milk and caffeine. With that diet, plus prescription medication, she's brought the painful, embarrassing bowel spasms of IBS under control.

"This change in my way of eating is for a lifetime," she says. "IBS doesn't go away. But my life is so much better now—I can plan things and do things."

Food: A Problem and a Solution

Once in a while we all come down with a little diarrhea, a tummyache or constipation. But you have IBS—and should see a doctor—if any of these telltale signs become chronic: changes in stool frequency, changes in stool consistency (from watery to hard, for example), excessive straining, passage of mucus and bloating of the abdomen.

Beyond discomfort and inconvenience, IBS can throw a monkey wrench into the smooth running of your life, causing sleepless nights, canceled social plans and disrupted intimacy with your partner.

"IBS is not life-threatening, but it can be a nuisance for some and a life-altering experience for others," says Dr. Gebhard. "No one really knows the reason it happens, but it seems to be abnormal spasms in the small intestine and colon. The wrong foods can set things off, and so can anxiety or tension or an important deadline at work."

News to Digest

Today, there's reassuring news for the one in five Americans with IBS: You can fine-tune your diet to relieve constipation, control diarrhea or soothe gas pains and bloating.

"Sometimes one or two changes will make a big difference—like cutting out soda pop if you can't digest the high-fructose corn syrup in it or avoiding caffeine, which can cause diarrhea," says internist Gerard Guillory, M.D., assistant clinical professor of medicine at the University of Colorado Health Sciences Center in Denver and author of *IBS: A Doctor's Plan for Chronic Digestive Troubles*. "The more we learn about IBS, the more we can pinpoint specific treatments."

When Renee Ozier went to see Dr. Guillory, for example, she learned that she has lactose intolerance, meaning that her body cannot digest milk sugar. She now avoids dairy products or uses low-lactose versions. In addition, she steers clear of beverages containing caffeine, which can bring on diarrhea. She's added more fiber to her diet and, on the advice of Dr. Guillory, varies her diet so she doesn't eat any food more often than about twice a week.

Your own food strategy for IBS, Dr. Guillory notes, will depend on whether you experience mostly constipation, diarrhea or gas and abdominal pain—or a combination of these. It will also be tailored to any individual food sensitivities or intolerances.

"I ask people to look at what they're eating and find patterns in their meal choices and how they're feeling," says Dr. Guillory. "It's the starting point."

Ozier agrees.

"Before I found this diet, I had doctors tell me that I simply needed to relax. But I always knew it was more than that," she says. "Tranquilizers didn't help my IBS. Meditation helped a little bit. But this is a bowel problem—my bowels do not work the way a normal person's do. That's what has to be addressed to handle IBS."

Table Manners for IBS

There's no cure for IBS, and sometimes food alone doesn't even provide total relief. Doctors sometimes recommend over-the-counter medications containing loperamide for diarrhea, fiber supplements to relieve constipation and prescription spasm-stopping medicines to block the clutching pain that many with IBS feel after eating. Relaxation exercises are often suggested, too.

Nevertheless, food comes first. And no matter what your IBS symptoms are, start with the following "table rules" to help ease a clenching gut.

Eat slowly. Chew your food carefully. Savor the flavor. Bolting meals can lead to overeating and then to indigestion, bloating and abdominal pain, says Dr. Guillory.

Eat on time. Sitting down to regular meals helps keep your digestive system on a schedule, says Dr. Guillory. Jennifer Nelson, who runs diet seminars for people with IBS, agrees. "An eating schedule helps curb the overindulgence that can come with skipping breakfast, grabbing a quick lunch and then filling up at dinner," she says.

Nurture yourself. Stress—brought on by anticipating an important appointment, for example, or making a business presentation—often triggers IBS symptoms. During times when you're under a lot of pressure, you can use food to nurture yourself rather than skipping meals to avoid pain and diarrhea or reaching for junk foods that could make food reactions worse, says Dr. Guillory.

"It really gets back to knowing what your safe foods are," he says. "Let's say you have a big business presentation to give at the end of a luncheon. Eat moderately and stick to the foods you can handle. If you're eating at home or at your desk, pull some homemade soup out of the freezer. There's something psychologically uplifting about getting control of what you eat and nurturing your body."

"Roughing It" the Burkitt Way

They called him the Bran Man. When British fiber pioneer Denis P. Burkitt, M.D., first urged his countrymen to dig into whole-wheat bread, oatmeal, mashed potatoes and other fiber-rich foods in order to prevent digestive problems, the skeptics chuckled.

But Dr. Burkitt's fiber revolution was unstoppable.

Back in the low-fiber era of white bread, listless salads and big beefsteaks, Dr. Burkitt's observations as a medical missionary in Africa as well as later research convinced him that Westerners needed more fiber. In comparing the health of rural Africans to that of Americans, for example, he found not only more constipation and obesity among the Westerners but also:

- 60 times more gallstones.
- 50 times more diverticular disease.
- 40 times more appendicitis.
- Nearly twice as much large-bowel cancer.

The reason? Fiber-depleted food.

His advice to fiber-starved Westerners? Stick with unprocessed foods, fiber-rich breakfast cereals like All-Bran or oatmeal, beans and vegetables such as cabbage, potatoes, carrots, peas, brussels sprouts and onions. The message still holds true today, as doctors recommend we fit in 20 to 35 grams of fiber daily.

"Most of us get closer to ten grams of fiber, and our health shows it," according to Steven R. Peikin, M.D., professor of medicine and head of the Division of Gastroenterology at the University of Medicine and Dentistry of New Jersey, Robert Wood Johnson Medical School at Camden. "We have diverticulitis, colon cancer, appendicitis, constipation, high cholesterol— all things that are almost unheard-of in places where the people eat high-fiber diets."

Special Relief for Constipation

If constipation is your main IBS complaint, getting adequate fiber and drinking plenty of water are the most powerful strategies you can employ for relief, says Dr. Guillory. It's virtually the same dietary program that works for the garden-variety constipation described earlier.

"Try for 30 to 60 grams of fiber a day," suggests Dr. Guillory. "If you can't get that much from food, add a fiber supplement—but take it at mealtime. If you take it before bed, you could be very uncomfortable—with a hard stool lodged in your colon and a big, gelatinous mass above it."

If you also experience bloating, excessive gas and abdominal pain, limit your intake of the water-soluble types of fiber, which are found in greater quantities in oat bran, beans and fruits such as apples.

"The goal is to have a soft, easy-to-pass stool," says Dr. Guillory. "The frequency of your bowel movements is not as important. Take it slowly—add an extra fiber serving, wait three to five days and then add another daily serving of fiber if you are comfortable. Doing too much, too fast with fiber can make you bloated and uncomfortable."

One word of caution: Be careful with wheat bran. While it's highly recommended to the general public for constipation relief, a study of 100 people with IBS at the University Hospital of South Manchester in England found that more than half had more pain, bloating and bowel disturbances after adding wheat bran to their diets. Only one in ten saw improvement.

Taming Food Reactions

Dairy products, wheat, citrus fruits and juices, chocolate, eggs and high-fat foods are often IBS troublemakers that cause diarrhea. Why? Sometimes the problem is a true food intolerance—your body may lack the enzyme needed to digest lactose, for example.

"But it can also be a food sensitivity—not an allergy or an intolerance but something that just bothers you," says Dr. Guillory. "The signs can include diarrhea as well as gas, bloating and pain."

Uncover your triggers by keeping a detailed food diary. In a notebook, make a note of what you ate and how much, when you ate it, the kind of day you were having—"calm and quiet," for example, or "rushed; big work deadline"—and any resulting bowel reaction. Remember to record everything you've eaten and be as specific as possible, including small additions like the margarine on your morning toast.

After two weeks of record-keeping, begin sleuthing for connections. Show the diary to your doctor for assistance, suggests Dr. Guillory. Then follow these steps to rein in food reactions that cause diarrhea.

Limit before you avoid. Nelson suggests limiting a problem food before cutting it out of your diet completely.

"I get concerned from a nutritional standpoint if someone cuts out entire food groups, such as all dairy products or all fruits," she says. "Don't eliminate a food completely unless you have frequent problems with it."

Dr. Guillory agrees—to a point. "Overall nutrition is important to keep in mind. If a particular food item consistently brings on symptoms, however, I would advise avoidance, at least until the connection can be established." If a particular food appears to bring on symptoms, try eating a half-size portion or eat it only with other foods at a meal, suggests Nelson. Try it prepared in a different way—eat cooked or canned fruit instead of fresh, for example. Or experiment with a different form of the troublesome food, such as yogurt instead of milk. If you still get no relief, Dr. Guillory says, consult your doctor or nutritionist before cutting out any food group entirely.

Be wary of sweet things. Fructose is the sweetener used in many soft drinks, and sorbitol is a sweetener found in many sugar-free products. Either of these may lead to cramps, gas, bloating and diarrhea if your body cannot completely absorb them, says Dr. Guillory.

"Read labels so you know what you're getting," he says. "And see how much you can tolerate. Some people are fine with one soft drink but have trouble after two or three."

Don't Let Food Bug Your Ulcer

Once doctors believed that cream and milk soothed the savage stomach ulcer. And spicy or acidic fare—from five-alarm chili to grapefruit juice—was blamed for igniting an ulcer's gnawing, burning agony.

But not anymore.

"We don't think *any* food can cause an ulcer," says David Peura, M.D., associate professor of medicine at the University of Virginia Medical Center in Charlottesville. "And while milk might make an ulcer feel better in the short run, it actually can stimulate production of more stomach acid, irritating that ulcer a few hours later."

Today, food plays a minor, though still important, role in taming ulcer pain, Dr. Peura says. But researchers have exploded the old myths that diet—and stress—cause those painful craters in the lining of the stomach or duodenum, the upper part of the small intestine.

The real culprit? Researchers have found that a tough, spiral-shaped bacterium called *Helicobacter pylori* is responsible for eight out of ten ulcers of the stomach and duodenum. The rest are the result of taking too many nonsteroidal anti-inflammatory drugs (NSAIDs) such as aspirin, ibuprofen and other drugs that relieve headaches, fever and arthritis.

If you have an ulcer, your doctor can have you tested for the presence of *H. pylori* and prescribe a triple therapy, which consists of two antibiotics to kill the bacteria plus Pepto-Bismol to protect the ulcer from the irritating effects of stomach acids.

If NSAIDs brought on your ulcer, your doctor will advise you to lay off those

---

Reconsider dairy. If milk, cheese, ice cream or any other dairy product gives you symptoms of IBS such as diarrhea and gas pains, you may have lactose intolerance, says Dr. Guillory. Limiting lactose-rich dairy products is the answer.

Keep your cuisine lean. Fat from any source—whether it's the saturated fat in a hamburger or the monounsaturated fat in olive oil—stimulates bowel contractions after a meal. "It's a major trigger for spasms, pain and diarrhea," says Dr. Guillory. "I advise patients to eat a low-fat diet for comfort. The bonus is, it helps with weight control, too."

Trim high-fat recipes the easy way by making substitutions. Try lean ground turkey instead of higher-fat ground beef. Pour skim milk instead of whole milk on your cereal or in your coffee. And you can often use low-fat yogurt in place of mayonnaise. Another idea: Use small amounts of flavorful grated cheese like Parmesan instead of large amounts of milder cheese that end up adding a lot to your daily fat count. Experiment with fat-free condiments, seasonings and flavorings, such as mustard, fresh herbs or

painkillers and help you find an alternative. "Tylenol works for many people," says Dr. Peura. Acid-suppressing drugs and antacids help quell the pain while healing takes place.

Where does food fit in? Dr. Peura says these food choices will also keep you more comfortable.

Eat regular meals. Food acts as a buffer against stomach acid, the liquid that burns ulcers because it's as caustic as battery acid. "Going for long periods without eating can be very painful," Dr. Peura says.

Avoid caffeine—and decaf, too. Set aside the java—regular and decaf—as well as cola drinks, tea and chocolate.

"Caffeine, and something else in decaf coffee, stimulates acid secretion, which can aggravate an existing ulcer," says Dr. Peura.

Stay on the wagon. While ulcer experts no longer blame alcohol for ulcers, a drink or two could irritate the one you've got, according to Dr. Peura. The protein in alcohol stimulates acid secretion, which makes beer even more irritating than a shot of spirits for some people. And if you have a bleeding ulcer, any drink puts you at higher risk for more bleeding.

"The combination of alcohol and NSAIDs is especially bad for bleeding ulcers," says Dr. Peura.

If it hurts, skip it. If you notice that cabbage, onions, a hot-pepper pizza or any other food makes your ulcer sting, steer clear. "There are individual foods that bother different people," Dr. Peura says. "They should simply stay away from them until the ulcer is healed."

lemon juice, instead of high-fat dips, sauces and dressings.

Add de- to -caf. The caffeine in coffee, tea, colas and some other soft drinks can stimulate a bowel movement, whether you want one or not, says Dr. Guillory. Skip the java jolt and go for decaffeinated varieties.

Watch for MSG. For a small percentage of people with IBS, the flavor-enhancer monosodium glutamate (MSG) may trigger pain and diarrhea, Dr. Guillory says. "If it seems to affect you, you have to do more than order your Chinese food without MSG," he says. "MSG is everywhere. You have to read labels and choose a lot of fresh foods as opposed to prepared foods."

Gallstones: A Preventive Role for Diet

Pain sears your upper abdomen, sending flames of agony up between your shoulder blades. Nausea may not be far behind. A gallstone—as big as a table tennis ball or as small as a grain of sand—is making your life completely and utterly miserable.

If this is your first gallstone attack, you may wonder whether this agony is actually a heart attack or some abdominal disaster. And even after the pain subsides, you'll find that you have something else to dread—its return. And return it may: The odds are better than one in three that your gallbladder will act up again within a year after the first attack. If it happens, your doctor may suggest that you join the half-million other Americans each year who have their gallbladders removed.

But what can you do to avoid gallstones in the first place—or prevent a second-wave attack? And what's the food connection?

While no clear link between diet and gallstones has been found, some experts are beginning to believe that the same type of low-fat, high-fiber eating plan that prevents heart disease—like the Ornish and Pritikin plans—will also forestall the growth of gallstones.

"I personally think that high-calorie, high-fat diets do cause gallstones," says Henry Pitt, M.D., director of the Gallstone and Biliary Disease Center at Johns Hopkins Medical Institutions in Baltimore. "A low-calorie, low-fat diet is part of the equation for prevention."

A Pesky Pump

The cause of this galling problem is a thumb-size little blob tucked beneath the liver on the right side of your abdomen. Your gallbladder is a pear-shaped pump that stores and concentrates oily green bile before squirting about a quart of it into the small intestine every day. That hearty dose of bile aids in digesting fats.

But that hyperproductive pump has a built-in problem that can be aggravated by body chemistry, weight, inefficient gallbladder contractions and possibly diet. When conditions upset the gallbladder's usually efficient operations, stones may form in its pool of stored bile. These hard, crystal-like particles are most often made of cholesterol and occasionally of pigments found in bile.

Stones are so common that at least ten million Americans already have them, and another million are likely to join the gallstone club every year, according to the NIH. Women, the elderly, Native Americans and Mexican-Americans are most likely to develop stones. By age 75, one in three women and one in five men have them.

Happily, most are "silent stones" that never bring on an attack. But if a gallstone lodges in the duct leading to the small intestine, the result is agony. Often the next step is surgery to remove the gallbladder or drug therapy to dissolve the offending stones. (And yes, you can live without your gallbladder—bile from your liver also dribbles directly into the small intestine.)

Fortunately, researchers are uncovering connections among lifestyle, eating habits and gallstones that may help you prevent an "attack of the stones."

Sidestepping Gallstones

People at higher-than-normal risk for gallstones include women who are pregnant, have had more than one child or are overweight and both men and women over age 60. If you're in any of these groups, you can take simple steps to cut gallstone risk, says Dr. Pitt.

Fight back with fiber. Water-soluble fiber, the kind found in beans and fruit, "is the dietary component frequently shown to help protect people from gallstones in some studies," says James E. Everhart, M.D., medical officer in the Division of Digestive Diseases and Nutrition of the National Institute of Diabetes and Digestive and Kidney Diseases at the NIH. Raising your daily intake to 20 grams or more may help. This is easier to accomplish if you're on a vegetarian diet or an Ornish- or Pritikin-style program that's low in fat and very high in fiber. (See chapters 7 and 8 for the specifics on these programs.)

Think lean. Try keeping fat intake to 30 percent of daily calories, suggests Dominic J. Nompleggi, M.D., Ph.D., assistant professor of medicine and surgery and director of nutrition support services at the University of Massachusetts Medical Center in Worcester. People who eat high amounts of fat seem to develop more gallstones, he says.

The same strategy is particularly good advice if you know you already have gallstones. Not only does a high-fat diet promote gallstone formation, but a big, fat-laden meal could actually stimulate a gallstone attack.

Maintain a healthy weight. Being overweight is a known risk factor for gallstones. In a major study of 88,837 women, researchers at the Harvard School of Public Health found that even slightly overweight women nearly doubled their risk for gallstones compared to women of normal weight. Obese women—those who were 30 percent or more over their ideal weight—were six times more likely to develop stones than normal-weight women.

Don't crash diet. If you go on a weight-loss program, it doesn't mean you should crash diet, or you'll find yourself in another high-risk group. People on very low calorie liquid diets—those getting about 520 calories a day—increase their risk of gallstones by 10 to 25 percent, says Dr. Nompleggi. Keeping your daily intake around 1,000 to 1,200 calories helps lower the risk, he says.

Avoid yo-yo dieting. Not surprisingly, your gallbladder may balk if you teeter back and forth between weight loss and gain. "Huge weight swings aren't good," says Dr. Pitt. "That's clearly a factor for gallstones."

Nosh regularly. Skipping meals raises the risk of gallstone formation, says Dr. Everhart. Plan for three well-spaced meals during the day or even divide lunch into two snacks if you know dinner will be late.

Reel in some fish. Researchers at Johns Hopkins Hospital in Baltimore found that omega-3 fatty acids—a type of fat found in cold-water fish like Atlantic herring, anchovies, salmon and sardines—seem to put the brakes on gallstone formation. After 17 gallbladder patients took fish oil capsules for

14 days, some types of crystals that become gallstones formed more slowly in their bile.

People in the study took 960 milligrams of omega-3 fatty acids three times a day. "That's a typical amount for a normal person to take," says Dr. Pitt, who led the study. "I think eating fish would work just as well."

Although the study was small, Dr. Pitt points out that fish oil is good for you for lots of reasons. "It's known to help fight heart disease. There are good reasons to take it," he says.

Winning Your Bouts with IBD

Cheryl Knapp had had enough.

By age 29, this Indianapolis woman had been hospitalized 48 times, undergone six surgical procedures and had all but eight feet of her small intestine and colon removed.

Her weight dropped to 85 pounds, making her dangerously thin for her five-foot-seven frame. And doctors were talking about a permanent feeding tube. "They told me I would die in five years," says Knapp. "I had tried everything, from medication and surgery to psychics and psychiatrists."

All this was thanks to Crohn's disease, a form of IBD in which the small intestine—and sometimes other parts of the digestive tract—becomes inflamed. As with other kinds of IBD, the inflammation associated with Crohn's disease leads to intense pain, diarrhea, bleeding, vomiting, fever and poor absorption of nutrients.

A tiny notice in a Texas newspaper introduced Knapp to the Specific Carbohydrate Diet, an eating plan devised for people with IBD. "I didn't think I was interested, because you have to cut out all grains and grain products like bread and pasta as well as potatoes and sugar, among other things," she says. "But when I was really sick, I decided, What do I have to lose?"

Sticking to this eating plan also meant cutting out processed meats and cheeses, chick-peas, bean sprouts, soybeans, milk, buttermilk, sour cream, yogurt, corn syrup, maple syrup and molasses. "I would eat a huge amount of fruit for breakfast and have tomatoes, eggs and lean ground sirloin for lunch every day," she says. "Dinner might be broiled chicken and zucchini cooked with a dab of olive oil."

Six weeks after starting the diet, Knapp was still taking medication to control inflammation and diarrhea, but thanks to the diet, she'd gained weight and was enjoying new-found freedom. "I could exercise again," she said. "I had no pain and felt, in general, like a new person."

A year and a half later, she was off the medication. What's more, her recovery gave her a "new lease on life." She earned her bachelor's degree in business administration and got a job with a publishing company. "I had forgotten what good health feels like," she says. "Now life has infinite possibilities."

Diets for IBD Relief

If you have IBD, "the dietary recommendations that apply to the general public aren't for you," says Stephen B. Hanauer, M.D., professor of medicine and clinical pharmacology at the University of Chicago Medical Center and co-author of *Inflammatory Bowel Disease: A Guide for Patients and Their Families*.

"If you have diarrhea with IBD, you must avoid laxative foods—like very large amounts of fiber in raw fruits and vegetables," he says. "Highly spiced foods and things like nuts and seeds can be very irritating if your bowel is inflamed."

But IBD is a painful puzzle. Doctors aren't sure what causes it, although they've found that IBD can run in families. Some experts think that a virus or bacteria may cause the body's immune system to respond with intestinal inflammation.

If you have IBD, you may experience diarrhea, abdominal pains, weight loss, rectal bleeding, swollen joints, anemia and a fever, says Dr. Hanauer. If you have a form of IBD called ulcerative colitis, the inner lining of your colon and rectum is inflamed. If it's Crohn's disease, the inflammation goes deeper into the intestinal wall, and while it usually affects the small intestine, it may creep to the stomach, esophagus and even the mouth.

But getting a firm diagnosis can take time, because this disorder mimics other intestinal problems. And there's no sure cure. Medication can help stop diarrhea, ease

Is It *IB* with a *D* ?

Diarrhea. Crampy pains. Bleeding. A fever. These are all sure signs that your bowel is in distress and disrupting your daily routine. You might suspect it's irritable bowel syndrome (IBS). But it could be another kind of innards problem called inflammatory bowel disease, or IBD. Only a doctor can say for sure.

"It's easy to mix up IBD with other digestion problems," says Stephen B. Hanauer, M.D., professor of medicine and clinical pharmacology at the University of Chicago Medical Center and co-author of *Inflammatory Bowel Disease: A Guide for Patients and Their Families*. "That's why you need medical tests to confirm It," including some or all of the following.

• Blood tests will show if you are anemic (due to loss of blood) or if your white blood cell count is high—a sign that your body is fighting off inflammation.

• A stool sample will reveal whether the problem is really an infection brought on by bacteria or a parasite.

• Using a flexible tube called an endoscope, your doctor will look inside your rectum and colon for signs of inflammation and bleeding. She may also snip a sample of tissue from the lining of the colon (don't worry, it's painless) to examine under the microscope.

• IBD can affect any part of your intestinal tract, so you may need an x-ray to show which sections are inflamed.

"When you know what the problem is, you can reduce the symptoms through diet and start healing the inflammation with the right medicine," Dr. Hanauer says.

pain and reverse some inflammation. Surgery can remove disease-damaged tissue. But once it settles in, IBD stays for good.

"Diet cannot cure IBD either, but it can reduce some symptoms like cramps, bloating and diarrhea," Dr. Hanauer says. "It's the first line of defense for mild IBD. And it can help people with more advanced cases."

A Carbohydrate-Limiting Plan

One diet plan that may ease symptoms is the Specific Carbohydrate Diet—the plan Cheryl Knapp tried.

Devised by the late Sidney Valentine Haas, M.D., this approach is a response to the fact that people with IBD often cannot digest and absorb the carbohydrates in grains, sweeteners and milk.

Dr. Hanauer's recommendations are very similar to the Specific Carbohydrate Diet. "When my patients with IBD have trouble tolerating certain foods, I tell them to stop eating them," Dr. Hanauer says. "Often that includes foods that use the sweetener sorbitol. I also see people who cannot tolerate milk and occasionally those who cannot tolerate the gluten in many grains."

What's left to eat?

Meat, fish, legumes, homemade yogurt and most cheeses. Most vegetables and fruits. Nuts and honey.

"This diet is a big adjustment, but it's worth it for people with IBD," says Elaine Gottschall, of Kirkton, Ontario, author of *Breaking the Vicious Cycle: Intestinal Health through Diet*, whose daughter had IBD at a very young age. "We eat butternut and acorn squash instead of potatoes. And we make our baked goods using ground nuts for flour and honey for sweetener, for example. It's unusual, but they're very delicious and won't cause a reaction," she says.

Help for Gluten Intolerance

You notice that your child is suddenly irritable and pale, with a big belly and odd-smelling stools. Or you find yourself losing weight, drained of energy and bothered by diarrhea and stomach pains.

For either you or your child, the gut-level trouble might be caused by your daily bread.

"At least 1 in 2,000 Americans has gluten intolerance," says Dr. Gebhard. "The telltale clues of gluten intolerance—which is also called celiac sprue—include weight loss, diarrhea and watery, frothy, oily stools. Often there are nutritional deficiencies, which may seem odd, because people eating the typical American diet get more nutrition than they need."

Nut muffins. Spaghetti squash. Honey.

Meet Elaine Gottschall's healing foods. They're just a few of the edibles featured on the Specific Carbohydrate Diet, a plan designed to end the painful and debilitating intestinal symptoms associated with inflammatory bowel disease (IBD).

"I've had hundreds of letters from people with IBD who say that the diet helped them get well," says Gottschall, a Kirkton, Ontario, woman whose book, *Breaking the Vicious Cycle: Intestinal Health through Diet,* outlines the food strategy she originally used to ease her daughter's IBD.

The theory is that, for some people, certain foods may encourage an overgrowth of intestinal bacteria. Limiting carbohydrates may decrease the number of harmful microbes in the intestine, thereby easing inflammation, says Ronald L. Hoffman, M.D., medical director of the Hoffman Center in New York City and author of *Seven Weeks to a Settled Stomach.*

Foods forbidden on the Specific Carbohydrate Diet include processed meats such as hot dogs and lunch meats; processed cheeses; canned vegetables; potatoes and yams; chick-peas, bean sprouts, soybeans, mung beans and fava beans; sweetened canned fruit; fluid milk and commercially produced yogurt; grain and grain products, including bread and pasta; and sweeteners such as sugar, molasses, corn syrup, chocolate and maple syrup.

What "safe foods" are left to eat? Fresh and frozen meats, most vegetables and fruits, unsweetened juices, natural cheeses, nuts, honey, weak tea and coffee, homemade yogurt and most dried fruit.

"You have to make some substitutions," Gottschall notes. "You can make very good muffins and baked goods with nut flours. Butternut and acorn squash are potato substitutes. Spaghetti squash is a great stand-in for pasta. This is really a very enjoyable diet, although it does take some time in the kitchen."

Gottschall says the diet works for roughly seven out of ten people with IBD (including those with Crohn's disease and ulcerative colitis). Those who do benefit can expect relief in about a month. "After at least one year or more, a person with IBD could start carefully trying some of the forbidden foods they've missed," says Dr. Hoffman. "If they are eaten in small quantities, there shouldn't be a problem."

What's on the Specific Carbohydrate Diet menu? Here's a sample day of healing meals.

Breakfast: A baked apple with honey and cinnamon; scrambled eggs; a homemade nut muffin with butter and homemade jam; weak tea, coffee, grape juice or apple juice.

Lunch: Tuna salad made with homemade mayonnaise, olives and dill pickle and served on lettuce; Cheddar cheese; homemade pumpkin pie with nut crust.

Dinner: Homemade spaghetti sauce made with tomato juice, ground beef, onions, garlic and herbs and served over boiled beans or spaghetti squash; freshly grated cabbage salad made with homemade mayonnaise or oil and vinegar; peas and carrots with butter; fresh fruit; tea.

When Wheat Was Scarce

It was a wartime mystery: Why did Dutch children diagnosed with celiac sprue—a debilitating disease that left them listless and underweight—thrive when food was scarce during World War II, only to relapse in peacetime?

Dutch researcher Willem Dicke, M.D., realized that the answer was grain.

"Dr. Dicke saw these children get well when there wasn't any wheat or other grains to eat during the war and then become sick again when there was grain after the war," says Leon Rottman, Ph.D., executive director of the Celiac Sprue Association (CSA) in Omaha, Nebraska. "It was a breakthrough—the start of the wheat-free diet. His research at the University of Utrecht in Holland established the first scientific connection between cereal grains and celiac sprue."

Today, thanks to more research, children and adults with celiac sprue know that they must avoid not only wheat but all grains that contain a protein called gluten—including oats, barley, rye, buckwheat, triticale and amaranth—in order to feel well and thrive.

Happily, a gluten-free diet doesn't mean giving up bread, spaghetti or baked desserts anymore. "These days, you can buy or make tasty breads, desserts and even pasta with alternative flours such as those made from rice, potato starch, soy, tapioca, corn, beans or acorns," says Jean E. Guest, R.D., a dietitian consultant for the CSA.

Against the Grain

If you have gluten intolerance, your body cannot absorb nutrients from the foods you eat. It begins, Dr. Gebhard says, with a genetic sensitivity to gluten, a substance found in many grains.

"Gluten proteins trigger the immune system to attack cells lining the small intestine," he says. "When these cells don't work well, you cannot absorb all sorts of sugars and proteins. That's why you can be eating well but still have a calcium deficiency or a deficiency of vitamin K, which helps your blood clot, or a deficiency of vitamin A, which helps with night vision and skin health."

Cutting gluten, says Dr. Gebhard, is the answer. Gluten is a protein in the wheat kernel, but it is also found in barley, rye, oats, buckwheat, triticale and amaranth.

"Then the healing can take place, which may require weeks or even months," he says. "Even when healed, a person with gluten intolerance should avoid all gluten; even small amounts can cause a reaction."

That means most commercial breads, noodles, cakes and crackers are off-limits. So are many salad dressings, canned soups and even distilled white vinegar, all of which can contain gluten additives.

What's the alternative? People with gluten intolerance often buy specially made breads through mail order, study the art of gluten-free baking and learn how to communicate their needs in restaurants and fast-food establishments, says Jean E. Guest, R.D., a dietitian consultant for the Celiac Sprue Association (CSA) in Omaha, Nebraska.

Safe, gluten-free substitutes for more familiar flours include flours made from rice, potato starch, soy, tapioca, corn, beans and acorns. "You have to work with these flours to get good mixtures and good products," says Guest. "The thing I tell my patients with celiac sprue is to contact the CSA—they have preparation hints, including bread recipes, that really help."

Living with Gluten Intolerance

But you can't make every meal from scratch. Successfully finding safe, gluten-free foods in supermarkets and restaurants requires knowing how to avoid obvious and hidden sources of gluten, says Dr. Gebhard. Here are ways to improve your gluten savvy.

Uncover hidden gluten. "In my opinion, the classic hidden gluten is malt flavoring, which typically comes from barley," says Guest. "Often it bothers adults with celiac disease more than it bothers children."

There may be gluten in wheat starch, food starch, thickeners used in commercial pies and pie fillings, preservatives in lunch meats and any ingredient labeled as an emulsifier, stabilizer, vegetable gum, hydrolyzed vegetable protein or hydrolyzed plant protein.

Where will you find these hidden sources of gluten? Watch out for cheese foods and spreads, some commercial salad dressings, instant coffee, commercial chocolate milk and hot cocoa mix, most canned and powdered soups, distilled white vinegar, soy sauce, ice cream that uses gluten stabilizers, self-basting poultry, some curry powders and gravy mixes, and condiments such as ketchup, mustard and horseradish that are made with distilled white vinegar.

Keep on reading labels. Even the recipes for "safe" products can change and may suddenly include gluten, says Guest.

"Keep reading ingredient labels or keep checking with a group like the CSA to find out what's in commercial products," she says. "Once I recommended a rice cereal to the mother of a child with gluten intolerance without realizing that the recipe had changed to include malt flavoring, which contains gluten. It was a lesson that you have to be very, very careful."

Initiate table talk. Dining out can still be a pleasurable experience, says Guest. "Choose a local restaurant that you like and go in during a slow time and talk with the manager about your needs," she suggests. "Find out which dishes are safe. Don't overlook issues like whether breaded foods are fried or grilled in the same place with unbreaded foods—a little gluten left over from breaded fish could end up on your grilled fish."

Call on the experts. The CSA compiles an annual list of gluten-free commercial products that's highly recommended by doctors and nutritionists. Ingredient information is provided by the food manufacturers themselves. "It's worth the small fee to have a list of safe products that you can take to the grocery store with you," says Guest, who helped review the CSA's "Cooperative Gluten-Free Commercial Products Listing."

Other CSA offerings include a restaurant card that explains your dietary needs to waiters, bread recipes and general dietary advice. For more information, contact the Celiac Sprue Association/United States of America at P.O. Box 31700, Omaha, NE 68131-0700.

19 Fatigue

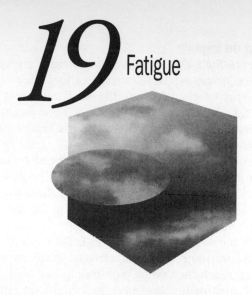

Eating Away Your Exhaustion

Sometimes fatigue is a good thing. Body builders push their muscles to the point of fatigue so they'll grow bigger and stronger. Playing with children and grandchildren yields a feeling of pleasant fatigue at day's end. And there's nothing more satisfying than resting your fatigued body after a day of planting your garden or painting your house.

But if you find yourself unable to get your weary bones out of bed when your major exertion was washing your hair the night before, fatigue isn't a good feeling. It's a problem.

At least you aren't suffering alone. Surveys show that in our whirl-wind world, fatigue is one of the most common reasons that people drag themselves to their family doctors. And the factors that contribute to fatigue are as varied as the millions of people suffering from it. Stress, depression, anemia, allergies, menopause, premenstrual syndrome and a host of other ailments can contribute to your shutdown, say experts. Or it could simply be that you're not getting enough sleep.

Of course, if you just have fatigue from missing a night's sleep or spending a hard week on a project, you'll probably recover with a little rest. But if the fatigue lingers and seems hard to shake off, you might want to consider the following advice from experts.

Running on Empty

Whatever the fatiguing factors—too much stress, too little shuteye, a viral infection, toxin exposure or some other factor— there's one ingredient in the recipe for fatigue that underlies most cases and often acts as the primary offender. That's poor nutrition, says Jesse A. Stoff, M.D., a physician in private practice in Tucson and author of *Chronic Fatigue Syndrome: The Hidden Epidemic*.

"Poor nutrition plays a huge role in fatigue on many different levels," says Dr. Stoff. "Most people are eating highly processed foods, foods that are grown in depleted soil and refined foods that have no nutritional value left. All of these things leave you deficient in the nutrients you need for optimal health and energy."

Even if the source of your lassitude isn't solely a nutritional deficit, a bad diet can contribute to your downward spiral, says Dr. Stoff. "You feel down, so you reach for a quick pick-me-up like sugar or caffeine, which not only has no nutritional value but actually depletes nutrients from the body. Before you know it, you're feeling worse."

One important aspect of beating most cases of fatigue is giving your diet a good spring cleaning by tossing the old energy-robbing foods and bringing in a fresh bunch of energizers, say the experts.

But that's not a remedy for everyone. If you've been battling fatigue so crippling that everyday tasks are impossible, you must see your doctor. You might have a flulike viral disease called chronic fatigue syndrome (CFS), which requires medical attention. (For more on CFS, see chapter 16.)

Otherwise, here are some dietary tips that the experts say can help pump up your flagging energy levels. Not surprisingly, many are the same tips that nutritionists have been giving us for years.

Do Some Iron-ing

"An underlying iron deficiency is a significant factor in fatigue among women," says Michael T. Murray, N.D., a naturopathic physician in Seattle and author of *Chronic Fatigue Syndrome: Getting Well Naturally*, who frequently finds he can clear up their fatigue just by supplementing with iron.

Anemia, which is often caused by iron deficiency and usually causes fatigue, is so widespread that women's health authority Susan M. Lark, M.D., a physician in private practice in Los Altos, California, and author of *Chronic Fatigue and Tiredness*, calls it one of the most common health problem among women of all ages.

The problem, she explains, is that women simply don't eat enough iron-rich foods, so they have depleted iron stores. Without iron, red blood cells can't do their job—transporting oxygen to all the places it needs to go in the body. The result: fatigue.

To put more muscle power in your diet, you can try eating more iron-rich foods. Liver is the best source, but you'll probably want to avoid it since all liver is exceptionally high in fat and cholesterol. Excellent nonmeat sources include Cream of Wheat cereal and tofu. Another good source is quinoa, a grain that can be cooked like rice. But the kind of iron they contain, called nonheme iron, is best assimilated if you eat it along with a good source of vitamin C. Having a glass of orange juice (high in vitamin C) with Cream of Wheat cereal (high in iron) makes an iron-building breakfast. "I also recommend that people with iron deficiencies take two 500-milligram capsules of hydrolyzed (liquid) liver extract a day," says Dr. Murray. "It provides the best iron without the fat and cholesterol."

Nixing the Caffeine Fix

The alarm goes off, sounding like a medieval torture device. You can barely garner the energy to slap the snooze button for a precious nine more minutes of sweet dreams. Just as you're drifting back into Slumberland . . . *b-e-e-e-e-e-e-p*. As you crawl out of bed and slog to the kitchen, your brain screams "Coffee!" That's what you need—a shot of coal-black Mississippi Mud.

Or do you?

That nerve-electrifying jolt of hot java might be what's draining your energy to begin with, says Dr. Murray.

"Caffeine steals B vitamins from the body and interferes with the absorption of essential minerals like iron," says Paul Cheney, M.D., director of the Cheney Clinic in Charlotte, North Carolina.

Without a sufficient amount of B vitamins, your body has a tough time converting the food you eat into usable energy, say doctors. And that lack of iron can lead to anemia, as your body experiences a shortage of oxygen-carrying red blood cells. The result: You feel like a dirty dishrag in an all-night diner.

This energy slope gets even more slippery when you consider how our bodies adapt to our favorite liquid pick-me-up, says Dr. Murray.

"Chronic coffee consumption causes big problems," says Dr. Murray, who practices near Seattle, the cappuccino capital of the United States. As your body adapts to caffeine, you need an increasing amount for stimulation. Ultimately, you may end up drinking so much coffee that it leads to insomnia and irritability, he says.

If you can't eliminate caffeine from your diet completely, it helps if you can start to limit consumption, according to Elizabeth Somer, R.D., author of *Food and Mood*. Somer recommends limiting your consumption to no more than 300 milligrams of caffeine a day, which is the amount you'd get in two eight-ounce mugs of coffee. Dr. Cheney agrees that this type of moderate consumption is acceptable for most people.

The Best Order for Energy

So you say you're eating healthy and you still feel like Atlas lugging around the weight of the world? Maybe you don't need to change your diet, just the order in which you eat it, says Elizabeth Somer, R.D., author of *Food and Mood*.

"Foods high in carbohydrates, whether they're breads or sweet desserts, increase levels of a brain chemical called serotonin, which is known to improve your mood or make you drowsy," says Somer. "On the other hand, high-protein foods like turkey, fish and yogurt trigger the release of the energizing brain chemicals dopamine and norepinephrine," she says.

Your strategy should be to eat your pastas and proteins with the ebbs and flows of your energy levels, advises Somer. "If you know you 'crash' after lunch, skip the heavy or high-carbohydrate midday meal and eat a light, protein-rich lunch, such as a tuna sandwich, fruit and skim milk, instead. Then, when you need to wind down at the end of the day, go for the spaghetti dinner."

When Sweets Deplete

Nothing goes better with a steamy cup of cappuccino than a gooey, toasty-warm cinnamon bun. A little sugar on top of the caffeine really gives you a boost—at least for the next 15 minutes.

Unfortunately, sugar, like caffeine, provides a false sense of energy while insidiously pulling you further down, says Dr. Murray.

And once it's inside your body, sugar makes a mess stickier than a cara-mel apple in July. Like caffeine, the sweet stuff de- pletes your body of B vitamins and essential minerals, which increases nervous anxiety and irrita- bility. That sugar also decreases energy and impairs immunity, say nutritionists.

Sweets also send your body into overdrive, especially your adrenal glands, which pro- duce the famous fight-or-flight hormone, adrenaline. If you've ever driven a little too fast past a police speed trap, you've felt the internal surge of adrenaline as your scared mind screams "I'm caught!" Too many of these surges, such as those from excess sugar, and you risk exhausting your adrenals—a major cause of fatigue, he says.

Too Much of a Sweet Thing

Excess sugar also has an impact on levels of insulin, the compound that helps regulate the supplies of blood sugar that flow through your body, according to Somer. "Eating sugar encourages your pancreas to produce extra insulin, which depresses your blood sugar, making you want more sugar and creating a roller coaster of sugar ups and downs, so you never feel good."

By one estimate, we eat our own weight in sugar each year—almost 130 pounds worth. That's a whopping amount of a substance that has a big impact on our energy and behavior. In fact, nutritionists say that sugar shouldn't exceed 10 percent of our daily intake of calories. If you're getting 2,000 calories a day, that means that only 200 should come from sugar—about what you get from one small slice of apple pie.

To stay within these limits, Somer recommends cutting back on sweets like cakes, cookies and doughnuts. Limit soft drinks to no more than one a day, she says. In general, try to skip foods that have sugar listed as the first, second or third ingredient on the label.

There's More to Fat than Meats

Between the tackles and Hail Mary passes of any Sunday afternoon clash of National Football League titans, you'll find a glut of commercials for antacids and other tummy tamers. Why? Well, if you've got a lot of armchair quarterbacks munching pepperoni pizzas and gnawing buffalo wings, the need for a tummy truce gets pretty powerful around the third quarter.

But maybe those commercials should feature alarm clocks, too. After all that fatty food, say the experts, fatigue follows as inevitably as night after day.

High-fat diets, as well as diets rich in meat—which are generally also high in fat—definitely help to perpetuate fatigue, according to Dr. Stoff. Their primary fatiguing force is that they're tough to digest and put significant stress on the liver.

If you have any doubt that the process of digestion is a full-body workout, just look around the living room following the typical American Thanksgiving feast. All those yawns and groans and figures sprawled in armchairs are a perfect picture of what happens when a high-fat meal pumps up digestion and leaves hearty eaters feeling drowsy. In fact, a high-calorie meal—whether or not it's high in fat—can have the same effect.

As far as fuel goes, trying to get a kickstart from a fatty meal is like trying to start a campfire with wet newspaper, says Somer. Your body doesn't want to burn fat. It wants to store it. You have to stoke your fires with pure kindling, like complex carbohydrates, if you want energy, she says.

Alcohol: More Snooze than Buzz

They don't call it a nightcap for nothing. Even though some people feel as if it gives them a buzz, alcohol is a sedative. Although the brew-guzzling guys and dolls in the beer commercials look spry and bright, alcohol ultimately brings you down, especially if you're already suffering from fatigue, say experts.

Vital Energy Nutrients

When the first vitamins were discovered back in the early 1900s, they were called *vita-amines,* meaning "vital to life." Eighty-some years later, we know that they're also vital for optimal energy.

"You don't have to be deficient to feel the effects," explains Allan Magaziner, D.O., director of the Magaziner Medical Center in Cherry Hill, New Jersey. "Just having low levels of certain nutrients can lead to fatigue. And most people don't get all the nutrients they need through their diets," he says.

Most experts recommend that people with fatigue take a good multi-vitamin/mineral supplement. These are the nutrients they say are most important for recapturing your energy.

B-complex vitamins. If you're feeling fatigued, experts agree, reach for B vitamins. The big reasons: B vitamins are largely responsible for healthy brain and nerve function as well as energy regulation. We burn up B vitamins most quickly when we're under stress. And most people don't eat enough beans and whole grains to get adequate amounts of B vitamins in their diets. Experts suggest taking 50 milligrams of B-complex vitamins two to three times daily.

Beta-carotene. A potent antioxidant, beta-carotene sweeps up cell-damaging free radicals that are produced due to everyday stress. These unstable compounds float among your cells and damage tissue structure, which leads to rapid aging. Getting rid of free radicals keeps your body healthy, which boosts energy, says Jesse A. Stoff, M.D., a physician in private practice in Tucson and author of *Chronic Fatigue Syndrome: The Hidden Epidemic.* Experts generally recommend getting between 10,000 and 15,000 international units of beta-carotene a day. Good food sources include orange, yellow or dark green, leafy vegetables and

---

On top of being a depressant, alcohol plays nutrient-thieving tricks like caffeine and sugar, leaving you low in precious B vitamins and essential minerals. Experts advise skipping all alcohol and sipping mineral water instead.

Food Allergy Fatigue

Along with the usual suspects that cause fatigue is a group of rogue foods that may be fine for some people but wreak havoc with others. Even some foods that have traditionally been the cornerstones of a good diet can run like a raging bull through the system of someone who's allergic to them.

The primary symptoms are often indigestion, bloating and diarrhea. But if you have food allergies, you're likely to feel fatigue because of these and related symptoms. Nutrition experts agree that allergies can tax the

fruits such as carrots, beet greens and cantaloupe.

Vitamin C. Like beta-carotene, vitamin C is a powerful antioxidant. It's also a proven immunity booster, says Dr. Stoff. Experts recommend at least 500 to 1,500 milligrams of vitamin C daily. Just be forewarned that high doses of supplemental vitamin C may cause diarrhea in some people. Good food sources include citrus fruits, broccoli and red bell peppers.

Vitamin E. Vitamin E is a free radical fighter, an antioxidant and an immunity booster. Experts recommend 400 international units daily. To add more E to your diet, reach for wheat germ, mangoes and apples, and cook with vegetable oil. People who are taking anticoagulants or have had strokes or bleeding problems should get a doctor's okay before taking vitamin E supplements in any amount.

Magnesium. Turning the tuna sandwich you ate for lunch into usable fuel for the body is part of magnesium's job as a pivotal mineral for energy production. Yet, unless you're eating plenty of beans, tofu, nuts and seeds or wheat germ, you may not be getting all you need. Experts recommend supplementing with 500 milligrams a day of an amino-chelated form, as indicated on the label. That amount is slightly higher than the Daily Value of 400 milligrams, so check with your doctor before taking it. Also, people with heart or kidney problems should not take supplemental magnesium.

Zinc. Zinc is an irreplaceable middleman on the energy production line. It helps your pancreas make insulin, and insulin in turn boosts the delivery of energizing glucose to your cells. Like the antioxidant vitamins, zinc also strengthens immunity, says Dr. Stoff. Experts recommend getting about 15 milligrams a day. Superior zinc sources include miso, wheat germ and beef.

---

system and cause fatigue in many people. So if some kind of food is giving your digestion fits, you need to get to the root of it to get your energy back.

One of the most common food culprits in the allergy department is milk. Although we've all been told that drinking milk results in strong bones and healthy teeth, for many it means bloating, intestinal gas, stomach cramps and fatigue.

Another common allergen is wheat, which can be difficult to digest and highly allergenic for some people, according to Dr. Stoff. Wheat intolerance can make you prone to intestinal problems such as bloating and gas as well as overall body problems such as fatigue and depression, he says.

If you're having any kind of symptoms related to digestion, be sure to see chapter 20 as well as the information on lactose intolerance on page 312 and gluten intolerance on page 326.

Resources for Healing

Books

Chronic Fatigue and Tiredness
Susan M. Lark, M.D.
Westchester Publishing

Curing Fatigue
David S. Bell, M.D., and Stef Donev
Rodale Press

Tired All the Time: How to Regain Your Lost Energy
Ronald L. Hoffman, M.D.
Simon & Schuster

Tired of Being Tired: Overcoming Chronic Fatigue and Low Vitality
Michael A. Schmidt
Frog, Ltd.

The bottom line is that if you're sick and tired of feeling sick and tired, it's time to listen to what nutritionists have been telling us for years, says Dr. Stoff.

"Eating vegetables and grains for most of your diet is optimum for health and energy," he says. Make complex carbohydrates about 50 to 60 percent of your daily intake, make protein 20 to 25 percent and keep fat intake to about 20 or 25 percent, advises Dr. Stoff.

While he believes a vegetarian diet is the ideal for most of us, he quickly acknowledges that a meatless world is too dull for many. "So stick to small amounts of skinless chicken and fish and enjoy life," he says.

20 Food Allergies and Sensitivities

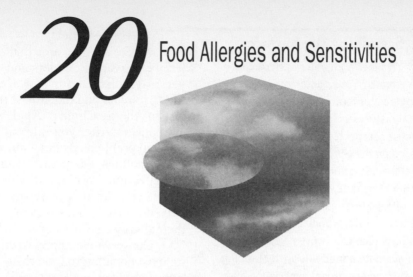

Was It Really Something You Ate?

Crunch a juicy Macintosh apple, and suddenly your lips itch. Drink a cool glass of milk, and red, itchy hives swell on your arms or legs. Or perhaps the tiniest chunk of peanut leaves you gasping for air. Sometimes the connection between what we eat and how we feel is crystal-clear.

But the link between food and feelings isn't always so obvious. You may secretly wonder, for example, if the cupcakes you downed at lunch contributed to the lethargy you battled in the afternoon, or if last night's fried rice brought on this morning's throbbing backache.

Food reactions like these can be so powerful—and so puzzling— that one in four Americans believes they're allergic to at least one food: They report uncomfortable responses to edibles as varied as grapefruit, garlic, cola, red wine, chocolate and pork. And yet only about 1 adult in 100 has a true food allergy.

"Food allergies are rare," says allergist Daryl Altman, M.D., director of Allergy Information Services in Hewlett, New York. "Right now, the bottom line for the people who have them is that you must avoid your problem food."

But the bottom line isn't as clear for the thousands whose food reactions aren't true allergies.

Scratching the Surface

Wondering if you're allergic to some foods? Your doctor may be able to pinpoint a food allergy with a personal history and skin tests. Diluted extracts of suspected trouble foods are placed on the skin, which is then scratched. If a bump rises on the spot within 15 minutes, you may be allergic.

Blood tests can also narrow the list of potential troublemakers. But no matter which test is used, your doctor will evaluate a food allergy by looking at your own postmeal experience and confirm it, if necessary, with another test called a double-blind placebo food challenge.

"I suggest that my patients keep a food activity and symptom scare diary for three weeks," says Marianne Frieri, M.D., Ph.D., director of the allergy/immunology training program at Nassau County Medical Center in East Meadow, New York, and associate professor of medicine and pathology at the State University of New York at Stony Brook. "When they bring it back in, we look for connections between allergic reactions, activity and specific foods."

Allergic—Or Not?

"There's a gray area that allergy experts don't understand yet," says allergist Steven Kagen, M.D., founder and director of the Kagen Allergy Clinic in Appleton, Wisconsin. "After you rule out medical problems that can mimic food reactions, like peptic ulcers and infections, you're left with people who are simply hypersensitive to certain foods—even if their allergy tests are negative."

Conservative allergists chalk up most nonallergic food reactions to hidden medical conditions, stress and psychological problems. More rarely, they say that the reactions can be attributed to additives and natural substances in foods that can produce headaches, hives and digestive distress that feel just like an allergy attack.

"Often the vague symptoms that people complain of are not food-related at all," says Carol G. Baum, M.D., director of the Department of Allergy and Clinical Immunology for Kaiser-Permanente's New York service area. "They may feel tired or have a foggy feeling. That's not a clear food allergy. They may really have a medical condition that needs attention or be very anxious or under stress. The problem is not food."

Looking Within

Many doctors with an alternative view of allergies would disagree with Dr. Baum. They insist that foods we eat every day—from whole-wheat bread to sweets, from oranges to corn—are responsible for fatigue, headaches, intestinal discomfort and breathing problems.

"There's a whole, huge range of delayed food allergies that most traditional allergists don't think exist or are important," says allergist William E. Walsh, M.D., founder of the Adult and Child Allergy Clinic in St. Paul, Minnesota. "But once you see the pattern and the way people improve when you take specific foods out of the diet, you see that something's really going on."

There are few medical studies that examine delayed food allergy, Dr. Walsh concedes. "We can't explain what's happening in the body," he says. "But we see the results when people change their diets."

Both sides do agree that if you're experiencing adverse reactions to food, you should start by seeing your doctor. The problem may very well be a real food allergy or a medical condition or reaction that mimics an allergy.

Finding the Troublemakers: True Allergies

If you have a true food allergy, your immune system overreacts to harmless proteins in the foods you eat.

"For some reason, the immune system of an allergic person sees these proteins as foreign invaders," explains Dr. Altman. "After your immune system is sensitized to that protein, there is an outpouring of the body's natural defense chemicals that can cause itching, sneezing, rashes, vomiting, asthma and diarrhea."

The reaction can be as mild as a rash, Dr. Altman observes, but stronger reactions are feared, particularly anaphylactic shock. That's when the reaction is so extreme that you can't breathe. Arteries dilate, dangerously dropping blood pressure. Your larynx and the bronchi of your lungs can also constrict, cutting off the oxygen supply. Unless there's immediate emergency treatment, anaphylactic shock can lead to coma and death.

Why food allergies strike when they do is a mystery. Many begin in childhood, but adults may suddenly find that their food is biting back. Oddly, some allergies vanish within a year or so if you steadfastly avoid trouble foods. But others—including the most life-threatening type—are yours for life.

Peanuts, fish and shellfish and tree nuts like almonds, Brazil nuts, cashews and pecans are the most common foods that cause allergic reactions in adults. But cow's milk, eggs, soybeans, wheat and, in rarer cases, barley, rice, citrus, melons, bananas, tomatoes, spinach, corn and potatoes can also cause reactions.

"If you know your reactions are mild, you might be able to get away with eating a little bit of the food—say, the amount of milk baked into a chocolate chip cookie," says Dr. Altman. "But if your reactions are severe, as some reactions to peanuts and seafood are, you have to learn how to read food labels in the supermarket and talk with chefs or restaurant managers to be sure your food is safe when you eat out."

Uncomfortable Cousins

Like a security guard alert for dangerous invaders, your immune system scans all the "foreign" stuff that enters your body—including the food you eat.

But, oops! Sometimes this guard gets muddled, mistaking substances in fruits and vegetables for allergy-producing pollens—with "interesting but unpleasant results," says Steven Kagen, M.D., founder and director of the Kagen Allergy Clinic in Appleton, Wisconsin. This type of reaction is called oral allergy syndrome (OAS).

"If you're allergic to birch pollen, for example, there are compounds on the outside of apples, peaches and pears that, to your immune system, look just like the proteins in birch pollen," he says. "Eat one, and it can set up a cross-reaction. Your lips may swell, your ears may tingle, or you may get cramps or indigestion."

Oddest of all, if you're allergic to cats, you may have a cross-reaction when eating pork, Dr. Kagen notes. And if you wheeze or break out in hives after eating avocados, bananas, kiwifruit or water chestnuts, you may also be allergic to latex. This is something you should mention to your doctor before any invasive surgical procedure, since the gloves as well as some surgical equipment used by doctors are made of latex.

When two or more foods gang up to cause problems, Dr. Kagen calls these cross-reactors food cousins. Here are some of them.

• Ragweed pollen and watermelon, cantaloupe, pumpkin, pumpkin seeds, squash, sunflower seeds and bananas.

• Grass pollen and tomatoes, carrots, celery, caraway, parsley, anise, beer, corn, oats, wheat, barley, lettuce, chives and potato skins.

• Birch pollen and celery, carrots, all stony, pitted fruits like cherries, plums, peaches and nectarines, and pears and apples.

"This doesn't mean you necessarily have to avoid these foods," Dr. Kagen says. But he advises people to be aware of possible cross-reactions and—if you've had bad experiences before—prepare for the worst.

Symptoms of a cross-reaction are itching and swelling of the lips, tongue, throat and roof of the mouth. Since anaphylactic shock, which is much more serious, also begins this way, you may not know whether you're having a mild or a life-threatening reaction. The first few times you have a cross-reaction, you may be uncertain about what is happening, so you should carry injectable epinephrine, suggests John W. Yunginger, M.D., professor of pediatrics at the Mayo Medical School and a consultant in pediatrics at the Mayo Clinic and Foundation in Rochester, Minnesota.

You should also get into the habit of slicing and microwaving any food that might cause an allergic cross-reaction. Microwaving the food on high power for one minute renders the compounds that are responsible for the reaction harmless, Dr. Kagen says. "This can dry out fruit, so soak it in water overnight to rehydrate it," he suggests.

When Forbidden Foods Are Hidden

You know what a peanut, a shrimp or an egg looks like. But spotting trouble foods isn't always that simple.

Peanuts may be hidden—as peanut butter—in the wrapper of an egg roll. There could be soy in the vegetable broth of your favorite canned soup. If you have a true milk allergy, you may react to casein or lacto-albumin-milk derivatives that are often found in baked goods.

Avoiding hidden allergens in foods takes some knowledge and practice, notes Patricia Kendall, R.D., Ph.D., professor of nutrition in the Department of Food Science and Human Nutrition at Colorado State University in Fort Collins. And if you must avoid major food groups, replacing lost nutrients requires savvy, too.

"If you're cutting out milk and all dairy products, you have to think about calcium," Dr. Kendall says. "You can get some from dark green, leafy vegetables and by eating fish with tiny bones, but you will probably also need a supplement."

Avoiding foods that cause allergies can mean a lot of label reading. But what are you really looking for when you start searching the fine print?

A list of hidden sources of common allergens in foods is available from the Food Allergy Network (FAN), which constantly updates its allergen-alert lists. Call 1-800-929-4040 for more information. Here's a partial list of foods and ingredients to avoid.

Wheat-free diet: Avoid bran, bulgur, couscous, cereal extract, cracker meal, gluten, high-protein flour, semolina and spelt.

Peanut-free diet: Avoid ground nuts, mixed nuts and cold-pressed peanut oil. The foods and ingredients that may contain peanut protein include baked goods, candy, chili, chocolate, egg rolls, hydrolyzed plant or vegetable protein, marzipan and nougat.

Egg-free diet: Avoid albumin, apovitellin, egg substitutes, globulin, mayonnaise, meringue, ovalbumin, ovomucin and ovomuccoid. A shiny glaze or yellow color often indicates the presence of eggs in baked goods.

Soy-free diet: Avoid miso, shoyu sauce, tamari, tempeh, textured vegetable protein and tofu. When you're checking labels, look for the following ingredients that may indicate the presence of soy protein: hydrolyzed plant protein, natural flavoring, vegetable broth and vegetable starch.

Milk-free diet: You'll need to watch out for all dairy products, such as yogurt, cheese, butter and cream, and their derivatives. Also avoid casein, caseinates, curds, hydrolysates, lactalbumin, lactoglobulin, nougat and whey.

To expand your range of safe, milk-free foods, check the labels on kosher products. "Kosher foods are helpful because they offer some substitute food choices," Dr. Baum notes. Kosher foods marked with a *D* contain dairy products. But even if they have some other marking (like a *K*, which simply means "kosher"), you should check the ingredients list to be sure, according to Dr. Baum.

Special Precautions for Food Allergies

Once you and your doctor have identified a food allergy, avoidance is a big part of the game. But even so, there are likely to be times when a sly allergen slips past your vigilance. For these situations, the scout law applies: Be prepared. Here are steps to help safeguard yourself from the most serious allergic reactions.

Carry a lifesaver. If you have a history of severe allergic reactions, toting a syringe loaded with epinephrine for self-injection could save your life by halting anaphylactic shock, Dr. Baum says. They're available by prescription only, but the peace of mind is well worth a doctor's visit.

"There are different brands with different features, but I like Epipen—it looks like a big pen with a safety cap. It's easy to use under stress," she says. "You just take off the cap and hold the 'pen' firmly against your thigh for ten seconds. The pressure-driven syringe injects the epinephrine."

Keep one at work, another in your car and a third in your purse or briefcase, doctors advise. Your doctor can tell you about training kits that will allow you to practice without giving yourself an actual injection so you can learn to use it quickly and correctly if you need it. And after you've used it, go immediately to the emergency room of the nearest hospital, Dr. Altman says.

"Injectable epinephrine only lasts for about 15 minutes in the body," Dr. Altman says. "It doesn't resolve the problem, but it does buy you time to get to the emergency room. Studies of deaths and near-deaths due to food allergy show that those who get epinephrine within the first 30 minutes of a severe allergic reaction are the ones who survive."

Insist on safe foods. Dining out? If your reactions are severe, it's essential for you to have a conversation with the chef before ordering.

"You need to know what's in the dish, and more," says Dr. Altman. "If you have a severe allergy, a little bit of peanut protein left on a spatula from another dish or a little bit of shrimp protein left in the deep-fryer oil could make you sick. Ask what else the utensils are used for."

Be careful with alcohol and exercise. A drink with your meal or a workout afterward could bring on a quicker, stronger allergic reaction, Dr. Altman says. "It's an individual thing you can watch out for," she says. "The most extreme case I've seen was a young woman who said that she can eat shrimp, and she can drink beer, but if she has them both at the same meal, she ends up in the emergency room with an allergic reaction."

Reactions to Additives

Researchers and doctors have increasing evidence that some people react to specific substances. Although these aren't exactly true food allergies, people do have allergy-like or pseudo food reactions. They and their doctors may have trouble pinpointing the troublemaking food or substance.

Among the culprits is a chemical called histamine. This is the same substance that is released from special cells in your body, called mast cells, during an allergic reaction.

From Roquefort cheese to mackerel and from ketchup to sauerkraut, some foods have naturally high levels of histamine or other reaction-causing substances, like mold or sulfites. Some people are actually sensitive to the mold or sulfites in food, while others experience problems because these substances cause a release of histamine in the body. "If you're sensitive to histamine, you could wind up with a headache, flushing, a warm or burning sensation or even pain. There's no way to tell that this isn't a true food allergy," says Marianne Frieri, M.D., Ph.D., director of the allergy/immunology training program at Nassau County Medical Center in East Meadow, New York, and associate professor of medicine and pathology at the State University of New York at Stony Brook. Sneezing, diarrhea and shortness of breath are also possible allergic reactions.

When histamine-rich foods were removed from the diets of 45 women and men—all with suspected histamine sensitivities—in a study at the Dermatologic and Pediatric Allergy Clinic in Vienna, Austria, three out of four felt much better. The number of headaches was cut in half, as was the amount of pain medication that participants needed. They also experienced less itching, congestion and shortness of breath—all problems associated with histamine-laden foods.

Unmasking the Masqueraders

Both conservative and alternative allergists agree that doctors should consider medical conditions, as well as emotional or psychological factors, before blaming food when you have symptoms of an allergy-type reaction. Why?

"If you have inflammatory bowel disease (IBD) or an ulcer or are under stress, you may have symptoms that feel like a food allergy. You may cut out more and more foods to try to feel better," says Marianne Frieri, M.D., Ph.D., director of the allergy/immunology training program at the Nassau County Medical Center in East Meadow, New York, and associate professor of medicine and pathology at the State University of New York at Stony Brook.

"As a result," she says, "you may avoid so many nutritious foods that you're malnourished or you lose weight. Some people come to me with huge lists of foods that they don't think they can eat anymore. And the original problem has not been resolved."

Conditions that may masquerade as allergies range from the discomfort of overindulgence to serious gastrointestinal problems like IBD. "The minute someone has indigestion, they don't think 'Oh, I ate too much.' They think, 'I'm allergic to that food.'" says Dr. Frieri. "So you have to be a detective."

What feels like a food reaction could also be a symptom of a stomach ulcer, a malfunctioning gallbladder or pancreas or a bacterial or viral infection, says Steven Kagen, M.D., founder and director of the Kagen Allergy Clinic in Appleton, Wisconsin.

The Havoc of Additives

If you know that additives cause uncomfortable reactions, your best course of action is to avoid them, according to experts at the American Academy of Allergy, Asthma and Immunology. But first you've got to know which foods they're hiding in. Here are some food additives that—very infrequently and in very few people—do wreak havoc, and the foods that they may be found in.

Aspartame. In rare cases, this low-calorie sweetener causes swelling of the eyelids, lips, hands or feet in those who are sensitive to it. It's widely used in sugar-free drinks and desserts.

Benzoates. These food preservatives are often found in cake, cereals, chocolate, dressings, margarine, powdered potatoes and dry yeast, among other foods. They have been known to cause allergic reactions in rare cases.

BHA and BHT. These compounds, which prevent oxygen absorption and are usually found in cereals and other grain products, can cause hives and other skin reactions.

Dyes and colorings. In rare cases, tartrazine, also called FD&C Yellow No. 5, can cause hives or asthma attacks.

Monosodium glutamate (MSG). Reactions to this flavor enhancer can include headache, nausea, diarrhea, sweating, chest tightness and a burning feeling at the back of your neck. But these reactions have been reported by people who eat large quantities.

Nitrates and nitrites. These preservatives, found most often in processed meats like bologna, hot dogs and salami, may cause headaches and hives in some people.

Parabens. Used as preservatives in foods and medicines under names such as methyl, ethyl, propyl and butyl paraben and sodium benzoate, parabens may cause redness, swelling, itching and skin pain in some people after skin contact.

Sulfites. These are widely used as preservatives in beers, wines, baked goods, teas, dried fruits, fruit juices, jams, jellies and canned vegetables. Sulfites may cause chest tightness, hives, abdominal cramps, diarrhea, lowered blood pressure, light-headedness, weakness and a faster pulse rate, as well as asthma attacks.

What foods did they give up? Sardines, anchovies and mackerel. Cheeses like gouda, Roquefort, camembert and Cheddar. Salami and dried ham. Pickled cabbage, spinach and tomatoes. And beer and wine. These are all foods in which histamine or sulfites may lurk, and once these are out of the diet, many histamine-sensitive people can take a turn for the better.

Histamine levels can be detected in blood plasma or urine, says Dr. Frieri. "If someone gets a headache all the time after eating sauerkraut or drinking beer, they may want to try cutting them out. If it doesn't alter your diet radically, it may be wise."

Tracking Down the Culprits

From coloring agents to preservatives to flavor enhancers, between 2,000 and 20,000 different additives are baked and blended into the foods we eat. But just how many cause adverse reactions and how frequently those reactions occur are questions that allergy experts can't answer.

"Additives in foods can cause problems, but it's very difficult to pinpoint and really prove as a problem," says Dr. Baum. "You have to be a detective to do it. I have patients bring in the lists of ingredients in foods that may be causing trouble. Sometimes we even call the manufacturer to find out what is in the food that isn't on the label."

Conservative allergists believe that additive reactions are unusual. But experiencing such a reaction can be more than unpleasant.

According to some studies, about 5 percent of people with asthma may have mild to life-threatening reactions to sulfites, used to preserve freshness in many foods and wines. Skin reactions can occur in people who touch foods containing preservatives called parabens. For some, links have been found between outbreaks of hives and the preservatives BHT and BHA. Among people who have frequent headaches, there's occasionally a link to nitrates and nitrites, preservatives that are often found in processed meats.

Among the most notorious of reaction causers is the widely used flavor enhancer MSG. For some, MSG may bring on headaches, sweating, tight muscles in your chest or neck and the feeling that your skin is crawling.

Subtracting the Additives

"An additive-free diet may help, but it's challenging," says Dr. Frieri. "You cannot eat prepared foods, for the most part. And there are even high natural levels of sulfites in avocados, raisins and dried apricots, for example."

What's left on the menu?

"Anything that's not processed," says Sherry Wilson, R.D., clinical dietitian at the Oklahoma Allergy and Asthma Clinic in Oklahoma City. With the exception of avocados, most fresh fruits and vegetables as well as organic, preservative-free breads and cereals should not cause a reaction.

What about meats? "Talk with your butcher," Wilson advises. "You shouldn't have meats that contain nitrates or nitrites, such as sausage, bacon or ham, but you could have pork chops, beef roasts or any other fresh meat."

Wilson suggests that you try this preservative-free eating plan for a month, and if your symptoms improve, slowly add processed foods one at a time to try to pinpoint which might cause a reaction. But she stresses that this trial-and-error approach is not for someone who's having very strong reactions.

Don't try this approach without a doctor's supervision if you have severe vomiting or diarrhea, eczema, asthma, swelling and itching, hives or any other strong food reactions. "There's too much risk then," Wilson says. "You need a board-certified allergist's help."

Food Your Body Balks At

If your body cannot digest a food, the results—diarrhea, bloating, stomach pain and gas—can *feel* like a food allergy.

One of the most common food intolerances of this type is the well-known lactose intolerance, which occurs when your digestive system lacks the enzyme that breaks down lactose, the sugar found in milk and other dairy products. Less often, the symptoms can be traced to gluten intolerance, in which your body cannot digest gluten, a compound found in wheat, oats and other grains. For more information about these kinds of food intolerances, see page 312 and page 326.

Allergies from Overload

If you favor a heavy diet of wheat—in your daily bread, pasta, breakfast cereal or baked goods—will your body eventually rebel?

Could regular fill-ups of orange juice, corn, milk or beef in some way overload your digestive system?

This is where traditional and alternative allergists part company. While traditionalists say no, alternative practitioners say that it happens all the time.

"I see some of the most common foods in the American diet causing problems for people," says Kendall Gerdes, M.D., an allergist in private practice in Denver. "It's not a view that traditional allergists would agree with. But when we remove certain foods from people's diets, they feel better."

There are no medical studies to back up this alternative explanation for unexplained food reactions. No laboratory tests prove that it even exists.

But allergists like Dr. Gerdes say that a litany of unexplained problems—such as fatigue, headache, difficulty concentrating, bloating, indigestion, diarrhea, gas, congestion, asthma and even

Resources for Healing

Organizations

American Academy of Allergy, Asthma and Immunology
611 East Wells Street
Milwaukee, WI 53202

Asthma and Allergy Foundation of America
1125 15th Street, NW, Suite 502
Washington, DC 20005

The Food Allergy Network
4744 Holly Avenue
Fairfax, VA 22030-5647

arthritis—can be triggered by overexposure to some of the most well-loved foods in our diets. Among the culprits he accuses are wheat, milk and corn. Less often, problems are caused by chicken, beef, chocolate, oats, rice, citrus and apple juice, according to Dr. Gerdes.

And some other doctors do agree. Dr. Walsh says that he believes people can slowly develop sensitivities to foods that they eat too often. The most frequent overindulgences? Citrus, MSG, low-calorie sweeteners, re-fined sugar, milk, corn and wheat.

Dr. Kagen says that some people are prone to food hypersensitivities that allergy tests miss. He believes the reaction is triggered when the mast cells release too much histamine too quickly.

When Bad Things Happen with Good Foods

The surprising thing, in Dr. Gerdes's view, is that the edibles that make us feel bad are the same ones that we've been taught are good for us, so we eat them often. And while they are nutritionally valuable, a steady diet of them may, in Dr. Gerdes's view, create a sensitivity.

In fact, some people may even be addicted to the foods that are asso-ciated with their allergies. This possibility, Dr. Gerdes notes, was proposed by the late Theron Randolph, M.D., a clinical ecologist and allergist, who observed the connection between food allergies and food addiction more than 40 years ago. When Dr. Randolph saw that many people were addicted to the foods they were allergic to, he began to ask what foods they loved, what foods they craved, what their refrigerators were filled with. Those were the foods they needed to take out for a week. Dr. Randolph then had his patients test for allergies by eating a large amount of each kind of food, a procedure known as challenging.

Today, Dr. Gerdes uses Dr. Randolph's methods. During the week of avoiding all of the suspect foods, it's common for patients to experience the same symptoms or feel worse for three to six days. When the addictive withdrawal is over and they feel better, they can eat a large amount of each of the foods to see which cause the symptoms to return. If the challenge causes problems to recur, they know that's the food to avoid.

After three months to two years of abstinence, people can usually enjoy the troublemaker again. "But only occasionally," Dr. Gerdes cau-tions. "More than once a week could make the problems return."

Menu Merry-Go-Round: Rotation Diets

To avoid allergies that can result from overloading with certain foods, some people have adopted a rotation diet. Wendy Reed is one of them.

Potatoes make Reed's knees ache. Milk puts her to sleep. Carrots, lamb and peanuts have unpleasant side effects, too. "There are certain foods I always avoid and other foods I can eat sometimes," says Reed, a

Families in Rotation

If you have multiple food sensitivities, a rotation diet can help calm your symptoms, says Terrill Haws, D.O., an alternative medicine specialist formerly with the Randolph Allergy Clinic in Arlington Heights, Illinois.

A rotation diet for food allergies is simple to follow. First you cut out offending foods. Then you vary your diet: Don't repeat foods from the same food family more than once every two days, and do not eat the same food more than once every four days.

But what's a food family? According to advocates of the rotation diet, each food family is a group of "related" edibles that may cause allergy-like cross-reactions.

Listed below are the most basic food families. Use this list to plan varied and enjoyable meals that won't lead to new allergy symptoms.

Plant Families

Banana: Bananas, plantains

Beech: Beechnuts, chestnuts

Buckwheat: Buckwheat, rhubarb

Carrot: Anise, caraway, carrots, celery, coriander, cumin, dill, fennel, parsley, parsnips

Cashew: Cashews, mangoes, pistachios

Composite: Artichokes, chamomile, endive, escarole, lettuce, safflower oil, sunflower oil, flower seeds, tarragon, yarrow

Goosefoot: Beets, chard, spinach

Gourd: Melons, cucumbers, gherkins, pumpkins, squash

Grape: Dried currants, grapes, raisins, wine, wine vinegar

Grass: Barley, corn and corn products, millet, oats, rice, rye, sugar cane, triticale, wheat, wild rice

Heath: Blueberries, cranberries, huckleberries

Laurel: Avocados, bay leaf, cinnamon

Legume: Alfalfa sprouts, beans, lentils, peanuts

---

patient educator at the Randolph Allergy Clinic in Arlington Heights, Illinois. "If I don't have potatoes for a month, I can have a serving and feel okay."

Headaches and bouts of fatigue sent Reed to the Randolph Clinic when she was still a high school student, and she took a job there after college. "If I had milk at school, I would have to sleep it off on a couch in the high school lounge," she says. "My parents and I wanted to straighten things out before I went to college."

That's when she found out about the rotation diet, a structured eating

Mint: Basil, bergamot, lavender, marjoram, oregano, peppermint, rosemary, sage, spearmint, summer savory, thyme, winter savory

Mulberry: Figs, hops (used in beer), mulberries

Mustard: Broccoli, brussels sprouts, cabbage, cauliflower, collards, horseradish, kale, kohlrabi, mustard greens, mustard seeds, radishes, rutabaga, turnips, watercress

Palm: Coconut, dates

Potato: Eggplant, peppers, potatoes, tomatoes, tobacco

Rose: Almonds, apples, apricots, blackberries, boysenberries, cherries, peaches, pears, plums, quinces, raspberries

Rue: Grapefruit, lemons, limes, oranges, tangelos, tangerines

Saxifrage: Currants, gooseberries

Sterculia: Chocolate, cocoa

Walnut: Butternuts, hickory nuts, pecans, walnuts

Animal and Fish Families

Bovine: Beef, buffalo, goat, lamb, milk and dairy products, mutton

Codfish: Cod, haddock, hake, pollack

Croaker: Sea trout, silver perch, weakfish

Crustacean: Crab, crayfish, lobster, prawn, shrimp

Duck: Duck, goose

Herring: Herring, sardines

Flounder: Flounder, halibut, sole, turbot

Mackerel: Albacore, bonito, mackerel, tuna

Mollusk: Clams, mussels, oysters, scallops, snails, squid

Pheasant: Chicken, chicken eggs, pheasant, quail

Salmon: Salmon, trout

Swine: Bacon, ham, lard, sausage, scrapple

NOTE: Most varieties of fish, such as bluefish, mullet, swordfish and whitefish, are in their own, separate families.

plan that eased the headaches and boosted her energy levels. "I could eat any one food only once every four days," she explains. "If I slipped up and had, say, chocolate chip cookies on the wrong day, I would feel it."

All in the Families

The rotation diet that Reed follows is still recommended by alternative allergy centers for people with sensitivities to many different foods, says Terrill Haws, D.O., an alternative medicine specialist formerly with the Randolph Clinic.

Try It for a Week

By rotating food choices, you can avoid eating foods from the same family that might cause allergic reactions. The objective is to avoid developing sensitivities to new foods yet still enjoy a diversified diet. Here's a sample week's menu on the rotation diet.

Sunday   Breakfast—Cooked buckwheat with honey; cantaloupe
         Lunch—Poached salmon; steamed broccoli
         Dinner—Baked orange roughy; rice; spinach
         Snack—Peanuts

Monday   Breakfast—Poached eggs; potato; peppermint tea
         Lunch—Yogurt; honeydew melon; sunflower seeds
         Dinner—Broiled steak; watercress; carrots
         Snack—Dates

Tuesday Breakfast—Sugar-free applesauce; walnuts, almonds and raisins; chamomile tea
         Lunch—Ham; lima beans; cabbage
         Dinner—Baked cod; baked yams; beets
         Snack—Brazil nuts

Wednesday Breakfast—Oatmeal; pineapple
         Lunch—Swordfish; zucchini
         Dinner—Chicken; mango; avocado
         Snack—Walnuts

Thursday Breakfast—Orange slices; filberts
         Lunch—Tuna; black-eyed peas; peaches
         Dinner—Salmon steak; sweet potato
         Snack—Chestnuts

Friday   Breakfast—Poached eggs; grapes
         Lunch—Eggplant with onions; banana
         Dinner—Lamb chops; potato; steamed broccoli
         Snack—Currants

Saturday Breakfast—Yogurt; grapefruit sections
         Lunch—Baked flounder; endive with wine vinegar, oil and basil; pears
         Dinner—Turkey; rice; spinach
         Snack—Raspberries

"After eliminating problem foods, we try to minimize the number of times you're exposed to any single food so it has less chance to affect you," Dr. Haws says. "If you're a person prone to food reactions, you don't want to trade one food sensitivity for another. If you avoided wheat but ate rice all the time instead, you might develop a reaction to rice. With a rotation diet, that won't happen."

The goals of a rotation menu plan are simple: Diversify your diet and rotate the foods, which means repeating them only at specific intervals. Putting it into practice is another matter. Devotees must plan meals carefully so that they don't repeat any particular food more than once in four days. Related foods from any of 137 different "food families" may be eaten every other day.

The food families range from obvious groupings to some fairly obscure and strange associations. In the Bovine Family are beef, mutton and dairy products, while the Grass Family includes wheat, sweet corn and sugar cane. The Mustard Family encompasses broccoli, cauliflower and turnips, among others. In the Carrot Family are carrots, celery and parsley, while members of the Goosefoot Family include beets and spinach.

How does the rotation menu work? Well, if you have mutton, corn and broccoli on Monday, you can't eat yogurt, wheat bread or cauliflower until Wednesday, because they're in the same families as the first group. And you can't dine on mutton, corn or broccoli again until Saturday, when a new four-day rotation cycle begins.

Don't Get Crossed

There is a reason that foods are distributed this way in the rotation diet. According to practitioners, the foods in related families may cross-react, causing the same symptoms you're trying to ease. While some people follow 7-, 8- or even 14-day rotation diets, Dr. Haws says a 4-day cycle is simple and effective.

The diet also stresses whole foods. A steak, for instance, is preferable to meatballs, which may contain wheat, eggs and other hard-to-identify ingredients in addition to beef.

"The four-day rotation diet is generally no more difficult to plan out than any other diet. You can succeed on this diet," says Dr. Haws. "Even though we may occasionally fall off the wagon, it's important to get back on and try again. And we have the framework here to help us get back on."

A Different Kind of Proof?

Lacking studies, alternative practitioners rely on their patients' success stories to prove that unexplained food reactions are real—an approach that traditional allergists do not support.

"I look for cause and effect," says Dr. Gerdes. "Critics say it's subjective. But it's direct observation. If avoiding a food makes you feel better and then challenging that food makes you worse, it's a direct effect that patients can understand," he says. "For most patients, the foods that need to come out are favorite foods. But in order to feel well again, people usually make the necessary changes."

21 Heart Disease and High Cholesterol

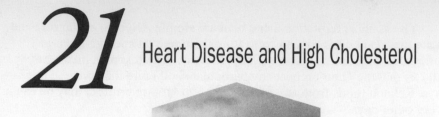

Beyond Low-Fat—The New Heart-Smart Eating

When it comes to preventing heart disease, you've stacked the odds in your favor.

You've said no to butter, banished premium ice cream from the freezer and traded in your old breakfast buddies—doughnuts and coffee, bacon and eggs—for oat bran and skim milk. You've embraced grilling, trim fat aggressively and have learned to savor the tart zing of raspberry vinegar on your salad (bye-bye, bleu cheese!).

Pat yourself on the back. Low-fat eating is the cornerstone of any heart disease prevention diet. But when it comes to food, researchers now say that there's more to preventing clogged arteries, chest pain, stroke and heart attacks than skipping the prime rib.

"One-third of the people who have heart attacks have normal blood cholesterol levels. So fixing cholesterol is not the whole answer," says James Anderson, M.D., professor of medicine and clinical nutrition in the Division of Endocrinology and Metabolism at the University of Kentucky College of Medicine in Lexington. "The foods we eat can provide other kinds of protection against heart disease. Eating low-fat is an important part of the story, but it's not the whole story."

What, then, is the rest of the story?

Although it's crucial to cut fatty foods—particularly animal fats—from your diet, the foods that you leave in your diet can be strong allies in the battle against the number one killer of men and women in America.

Researchers have found that by reaching for olive oil, soy, garlic, fruits and vegetables and grape juice—or for the water-soluble fiber found in foods like beans, oats and apples—you can reduce your risk of heart disease by nearly 25 percent.

Combining these strategies, says Dr. Anderson, magnifies your protection from the ailment that's responsible for the deaths of a half-million Americans every year and for the discomfort, worry and limits imposed on the lives of another five million who have chest pains or other symptoms of heart disease.

Two of the alternative diets described in this book—the Ornish diet and the Pritikin diet—have proven especially effective at reducing the risk of heart disease (see chapters 7 and 8 for more information about these plans). But even if you don't go whole-hog for these alternatives, there are many changes that you can make in your regular eating habits that can significantly lower your risk, research shows.

New Science for an Old Story

In fact, the heart-smart eating that researchers are now "discovering" has long been a way of life for many who follow alternative ways of eating, from vegetarianism to macrobiotics to many of the world's traditional peasant cuisines.

Test-tube science and real-life experiences have revealed the healing and protective potential in these delicious alternatives. Although we've described some of those benefits in other chapters, here's a summary of alternative diets that seem to help our hearts.

• Macrobiotics, a strict vegetarian eating plan, has been credited with reversing heart disease for skeptics such as Benjamin Spock, M.D., renowned author of *Dr. Spock's Baby and Child Care*.

"A macrobiotic diet is low in fat and high in fiber," says Dr. Anderson. "But it's also rich in antioxidants and other compounds, called phytochemicals, found in grains, soy and vegetables. These compounds can prevent blood clots and slow the clogging of arteries as well as 'tone up' diseased arteries."

• Vegetarians have lower rates of heart disease, lower blood cholesterol levels and lower body weights. Why? It could be because their diets are richer in fiber, unsaturated fats, minerals and antioxidants.

In rural China, people who eat traditional vegetarian fare—grains, fruits and veggies—have very low rates of heart disease and healthy blood levels of cholesterol, researchers with the China Project on Nutrition, Health and Environment found. In contrast, Chinese who live in big cities and eat a more Westernized diet replete with meat, eggs and dairy products have higher rates of heart disease.

• While enjoying a varied diet that includes olive oil, fresh fish, pasta and a wealth of fresh produce, dwellers on the Mediterranean island of

Crete reduce their risk of fatal heart disease by more than 70 percent.

"The Mediterranean diet contains an abundance of whole grains, fresh fruit and vegetables and olive oil, which is high in monounsaturated fat that's important for a good blood cholesterol profile," says Walter C. Willett, M.D., Dr.P.H., professor of epidemiology and nutrition at Harvard University School of Public Health and a proponent of the health benefits of Mediterranean eating. "There's plenty in the Mediterranean diet that can be adapted for Americans concerned with heart disease."

An Alternative to Disease

But you don't have to clear the cupboard or move to Crete to take advantage of the dietary alternatives to heart trouble.

"There are just too many people who are placed on cholesterol-lowering drugs who do not have to be doing that yet," says Robert Nicolosi, Ph.D., professor of clinical science and director of cardiovascular research at the University of Massachusetts in Lowell and a former member of the American Heart Association's (AHA) nutrition committee.

"If instead people modify their diets to lower the fat, raise the fiber and include other important nutrients with pharmaceutical-like activities, many won't have to use drugs, or they can at least delay them or use lesser amounts," he says. "Diet is a way for people concerned with heart disease to be in better control of their health."

Of course, food influences only some factors in the heart disease equation. A new way of eating can reduce your risk of heart disease by lowering total cholesterol levels, dropping high levels of "bad" low-density lipoprotein (LDL) cholesterol, preserving "good" high-density lipoprotein (HDL) cholesterol and keeping your body weight within a healthy range. But for both men and women, the risk of heart disease also rises as you age (it's higher for men over 45 and women over 55) and if you smoke, have a family history of early heart trouble, have diabetes, are not physically active or have high levels of stress.

"Still, what you eat is extremely important," says Ronald Krauss, M.D., chairman of the AHA nutrition committee and a researcher in the life science division of the Lawrence Berkeley Laboratory at the University of California at Berkeley. "What you choose and how much it can help depend on your health history and how you respond to dietary changes."

First Things First

Ray Kurzweil is one smart guy. He's among the world's leading authorities on artificial intelligence, runs a successful company, Kurzweil Applied Intelligence in Waltham, Massachusetts, and has, at last count, nine honorary doctorates.

But his diet and his genes nearly did him in.

"My father died of a heart attack when he was 58," he says. "I lived under a cloud. I had the sense that I would never live to see my own son reach the age of 32."

In late 1987, this creative and highly motivated engineer began using his brainpower to lower his risk of heart disease.

Kurzweil's blood cholesterol levels looked grim. His total cholesterol was 234 mg/dl (milligrams per deciliter) and was a risk factor all by itself. (Below 200 mg/dl is considered healthy, and 200 to 239 is borderline-high, while 240 and above is high-risk.)

But total cholesterol didn't tell the whole story.

At that time, doctors rarely measured LDL cholesterol, the type that can clog arteries and raise the risk of heart disease, so Kurzweil doesn't know how high his LDL level was. But chances are good that it too was in the danger zone. A healthy LDL level is 130 mg/dl and below.

Kurzweil's level of HDL, the good guys that remove cholesterol from LDL particles and transport it to the liver for reprocessing and excretion, was a dangerously low 27. (An HDL level under 35 is a risk factor for heart disease, while a level above 60 is considered protective.)

"I changed my way of eating almost overnight," he says. "First a low-fat diet recommended by the American Heart Association improved my cholesterol levels somewhat. But it wasn't enough for me. So I did a lot of research, talked with my doctor and adopted a diet that gets just 10 percent of calories from fat—a very low fat diet."

He added exercise and started walking 20 miles a week. He began practicing stress management, too.

By January 1989, his total cholesterol dropped to 110 and his HDL rose to 44. His LDL was a healthy 57. Eager to tell the world about his success, he wrote a book, *The 10 Percent Solution for a Healthy Life*.

"I don't worry about getting heart disease at all anymore," he says. "I'm quite confident that I won't. I feel the cloud has dissipated. Too bad I can't go back in time and give that knowledge to my father."

Too Much of a Good Thing

For a small percentage of women and men, high cholesterol levels and clogged arteries are genetic problems that are virtually unrelated to diet. But most of us are like Ray Kurzweil: While family history plays a role, we're sliding toward heart disease because we're eating too much fat, Dr. Nicolosi says.

Your body needs some fat and cholesterol. They are necessary for manufacturing cell membranes, storing energy and insulating your internal organs. Your body also needs fat to absorb the fat-soluble vitamins (A, D, E and K), maintain healthy hair and skin and construct hormone-like compounds that control important body functions.

And the Meat Goes On . . .

Don't pass the steak—dig in.

Long condemned as a villain in the battle against heart disease, red meat is now seen by nutrition experts as an acceptable—and enjoyable—part of a low-fat diet. "If you choose lower-fat cuts, trim all visible fat and grill or broil without added fat, we've found that beef has about the same effect on blood cholesterol as chicken," says Lynne Scott, R.D., director of the Diet Modification Clinic at Baylor College of Medicine in Houston.

For five weeks, Scott and other Baylor researchers fed a low-fat diet that that featured either chicken or beef to 38 men who had high levels of blood cholesterol. The beef was a small strip loin steak, and "the guys loved it!" Scott reports.

So did their hearts: Men on both diets saw total cholesterol and LDL (low-density lipoprotein) cholesterol levels drop.

But don't reach for the prime rib. Scott emphasizes that small portions, aggressive fat removal and simple cooking make beef a heart-healthy choice. For example, three ounces of top round, well-trimmed and broiled, weighs in with almost two grams of saturated fat and five grams of total fat—leaner than skinless, dark-meat chicken.

In contrast, three ounces of extra-lean hamburger has nearly 2½ times the fat of the top round with all the fat trimmed off. Here's how the leanest cuts of red meat stack up against equal three-ounce portions of equal three-ounce portions of chicken and fish.

But most Americans go overboard, getting about 34 percent of total calories from fat, an amount that's slightly higher than the 30 percent that the AHA recommendeds. But many heart experts advocate diets that get 20 percent or even 10 percent of their calories from fat, which makes the AHA's recommendations seem like overload. The 20 percent or 10 percent goal is much more feasible for people on an Ornish, Pritikin, macrobiotic, vegetarian or similar alternative diet, for example, than for those who cling to the mainstream American diet while trying to cut a little fat here and there.

Research also shows that we overdo it on saturated fats, which are found in animal products such as meat, cheese, whole milk and butter. Coconut and palm kernel oils are also high in saturated fat.

Since all fats are calorically dense (with nine calories per gram), we can also take in too much unsaturated fat, the kind found in fish and plants.

Meat	Total Fat (g.)	Saturated Fat (g.)
Beef (choice grade, all fat removed, broiled or braised)		
Top round	5.0	1.7
Top sirloin	6.7	2.6
Bottom round	7.5	2.5
Chuck arm pot roast	7.5	2.7
Ham (roasted)		
Lean ham, cured	4.7	1.5
Arm picnic	6.0	2.1
Regular ham, cured	7.7	2.7
Poultry		
Turkey, no skin, light meat, roasted	2.7	1
Chicken, no skin, light meat, roasted	3.9	1.1
Turkey, no skin, dark meat, roasted	6.2	2.1
Turkey with skin, light meat, roasted	7.1	2
Chicken, no skin, dark meat, roasted	8.3	2.3
Lean ground turkey	8.4	2.5
Chicken with skin, light meat, roasted	9.3	2.7
Fish and Seafood		
Lobster, boiled	0.5	0.1
Cod, baked	0.7	0.1
Haddock, baked	0.8	0.1
Shrimp, boiled	0.9	0.2
Crab, boiled	1.3	0.1
Tuna, water-packed	1.5	0.3
Swordfish, baked	4.4	1.2
Salmon, canned	5.1	1.3

The unsaturated fats include monounsaturates, which are abundant in olive, canola and peanut oils, and polyunsaturates, which are in rich supply in corn, safflower and sesame oils.

"Fat itself is not bad if consumed in moderation," Dr. Nicolosi notes. "But eat too much, particularly too much saturated fat, and the balance tilts."

Good Fat, Bad Fat

How do too many forkfuls of cheesecake become too much cholesterol in your bloodstream?

Too much saturated fat interferes with the liver's task of breaking down LDL cholesterol. "Saturated fat reduces the number and activity of fat receptors in the liver," Dr. Nicolosi says, "so more LDL stays in circulation."

The longer these LDL particles circulate, the greater the odds that they'll lodge in artery walls and form plaque, especially if those walls have

Still Good for What Oils You

For years, nutritionists and heart disease experts have championed olive and canola oils as the most heart-healthy of all vegetable oils. But not all researchers agree.

"These monounsaturated oils don't seem to lower the good HDL (high-density lipoprotein) cholesterol the way polyunsaturates like corn, safflower and sesame oil can," says Lynne Scott, R.D., director of the Diet Modification Clinic at Baylor College of Medicine in Houston. "I recommend olive oil for things like salads and milder-tasting canola for baking, to take the place of butter and lard." Monounsaturates may also protect LDL cholesterol from oxidation, a chemical change that can lead to clogged arteries and heart attacks.

Other researchers cite different findings. When a Stanford University researcher analyzed 20 oil studies, he found that polyunsaturated and monounsaturated oils were equally effective in preserving heart-healthy HDL. "There were no detectable differences in total, LDL or HDL cholesterol," notes Christopher Gardner, Ph.D., a nutritional scientist at the Stanford Center for Research in Disease Prevention in Palo Alto, California.

Even though he would not commit to choosing one type of oil over the other for cholesterol-lowering effects, Dr. Gardner notes that each type does have its own merits. "Monounsaturates may lead to less destructive oxidation in the body, and polyunsaturates may have a more beneficial impact on blood coagulation," he says. "So there may be different reasons to recommend one over the other."

---

been damaged by toxic by-products of normal cell activities. As this plaque builds—a process that doctors call atherosclerosis— artery passages become narrower.

This narrowing can restrict the flow of blood and oxygen to the heart, causing chest pain and even damage to the heart muscle. If the plaque breaks open, blood clots may form, further blocking the artery and starving the heart of needed oxygen. In a heart attack, this "starved" heart muscle dies.

Saturated fat also stimulates the liver to produce very low density lipoproteins (VLDL), which can become harmful LDL.

Substituting unsaturated fats—by dribbling a teaspoon of olive oil on your salad, for example, instead of dousing it with creamy ranch dressing that contains saturated fat—can increase the number of LDL receptors in the liver and pump up their activity level, Dr. Nicolosi says.

"Whenever you consume small amounts of monounsaturated fats or polyunsaturated fats like corn, safflower or cottonseed oil in place of saturated fats, you're ensuring that more LDL will be processed by the liver," he says.

But there's a second reason to choose unsaturated fats.

While foods cannot significantly raise HDL, monounsaturates—and possibly even polyunsaturates—are edibles that can preserve your current HDL level while LDL levels are dropping on a cholesterol-lowering diet. (The only way to actually raise your HDL is through exercise and moderate alcohol consumption, although the latter is recommended cautiously.)

But please, don't guzzle the canola. The key is to replace saturated fats with small amounts of unsaturated fat and to consume all fats in moderation, Dr. Nicolosi says. All fats and oils contain a hefty 120 calories per tablespoon, making it easy to overindulge and gain weight. And weight gain in itself can raise LDL levels.

Low, Lower, Lowest

How low must you go to reap the benefits of heart-smart, lean cuisine?

While heart disease experts have debated the question for years, they do agree on this: Keeping saturated fat under 10 percent of total calories is vital for maintaining healthy cholesterol levels. To lower high blood cholesterol, dropping "sat fats" below 7 percent is vital.

But disagreement is lively when it comes to the question of how much *total* fat is healthy. Total fat is the sum of all the saturated and unsaturated fat you eat in a day. What's best? Here's what heart specialists have to say.

The 30 percent view. The AHA recommends that all Americans over the age of two get no more than 30 percent of daily calories from fat. The AHA recommendations are also specific about the maximum amount of saturated fat you should be getting. If you have heart disease or are at high risk, a Step II diet with less than 7 percent of calories from saturated fat is recommended. If not, a Step I diet with 8 to 10 percent saturated fat is the goal.

Over time, this way of eating could reduce your blood cholesterol levels by 10 to 50 points, according to the AHA.

The 20 to 25 percent view. Many heart disease experts, including Dr. Nicolosi, believe that a leaner plan that gets just 20 to 25 percent of total calories from fat is the route to heart health.

"When we first proposed the 30 percent idea, Americans were consuming 40 to 45 percent of calories from fat, so 30 percent seemed radical," Dr. Nicolosi says. "Today, we're getting close to the 30 percent goal, but high cholesterol and heart disease are still major problems. And people are being lulled into a false sense of security, thinking that if they eat some low-fat foods, they cannot get fat or face heart disease."

A 20 to 25 percent plan is just right, he says. "Thirty isn't low enough."

The 10 percent view. Radical fat slashers like Dean Ornish, M.D., and heart specialists at the Pritikin Longevity Center in Santa Monica, California, say ultralean cuisine can actually reverse heart disease.

"This is a natural, no-added-fat diet," says Monroe Rosenthal, M.D., medical director of the Pritikin Longevity Center. "Why 10 percent? It's not a magic number. Our founder, Nathan Pritikin, found that if you eat just fruits, vegetables, whole grains, a small amount of skim dairy products and the occasional small serving of meat, that's the amount of fat you're eating.

The Sneaky Fat

Is margarine really better than butter?

For years, the answer was yes. Full of artery-clogging animal fat, butter was, in the view of heart experts, the fast lane to a heart attack. Margarine, in contrast, was deemed safer thanks to its vegetable oil base.

Now studies show that at least some margarine—and many other processed foods that contain trans-fatty acids—may be as bad as butter.

"Trans-fats are vegetable oils converted into solid fats, also called partially hydrogenated fats," explains Walter C. Willett, M.D., Dr.P.H., professor of epidemiology and nutrition at the Harvard University School of Public Health. "These fats are solid at room temperature, like animal fats. But in your body, they may be significantly worse."

Unlike other vegetable oils, trans-fats raise bad LDL cholesterol and lower good HDL—trends that could raise your risk for heart disease. In fact, when Dr. Willett and other researchers followed the diets of more than 80,000 nurses for eight years, they found that women who ate the most trans-fats raised their risk of heart disease by a significant amount. Women who ate four teaspoons of margarine a day had a 60 percent higher risk of heart disease than women who consumed margarine less than once a month, Dr. Willett's team found out.

"If you're really concerned about your health, you want to stay away from both trans-fats and saturated fats as much as possible," Dr. Willet says. Here are some ways to accomplish that.

• Look for liquid margarine or avoid margarine altogether.

• Use a little olive oil, sesame oil or peanut butter on your bread instead of margarine, suggests Dr. Willett. Occasionally, even a little butter is fine.

• Read ingredient labels and pass up items that contain partially hydrogenated vegetable oil. These trans-fats are used in many processed foods, including baked goods.

• Skip the deep-fryer. Fried foods, from doughnuts to french fries, are rich sources of trans-fats.

There is no added fat in this diet—no oil in the salad dressing, no cream sauces, no avocados or nuts."

Dr. Rosenthal's philosophy? "If you want great results, eat a great diet. If you want not-so-great results, eat a not-so-great diet. You really have to go below 20 percent of calories from fat to make a difference. Our program dramatically reduces cholesterol levels and heart disease as well as health problems like obesity and diabetes."

The bottom line? "People should follow an aggressive low-fat diet when the risk merits it," says Dr. Krauss. "Those with known heart disease and those at extremely high risk because of factors like an unfavorable cholesterol profile or family history of heart disease ought to be given the benefit of a more fat-modified diet."

But, Dr. Krauss notes, it may not be realistic or necessary for the entire population to follow an extremely low fat diet. "A super low fat diet is difficult to adhere to," he says. "Suggesting it for everyone is suggesting a big change that's not going to happen easily."

Can You Take a Yolk?

If high blood cholesterol levels are the enemy, wouldn't the best defense against heart disease be to avoid cholesterol-laden foods?

Yes and no. The AHA suggests that we all eat no more than 300 milligrams of cholesterol a day—about the amount in one egg yolk and a 3½-ounce piece of skinless, roasted chicken—and that those at higher risk for heart disease curb cholesterol consumption to less than 200 milligrams daily.

"But watching cholesterol is only part of the picture. Saturated fat has a much bigger impact on blood cholesterol levels than dietary cholesterol does," says Wahida Karmally, R.D., director of nutrition at the Irving Center for Clinical Research at Columbia-Presbyterian Medical Center in New York City. "Even if you consumed no cholesterol, your body would still manufacture its own."

In fact, most of the cholesterol traveling in your bloodstream comes from your liver, not from this morning's over-easy eggs.

Karmally and other researchers are also discovering that some of us can tolerate more dietary cholesterol than others. Genetic differences, age, body weight, exercise habits, fruit and vegetable intake and even menopausal status (premenopausal women enjoy some hormonal protection from heart disease) all partly explain why some people absorb more of the cholesterol they eat than others do.

In two studies at Columbia-Presbyterian Medical Center, Karmally and other researchers found that healthy young women and men who consumed three to four eggs a day as part of a low-fat diet saw modest rises in total cholesterol and LDL.

"The increase was modest but significant," Karmally says. "While it's true that some people are more sensitive to dietary cholesterol than others, there is no simple test that will help you find out how you respond. So at this point, we're suggesting that everybody stick with the four eggs a week limit suggested by the American Heart Association."

But if you eat a low-fat diet with few animal products, you may be able to enjoy eggs more often, she adds. "If you are a vegetarian or eat very small amounts of meat, fish or chicken, you may be able to have an egg a day, as long as you know that there's cholesterol in all animal foods."

It's also hidden in baked goods and many quick-cooking foods, from frozen entrées to ice cream and from cake mixes to cheese products. "And

(continued on page 366)

Hitting Some New Lows

Want to know how to streamline your cuisine? Here's how diet experts Penny Kris-Etherton, R.D., Ph.D., professor in the Department of Nutrition at Pennsylvania State University in University Park, and Diane Grabowski-Nepa, R.D., chief nutritionist at the Pritikin Longevity Center in Santa Monica, California, converted a typical day's meals into a range of heart-healthy choices that get either 30, 20 or 10 percent of calories from fat. Each menu totals about 1,870 calories.

30 Percent Calories from Fat

Breakfast ½ medium plain bagel with 1 teaspoon margarine and 1 teaspoon jelly
1 cup shredded wheat cereal
Small banana
8 ounces skim milk
8 ounces orange juice
Cup of coffee with 1 ounce skim milk

Lunch ½ cup canned, low-sodium minestrone soup
Roast beef sandwich made with 2 slices whole-wheat bread, 2 ounces lean roast beef, ¾ ounce low-fat, low-sodium American cheese, lettuce, 3 slices tomato and 2 teaspoons margarine
Apple
Water

Dinner 3 ounces flounder, cooked in 1 teaspoon vegetable oil
½ medium baked potato with ½ teaspoon margarine
½ cup green beans with ½ teaspoon margarine
½ cup carrots with ½ teaspoon margarine
White dinner roll with 1 teaspoon margarine
½ cup frozen yogurt
8 ounces unsweetened iced tea

Snack 3 cups popcorn with 2 teaspoons margarine

20 Percent Calories from Fat

Breakfast Medium plain bagel with 1 teaspoon nonhydrogenated peanut butter and 1 teaspoon jelly
1 cup shredded wheat cereal
Small banana
8 ounces skim milk
8 ounces orange juice
Cup of coffee with 1 ounce skim milk

Lunch ½ cup canned, low-sodium minestrone soup

Roast beef sandwich made with 2 slices whole-wheat bread, 2 ounces lean roast beef, ¾ ounce nonfat, low-sodium American cheese, lettuce, 3 slices tomato and mustard

Apple

Water

Snack 8 ounces nonfat yogurt

Dinner 3 ounces flounder, broiled without oil

½ medium baked potato with ½ teaspoon nonfat sour cream

½ cup green beans with ½ teaspoon olive oil

½ cup carrots with ½ teaspoon olive oil

Whole-wheat dinner roll with 1 teaspoon jelly

½ cup frozen yogurt

8 ounces unsweetened iced tea

Snack 3 cups air-popped or nonfat microwave popcorn

10 Percent Calories from Fat

Breakfast Plain bagel with 2 tablespoons nonfat cream cheese and 1 teaspoon sugar-free all-fruit jelly

1 cup shredded wheat cereal

¾ cup fresh berries

Cup of herbal tea or coffee with 1 ounce evaporated skim milk

Lunch ½ cup nonfat, low-sodium minestrone soup

Chicken or turkey sandwich made with 2 slices whole-wheat bread, 2 ounces sliced chicken or turkey, 1 slice nonfat American cheese, lettuce, 3 slices tomato and mustard

Apple

Large salad made with 1 cup vegetables and nonfat dressing

Snack 8 ounces nonfat yogurt

Nonfat oat bran muffin with blueberries

Dinner 3 ounces flounder, broiled without oil

Baked potato with 2 tablespoons nonfat sour cream

½ cup green beans

½ cup carrots

Whole-wheat dinner roll with 1 to 2 teaspoons sugar-free apple butter

½ cup nonfat frozen yogurt

Snack 3 cups nonfat microwave popcorn

Liposuction for Hamburger

Meat loaf. Meatballs. Meat tacos. If you hanker for the hearty flavor of ground meat but can't imagine consuming all that fat and cholesterol, then a biophysicist at Boston University School of Medicine has good news: With a pot, a strainer, some oil and boiling water, you can rinse away 90 percent of the saturated fat and up to half the cholesterol, leaving behind meat nearly as lean as a skinless chicken breast.

"I developed this in my kitchen and had it tested in the lab, and it's the only way I cook ground meat anymore," says Donald M. Small, M.D. "I think it's especially good news for men. Studies show that red meat is the main source of saturated fat and the second biggest source of cholesterol in their diets."

Here's the Small method for defatting a pound of hamburger: In a pan or teakettle, bring at least one cup of water to a boil. Meanwhile, add the meat and one cup of vegetable oil to a large saucepan and heat until the oil bubbles, gently mashing the meat into small pieces in the pan. Cook for ten minutes, then pour the oil and meat into a strainer placed over a large heatproof bowl. Immediately pour about one cup of the boiling water over the meat. This method can be adapted for use with up to several pounds of ground meat, if necessary.

"You can use this in meat loaf, stuffed grape leaves, spaghetti sauce, tacos or any recipe that calls for ground meat," says Dr. Small. "If you want to recapture some of the meat flavor that's washed away by the water, use a gravy separator or turkey baster to pull the broth— not the fat—out of the bowl, and add it to your spaghetti sauce."

Why use oil to remove the fat? "Fat and cholesterol dissolve in oil but not in water," Dr. Small explains. "As long as you wash all the oil out at the end, you won't be adding fat or calories to the meat. In fact, the meat will have all the protein calories but less than a quarter of the fat."

One word of culinary caution: This method doesn't make the best meat for burgers on the grill, Dr. Small notes. "I've tried binding the meat together with all sorts of things, and it's just not the same," he says.

---

any time you add eggs to a dish, remember that you're getting cholesterol," Karmally adds. "Two eggs in a quiche that feeds five is 80 milligrams per serving—almost as much cholesterol as in a small piece of chicken."

Feeling Your Oats, Peas, Beans and Barley

Remember the oat bran craze?

In the 1980s, the powdery, ground-up outer layer of the oat grain was all the rage in the battle against heart disease. It starred as an addition to cereals and muffins, as a soup thickener and casserole topping. Entire diet books were devoted to this humble product.

And for good reason. Rich in a kind of soluble fiber called beta-glucan, oat bran was found to lower total cholesterol by as much as 23 percent in people who ate between four and eight ounces for two to three weeks. LDL levels dropped as much as 24 percent.

These days, you don't have to find a million and one uses for oat bran in order to fit in soluble fiber.

"Beans, barley and fruits and vegetables are all good sources," says Dr. Anderson. "You don't have to stick with oat bran. About one-quarter of the fiber in most fruits and vegetables is the soluble fiber that helps fight heart disease."

Mopping Up Cholesterol

Think of fiber as a kitchen sponge. The loose-knit structure of fiber molecules permits them to grab and hold other molecules on the journey through your digestive system. Soluble fiber picks up water molecules and apparently much more.

Researchers are still scratching their heads over how this fiber sponge whisks LDL cholesterol out of the body, but many believe that it binds with bile acids in the intestines and escorts these cholesterol-laden compounds out. Your body must then recruit more cholesterol to make more bile acids, reducing cholesterol levels in the bloodstream.

Another theory is that by eliminating bile acids, fiber reduces the amount of fat absorbed into the body. Less fat means less LDL cholesterol.

Still others point out an indirect effect: A filling, high-fiber diet is probably also lower in saturated fat and would drop cholesterol levels simply because you're eating less fat.

"You need to get at least 10 to 15 grams of soluble fiber a day, as part of a diet that gets at least 30 grams of total fiber, to see any benefit," says Dr. Anderson. "Adding a half-cup of beans or a bowl of oat bran will really help."

Rich sources of soluble fiber include kidney beans, with three grams of soluble fiber in a half-cup serving; an unpeeled apple, with one gram; an orange, with one gram; carrots, with one gram per half-cup; oat bran, with three grams per cup of cooked cereal; oatmeal, with two grams per cup of cooked cereal; pearl barley, with two grams per three-quarters of a cup; and cooked sweet potato, with two grams per half-cup.

When you eat soluble fiber in fruits, vegetables and grains, you're getting a package that also contains vitamins, minerals and other nutrients, notes fiber researcher Helenbeth Reiss Reynolds, R.D., a spokesperson for the American Dietetic Association.

But if you cannot get enough soluble fiber or find that you fall short some days, Dr. Anderson suggests trying a fiber supplement made with psyllium, such as Metamucil. "I take it in the morning, mixed with water, and then have some psyllium wafers in the evening," he says. "That adds about seven grams of soluble fiber to my day."

Dining with Heart

Corn-crab soup. Salmon with molasses glaze. Fillet of beef with bleu cheese and toasted pecans.

In Philadelphia, that's heart-healthy eating.

"People eat out so often these days, we wanted to help them find great food that was also healthy," says Cheryl C. Marco, R.D., coordinator of the Dining with Heart program at Thomas Jefferson University Hospital. "You can have food that's fun and exciting without consuming too many calories or too much fat and sodium. The 40 restaurants in our program are proving it."

Among them is Carolina's Restaurant and Bar, where chef Paul Verica's low-fat creations include poached salmon with jalapeño ginger broth, pork tenderloin crusted with winter herbs, and venison with wilted spinach, sweet potato chips and a blackberry demiglaze.

"The attitude that healthy food can't taste good is wrong," Verica says. These are some of his palate-pleasing, heart-healthy cooking suggestions.

Watch the portion size. Even beef and pork can be low in fat and calories if you choose lean cuts and keep portion sizes to three to six ounces, depending on the cut.

Spritz on the oil. Very small amounts of olive oil, or even butter, add flavor without much fat. Or try using an olive oil spray.

Use small amounts of strong-tasting ingredients. "We use feta cheese crumbled in our Mediterranean salad," Verica says. "It's just an ounce, but it adds so much flavor."

Add flavor with broth or juice. Instead of using heavy, fat-laden sauces, serve meat dishes with a strong-flavored broth or even a thick juice. "A pear juice, made by pureeing a fresh pear, then thinning the puree with water or chicken stock, is delicious with pork," he says.

Cook without fat. Poach chicken or fish in stock or herbed water. Or, for meats with some fat, simply use a very hot pan.

Know no limits. Even foods that at first glance seem astronomically high in fat can often be transformed into a lower-fat dish. "I'm working on a duck recipe right now," Verica says. "If you remove the skin and grill or broil it to get the fat out, it's okay."

Go for bold flavors. Delight your taste buds with fresh ginger, cumin, lime or complex Indian spices. "Look for bigger, bolder flavors," he says. "You've got to try new things. Otherwise your mouth will be bored."

Fiber has an added bonus that can help you lose weight or maintain a healthy weight. "It fills you up," notes Reynolds. "You feel fuller for a longer period of time, so you may not have the urge for a snack."

One reminder: Add a little fiber each day to avoid bloating and gas.

Increase your intake of water and other fluids at the same time, aiming for eight (eight-ounce) glasses a day, to keep the fiber moist and moving.

Why Your Arteries Love Fruits and Vegetables

When the diets of more than 80,000 nurses were studied for eight years, scientists found a compelling link: The risk of heart disease was 34 percent lower among women who consumed the most vitamin E than among those who consumed the least. It fell 22 percent for those who got the most beta-carotene, the compound that gives carrots, squash and melons their orange hue. And it dropped 20 percent for those whose diets contained the most vitamin C. Overall, the risk of heart disease was 46 percent lower for the women with the highest intake of all three nutrients.

What is it about vitamins E and C and beta-carotene? They're among the most abundant antioxidants, a huge family of natural substances that appear to disable the chemical process that turns LDL cholesterol into an artery clogger.

Antioxidants, researchers say, also trap free radicals, toxic substances that are produced naturally in the body and can damage cells and contribute to the clogging process.

When researchers at Johns Hopkins University in Baltimore measured carotenoid levels in the blood of 123 people who had had a myocardial infarction, or heart attack, and 246 people without heart problems, the antioxidant-heart link was found to be especially relevant for people who smoke.

Those with the lowest levels of beta-carotene more than doubled their risk of heart attack. Those with the lowest levels of lycopene, an antioxidant found in tomatoes, increased their risk 30 percent. And smokers had the lowest blood levels of carotenoids and the highest risk of having a second heart attack.

Strawberries or Supplements?

Getting antioxidants from foods like carrots, oranges, spinach and grains is best, says Michael Gaziano, M.D., director of cardiovascular epidemiology at Brigham and Women's Hospital in Boston. While he suggests that five servings a day is a good start, other heart experts advocate adding supplements.

"Fruits and vegetables have been consistently protective," says Dr. Gaziano. "Exactly what substances in the fruits and vegetables are at work is something we don't know. There are thousands of antioxidants and 600 different carotenoids alone. The benefits may come from a combination of substances."

Vitamin E is found in vegetable oils, cereal grains, nuts and green vegetables. For beta-carotene and other carotenoids, try carrots, squash, melons, spinach and broccoli. For vitamin C, top choices are citrus fruit, cranberry juice, strawberries, guava, papaya, kiwifruit and black currants.

In addition, apples, onions and black tea seem to be packed with a

Quick Picks for a Healthy Heart

In a rush? You can still do your arteries a favor with these fast, heart-healthy choices.

Black tea. A rich source of flavonoids that can help prevent artery-blocking blood clots.

Boneless, skinless chicken breasts. They're quick-cooking, and white meat and no skin make them low in saturated fat.

Canned beans. Beans can add a quick helping of soluble fiber (generally, about three grams per half-cup serving). As a fast and meatless entrée, heat up a can of black beans mixed with a can of black bean soup and serve over brown rice with a side salad.

Fresh fruit. Fruit is a quick snack that's full of fiber and antioxidants. Top sources of beta-carotene include apricots (fresh or dried), cantaloupe and mangoes. For vitamin C, choose citrus fruits, strawberries, melons, kiwifruit, blackberries or raspberries. Pears, apples and berries are also high in soluble fiber.

Frozen fruit and vegetables. Antioxidant-packed choices include carrots, broccoli, okra and collard greens for vitamin A and frozen cranberry, grape, grapefruit or orange juice for vitamin C.

Grape juice. While fruit juices lack the fiber found in fresh fruit, purple grape juice is another rich source of flavonoids.

Low-fat processed meats. If you hanker for bacon, sausage, bologna or hot dogs, choose a low-fat variety.

Nonfat frozen yogurt, sorbet and frozen fruit juice bars. Low-fat and fat-free dessert selections can keep you from the temptation—and the saturated fat overload—of premium ice cream.

Nonfat yogurt. A fat-free snack with the bonus of bone-building calcium. Add raisins or fresh fruit for fiber and antioxidants.

Nonstick cooking spray. The spray greases pans for everything from muffins to a vegetable sauté with a fraction of the calories in a dollop of cooking oil.

Plain frozen fish fillets. Cook them quickly in the oven or microwave. Most

---

group of protective antioxidants called flavonoids. In a study of 805 men ages 65 to 84 living in Zutphen, the Netherlands, Dutch researchers found that those who ate the most of these common foods had the fewest heart attacks and lowest risk of death from coronary heart disease.

What if you can't fit in five servings of antioxidant-rich produce every day? Experts, including a panel of scientists called together by the Alliance for Aging Research, based in Washington, D.C., suggest that supplements can be a good nutritional backup.

"I tell patients in our preventive cardiology clinic who want to take supplements to stay on the low end," Dr. Gaziano says. "I suggest 100 to

varieties contain less fat than either red meat or chicken.

Prewashed, precut, bagged vegetables. Go for baby carrots for beta-carotene. Broccoli and dark, leafy greens like spinach are rich in both vitamin C and beta-carotene.

Quick-cooking barley. Use it as a side dish that's packed with soluble fiber and ready in less than 15 minutes.

Ready-to-eat whole-grain oat cereal. Pull out the box and pour on the skim milk for an instant breakfast. Or toss a handful into a plastic bag for a mid morning snack. A 1¼-ounce serving has three grams of soluble fiber.

Soy milk. Chocolate soy milk makes a tasty snack, and vanilla is good in baking or for French toast. Soy contains plant estrogens that fight heart disease.

Soy snack bars. One crunchy bar contains a healthy dose of soy protein and plant estrogens.

Textured vegetable protein (TVP). It sounds weird, but it cooks up like ground beef. Look for dried granules of TVP in health food stores and use it in place of ground meat in spaghetti sauce, lasagna, tacos, soups and stews. It's a good source of artery-protecting isoflavones.

Tofu. Sizzle cubes of tofu in a frying pan or wok with a smidgen of oil and a few of your favorite veggies, then serve over rice. (Look for blocks of isoflavone-rich tofu in the produce aisle of the supermarket.)

Veggie burgers. These burgers are quick-cooking, low in fat and high in fiber. Versions that contain soy protein concentrate, however, are low in heart-smart plant estrogens.

Wheat bran. It's not just for breakfast any more. Sprinkle it on casseroles and vegetable dishes as a crunchy topping or add it to muffins, waffles and pancakes.

Wheat bran and oat bran muffins. Both are packed with fiber. Choose small or medium-size muffins to avoid a calorie overload.

Whole-wheat bread. Whole-grain products are higher in fiber than those made with white flour and are rich in vitamin E, another heart-smart antioxidant.

---

200 international units of vitamin E, 250 milligrams of vitamin C and 5 to 10 milligrams of beta-carotene."

Remember, he says, that supplements cannot cancel out other risk factors for heart disease. "You can't take supplements in place of eating a healthy, low-fat diet or in place of exercising or in place of quitting smoking," he says. "Those lifestyle changes are clearly proven to benefit your heart."

Grape Ways to Block Heart Disease

It wasn't an office party. Inside the Coronary Artery Thrombosis Research and Prevention Laboratory at the University of Wisconsin in

Madison, director John D. Folts, Ph.D., and his colleagues took turns drinking grape juice and then drew each other's blood.

"After drinking grape juice, we looked at the platelet activity in our blood and found that it was slowed down by the grape juice," Dr. Folts says. "This may help prevent heart disease in several ways."

Disk-shaped platelets are the blood's clotting experts. But they also contribute to atherosclerosis and, when forming blood clots in narrow arteries, to heart attacks. Dr. Folts believes that quercetin, one of the flavonoids found in red wine, grape juice and many fruits and vegetables, makes platelets less "sticky" and less likely to form clots.

Flavonoids like quercetin may also be the key to understanding the so-called French Paradox—the fact that the croissant- and pâté-loving French have one-third the heart attack rate of Americans, despite the fact that they eat more saturated fat. "It could be the flavonoids in the wine that the French drink," Dr. Folts says. "And our research has found that you don't have to drink wine to get the benefits. Grape juice works, too."

How much grape juice?

"It takes about three glasses to get the effects of one glass of red wine," Dr. Folts says. "But there are lots of ways to get flavonoids in your diet. I drink black tea instead of coffee now. There are flavonoids in apples, broccoli and kale, too. If you get six to eight servings of fruit and vegetables a day, you're probably getting enough."

In fact, Dr. Folts—the researcher who discovered the anti-clotting properties of aspirin—thinks crunching and sipping flavonoid-rich foods and beverages may prove to be a better anti-clotting strategy than taking half an aspirin a day. "This is because flavonoids have other things going for them," he says. "They're also good antioxidants."

Soy, the All-Star Bean

Soy, the humble legume found more often in livestock feed than on dinner tables in the United States, is fast emerging as the versatile all-star of the heart-protection team.

With special abilities to sweep cholesterol from the bloodstream, soy seems to boost the already substantial health benefits of a low-fat diet. This tasty plant protein appears to protect against heart disease in two additional ways, by shielding LDL from oxidation and by halting the chain of events inside your arteries that can lead to coronary blockages.

How powerful is soy?

When researchers at the University of Kentucky reviewed the results of 38 soy studies involving 743 men, women and children, they found that people who consumed about 12 ounces of soy daily saw dangerous LDL cholesterol fall by 12.9 percent. At the same time, total cholesterol fell 9.3 percent, triglycerides dropped 10.5 percent, and beneficial HDL edged slightly upward.

Soy seems to rev up LDL receptors that draw bad cholesterol out of circulation and send it to the liver, where it is broken down before being excreted. There are benefits for people who don't have high cholesterol or heart disease, too. Soy also appears to prevent the growth of new smooth muscle cells inside arteries and to stop blood platelets from sticking together, both of which lead to atherosclerosis.

By protecting LDL from oxidation, soy seems to have the ability to halt atherosclerosis before it can begin. In addition, soy appears to keep artery walls flexible.

"In heart disease, artery walls constrict when they should dilate, or expand," Dr. Anderson says. "That's dangerous if you have plaque in your arteries already. With soy, artery walls tend to dilate when they're supposed to."

New Praise for an Old Bean

Grown in China for more than 5,000 years—where its name, *ta-tou*, means "greater bean"—soy was first significantly connected to lower cholesterol levels by American heart disease researchers in the 1960s. They discovered that prisoners who ate a soy-rich diet had lowered blood cholesterol. But those findings gained little public attention at first.

Today, many of the answers to the soy mystery are emerging in Italy, where this legume is the subject of serious research and where it is also widely prescribed to adults and children who have an inherited high cholesterol condition.

Just how hard-working soy clears cholesterol and protects arteries is still a mystery, says Dr. Anderson, who analyzed the soy studies. But evidence points toward two plant hormones called genistein and daidzein. "These hormones, called isoflavones, seem to be the active ingredients," says Dr. Anderson. "We know this because in laboratory studies, soy without the isoflavones did not have a beneficial effect, and soy with the isoflavones did."

Taking It to Heart

Where can you find this versatile bean? In blocks of tofu, boxes of creamy soy milk, granules of ground-beef-like textured vegetable protein (good in chili or tomato sauce) and even snack bars. These days, new soy products, including low-fat tofu, soy-filled veggie burgers and even soy-based Italian "sausage," redolent of garlic and basil, are popping up in the supermarket.

To reap soy's full benefits, Dr. Anderson suggests that someone with high cholesterol (240 or over) may want to consider replacing most animal protein with soy protein. "If someone has high cholesterol, about 20 to 25 grams of soy protein a day would have major benefits," he says." You can get that from soy drinks, like chocolate soy milk, or from soy snack bars. I eat one every afternoon that has 9 grams of soy protein in it."

Even a few servings a week may be helpful, he adds. But it's important to choose soy products that are rich in plant hormones. Products that contain concentrated soy protein, which is often found in veggie burgers, are lower in isoflavones, he notes.

Pungent Protection

Baked garlic spread on rounds of crusty French bread. Salad greens dressed with a shimmer of olive oil and a healthy sprinkle of chopped garlic. Chicken roasted with garlic and herbs. The stinking rose, as aficionados have nicknamed this pungent bulb, lends spice to almost any portion of a meal.

Yet garlic is more than a taste treat—and more than a telltale scent to cover up after a garlic-laden repast. When researchers at New York Medical College in Valhalla reviewed five studies of garlic's effect on blood cholesterol, they found that the equivalent of a half-clove to a clove a day could lower total cholesterol by 9 to 12 percent.

"As a physician practicing classical, traditional medicine, I have to say that most evidence does point to health benefits from garlic—not only by lowering cholesterol but also apparently by preventing blood clotting," says Stephen Warshafsky, M.D., assistant professor of medicine at New York Medical College and one of the researchers who looked at the garlic studies.

The analysis confirmed what other studies have pointed toward for more than two decades: Garlic is a heart-smart seasoning.

A Clove a Day . . .

Garlic's power seems to come from the same source that delivers its spicy taste and smell—volatile sulfur compounds such as allicin. Slice, chop or crush a clove and you'll smell this sharply scented substance.

"The truth is, nobody knows precisely how it works," Dr. Warshafsky says. "Garlic is a complex mixture of many compounds."

While the studies used garlic capsules, powder or a liquid extract, eating up to a clove a day of raw or cooked garlic is also beneficial, Dr. Warshafsky notes. "In theory, fresh garlic should work as well as a capsule. As for cooked garlic, I've seen studies from India that show that even fried garlic has an effect.

"I incorporate it into most of my foods," he says. "If I make pasta or marinades for fish or beef or chicken, I include chopped or crushed garlic. If I have a salad, I add a little chopped garlic. Luckily, I really enjoy the taste."

Of course, if you don't like the taste or don't care to exhale garlic breath, a garlic supplement will do. Doses found effective in the studies were a total of 600 to 1,000 milligrams of dry garlic powder a day.

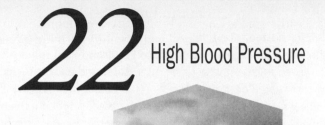

22 High Blood Pressure

Pressure-Sensitive Eating

Overheard at the supermarket:

"Corn chips?"

"No way—too much salt."

"Salami?"

"Okay, but only if it's low-sodium."

"Well, how about a shaker of salt substitute?"

"Good idea. You know, this low-sodium diet for my high blood pressure is a huge adjustment."

"Yeah, but the doctor says it's worth it."

Whether your blood pressure is a slightly elevated 140/90 or a "through the roof" 300/140, taming it is worth any effort, says Michael Alderman, M.D., professor of medicine and public health at Albert Einstein College of Medicine of Yeshiva University in the Bronx.

Why? Every year, this devious killer (also called hypertension) is responsible for 150,000 stroke deaths, a half-million heart attack deaths and thousands of cases of kidney disease.

All high blood pressure is dangerous, according to Dr. Alderman. "You want to do all you can, as soon as you can, to bring high blood pressure down to normal. For many people, that means medication. But diet and other lifestyle changes can sometimes be effective, too."

Ease the Pressure—Fast!

Call it the no-food solution.

No breakfast. No lunch. No dinner. When 51 women and men with high blood pressure fasted on water alone for 5 to 30 days, their blood pressure readings plummeted from perilous to perfect—and still registered as healthy more than two years later, according to research performed at the Center for Conservative Therapy in Penngrove, California.

"People were able to get off medication and stay off medication," says Alan Goldhamer, D.C., director of the center. "But it wasn't with fasting alone—afterward they ate whole, natural foods with no animal-based products like meat, cheese or milk, no added sodium and no added fat. They also began exercising and learned relaxation techniques."

Fasting, in Dr. Goldhamer's view, is both a powerful blood pressure tamer and a quietly dramatic "gateway" to new, health-promoting habits.

"The body goes through physiological changes in fasting," he says. "Some sodium and water are eliminated, which reduces blood volume and blood pressure. And body fat—including, I believe, fats that are clogging arteries—is burned as fuel. So the blood has more room inside your arteries."

But don't try this at home. "A medically supervised fast is best," Dr. Goldhamer says. "That way, a doctor will be monitoring your health. A decision can be made at the right time to stop blood pressure medication. It's safer."

Still, even those who don't have the time, money or inclination to undergo a medically supervised fast have seen their blood pressures drop after adopting the center's recommended healthy lifestyle plan, he adds.

"A fast alone won't fix high blood pressure. The only long-term solution is a nutritious vegetarian diet, regular exercise, relaxation and getting enough sleep," cautions Dr. Goldhamer. "You have to feed your body whole foods and keep stress from building up." (For more information on fasting, see chapter 11.)

Hypertension researchers, who study the diets, lifestyles and medications of people who have high blood pressure, say that getting enough calcium, magnesium, potassium and vitamin C may be the nutritional strategy that your body needs to put the damper on raging blood pressure. Avoiding sodium, while crucial for those with salt sensitivity, may not be important for everyone.

"Blood pressure control is no longer a single-nutrient issue," says David McCarron, M.D., director of the National Institute of Diabetes, Digestive and Kidney Disease clinical nutrition research unit at Oregon Health Sciences University in Portland. "For some people, salt may not be the real issue at all."

Taking the Low Road

Silent and stealthy, high blood pressure wears out your blood vessels, thickens your heart muscle, scars your kidneys and degenerates the retinas of your eyes. What's worst of all, elevated blood pressure may prompt blood vessels in your brain to leak, burst or clot, usually without giving you a single outward sign until the damage is done.

All told, the blood pressure of nearly one in four Americans is in the danger zone. Risk rises with age. You're also at greater risk if you're African-American, if you have diabetes, or if you have a family history of high blood pressure.

Discovering whether or not you have high blood pressure is simple: A nurse or doctor slips a blood pressure cuff around your upper arm, then inflates and rapidly deflates it, all the while listening intently to your pulse.

The pressure gauge linked to the cuff supplies two important numbers. The first measurement, called systolic pressure, indicates the pressure on blood vessel walls when the heart beats. The second number is diastolic pressure, the pressure between beats. At 140/90, you've officially joined the hypertension club, although hypertension experts say the risk of heart disease and stroke may actually begin to rise at 120/80.

But what can you do to keep high blood pressure in check?

The Vegetarian Approach

One of the best counteroffensives, according to some experts, is a vegetarian diet. They say that getting sufficient vitamin C and plenty of fiber may help. A good source of these nutrients is a menu that puts fruits, vegetables, whole grains and beans on center stage and relegates animal fats to a bit part—or no part at all, says Chris Melby, Dr.P.H., associate professor of nutritional science and director of the Human Energy Laboratory at Colorado State University in Fort Collins. So be sure to read about vegetarian diets if you want to enlist nutrition to help lower blood pressure (see chapter 1).

In a study of 167 African-American women and men, Dr. Melby found that those following vegetarian diets had the least hypertension and the lowest blood cholesterol levels.

"I think the potential benefit of the vegetarian diet is the mix of nutrients in the fruits, vegetables, whole grains and legumes," says Dr. Melby. "Researchers cannot find any single nutrient that seems responsible. In all likelihood, the higher intakes of fiber, vitamin C, potassium and magnesium may be important. Also, the lower prevalence of obesity among vegetarians contributes to their lower risk for developing high blood pressure."

You may be able to get the benefits of a vegetarian diet even if you're not strictly vegetarian. While many studies show that vegetarians have lower rates of high blood pressure than meat-eaters, Dr. Melby says that at least one revealed that vegetarians who added small amounts of lean meat to their diets did not show a rise in blood pressure.

And even if you don't "go vegetarian," make sure that you get enough vitamin C in your diet. Why? A study at Colorado State University found an association between higher blood levels of vitamin C and lower blood pressure. Further research is needed to help determine whether or not increasing vitamin C intake can actually lower blood pressure, notes Dr. Melby. In the meantime, it can't hurt to raise your daily ration of vitamin C by enjoying rich sources such as cherries, black currants, orange juice, red bell peppers, cranberry juice cocktail, strawberries, kiwifruit, cantaloupe, brussels sprouts and broccoli.

Sip Slowly, Dine Lightly

Apart from following a vegetarian or near-vegetarian diet, there are two other diet strategies that often help lower blood pressure—losing weight and drinking alcoholic beverages in moderation.

Consider weight loss. Whittling away just 10 pounds can lower your systolic reading by 10 points and your diastolic by 5—enough to whisk a person with mild hypertension out of the danger zone. Losing 22 pounds can accomplish even more, reducing systolic blood pressure by more than 15 points and diastolic by more than 13 points.

"Reducing body weight is probably the single most effective intervention you can make against hypertension without using drugs," says William J. Elliott, M.D., Ph.D., director of the Section of Clinical Research in the Department of Preventive Medicine at Rush-Presbyterian-St. Luke's Medical Center in Chicago. "It probably has even more impact than reducing salt intake. (To permanently lower your weight without dieting, see chapters 7 and 8.)

Hypertension experts agree that limiting alcoholic beverages also puts the brakes on revved-up pressure. For those who want to maintain healthy blood pressure, moderate sipping is a good strategy to remember.

"For hypertension control, limiting yourself to two drinks a day for a man or one drink a day for a woman is best," Dr. Alderman says. "Moderate drinking is all right. I think there's good evidence that a little bit of alcohol is good protection from heart disease."

One drink, by the way, is an ounce of the hard stuff, a 12-ounce glass of beer or a 5-ounce glass of wine.

A Grain of Salt

What about salt?

The National Academy of Sciences suggests that everyone limit sodium consumption to 2,400 milligrams a day. That's the amount in one level teaspoon of table salt and only about half of the 4,000 milligrams that

Fend Off Pressure's Partners

If you have high blood pressure, you may be one of the millions of Americans with a related, "tag-along" health problem or two. Like high blood pressure, those related problems often can be improved if you adopt new eating strategies or choose the right alternative diet to replace your current one.

In fact, overweight, high cholesterol and the tendency toward diabetes often accompany high blood pressure. "So often, actually, that they're called the deadly quartet," observes William J. Elliott, M.D., Ph.D., director of the Section of Clinical Research in the Depart-ment of Preventive Medicine at Rush-Presbyterian-St. Luke's Medical Center in Chicago. "In each case, what you eat can be part of the solution."

Here's why it's important to give these tag-alongs the slip.

Overweight. About one in three people with high blood pressure is also lugging around extra pounds. "The most effective high blood pressure intervention without taking pills is to reduce weight," Dr. Elliott says. And reducing weight can help reduce the risk of diabetes and high cholesterol, too.

Diabetes. One in three people with diabetes also has high blood pressure—a combination that accelerates the risk of kidney damage and eye problems as well as heart attack and stroke.

A low-fat, low-calorie, high-fiber diet improves both conditions, experts note. Adding foods that are rich in potassium and going light on the salt also help reduce blood pressure in people with diabetes.

High cholesterol. In one study of 11,199 New Englanders, 3 out of 20 people had both high blood cholesterol levels and high blood pressure.

In addition, a team of Italian researchers found that the "bad" LDL (low-density lipoprotein) cholesterol circulating in the blood of people with hypertension seems especially susceptible to chemical changes that lead to clogged arteries.

How can you fight back? Lose weight and exercise, the New England researchers suggest.

---

most Americans consume daily. Other experts say that the role of sodium—one of table salt's main ingredients—in raising blood pressure may be an issue only for people who are salt-sensitive.

"There's no question that some people are very sensitive to sodium and that eating less salt helps lower their blood pressure," says Dr. Alderman. "But we don't have any evidence that a low-sodium diet is good for everybody."

There might be another possibility, researchers say. Perhaps we're all salt-sensitive to some degree.

"If you have a high salt intake, you're at greater risk for high blood pressure," says Dr. Elliott. "The biggest worldwide study of hypertension, called INTERSALT, proved that. That study looked at people in 53 places, and the connection was quite clear. In the Amazonian rain forest, people who eat almost no salt have very low blood pressure. But in Hokkaido, Japan, where salt intake is among the highest in the world, the rate of hypertension is high."

Although there are no simple, inexpensive tests to prove salt sensitivity, it's possible that up to half of those with hypertension may be exquisitely responsive to salt. You and your doctor may be able to use dietary trial and error to see if salt's a factor for you, says Dr. Elliott.

"If you have high blood pressure and find out you're salt-sensitive, you'll want to do something about it," he says. "For such people, reducing salt intake is effective."

To cut back, target the salt shaker first, then go after the "salt mines" like anchovies, sauerkraut, salami and salty snack foods, including potato chips. And try to dodge the processed foods that account for more than 70 percent of our daily salt intake. Even though canned foods like beans and frozen foods like peas and corn may not seem salty, nearly all have added sodium, unless the label specifically says "salt-free" or "sodium-free," so read labels carefully.

One word of caution: In an eight-year study of 2,937 hypertensive men, Dr. Alderman and other researchers at Albert Einstein College of Medicine and Cornell University Medical College in Ithaca, New York, found that those with the lowest salt intakes had the highest rates of heart attack. "Caution would dictate that if you're taking hypertension medicine, you may not want to follow a low-salt diet," Dr. Alderman says. By consulting with your doctor, you can judge whether a low-salt diet is right for you.

Minerals That Make a Difference

Could a humble bowl of bran cereal, doused with skim milk and topped with a sliced banana, help tame dangerous high blood pressure?

Possibly, because this basic breakfast is rich in magnesium, calcium and potassium, three minerals that researchers say seem to play important supporting roles in the battle to lower high blood pressure.

"When you get enough calcium, magnesium and potassium, the effect of salt on blood pressure is much, much smaller," says Dr. McCarron. "When you don't, the effect of salt seems to be much greater."

But this mineral triumvirate does more than counteract the salt shaker's effects. In laboratory studies, Dr. McCarron says, these minerals reduce blood pressure by keeping blood vessels relaxed and more able to open up, giving your blood more room.

Dr. McCarron isn't alone. Here's what other researchers have learned about these three minerals.

Calcium

When researchers at the Centre de Recherche Hotel-Dieu de Montreal reviewed dozens of studies on the calcium-hypertension link, their conclusion was that getting enough calcium in your diet can help prevent high blood pressure.

How much calcium? In the researchers' view, getting at least 800 milligrams a day—or 1,200 milligrams if you're pregnant—should be sufficient. The best sources are dairy products and other calcium-rich foods.

The strongest proof? Large population studies. When researchers looked at the diets of 3,886 male Taiwanese workers, they found that significantly more of those with normal blood pressure took in at least 500 milligrams of calcium a day.

And when researchers from the Chinese Academy of Medical Sciences asked 2,762 Chinese men and women about their eating habits, they, too, found less high blood pressure among those who consumed the most calcium-packed edibles.

Other researchers recommend calcium levels higher than the 800 to 1,200 milligrams suggested by Dr. Pavel. Dr. McCarron recommends about 1,000 milligrams a day for most of us. And research shows that pregnant and nursing women need 1,200 to 1,500 milligrams to help build the baby's bones and possibly to prevent preeclampsia, a dangerous type of high blood pressure that can develop when you're expecting, according to the National Institutes of Health in Bethesda, Maryland.

Look for calcium in nonfat and low-fat dairy products, including skim milk, nonfat yogurt and part-skim mozzarella cheese. Other calcium-rich choices include collard and turnip greens, spinach, broccoli, canned sardines or salmon (eaten with the bones), almonds, calcium-fortified breakfast cereals and calcium-fortified citrus juices, according to the Calcium Information Center at Oregon Health Sciences University.

Potassium

Not too many minerals make headlines. But potassium did, after researchers in Naples, Italy, found that some people who ate plenty of potassium-rich foods could eventually cut their doses of hypertension medicine in half. Participants increased their daily consumption from about 2,760 milligrams to about 4,460 milligrams (about 1,000 milligrams more than the Daily Value, or DV), mostly by eating more fruits, vegetables and beans.

"There's some reason to believe that a high-potassium diet helps lower high blood pressure," Dr. Elliott notes. "In people with normal kidney function, extra dietary potassium doesn't hurt—and may help—blood pressure, particularly in African-Americans. So if your kidneys are okay, I'd say it's fine to try it."

Enjoy two or more servings of potassium-packed fruit and vegetables every day to keep your levels of this important mineral high, suggests Dr. McCarron. While most of us consume less than 2,700 milligrams a day, it's estimated that we need about 3,500 milligrams a day for good health. Rich potassium sources include baked potatoes, bananas, winter squash, spinach, kiwifruit and orange juice.

Foods to Mine for Lower Pressure

You'll fight high blood pressure every time you choose one of the foods listed below, which are rich in magnesium, potassium and/or calcium. But adding these foods to your menu won't do it alone. Make sure they're part of a meal plan that goes easy on sodium and helps you achieve or maintain a healthy weight. The table shows the percentage of the Daily Value for the critical nutrients that you get from each food.

Food	Portion	Nutrient	Amount (mg.)	% Daily Value
Almonds	1 oz.	Magnesium	86	22
Apricots, dried	10 halves	Potassium	482	13
Avocado	½ medium	Potassium	602	17
Banana	1	Potassium	451	12
Clams, steamed	20 small (about 3 oz.)	Potassium	565	16
Lima beans	½ cup	Potassium	485	13
Mackerel	3 oz.	Magnesium	83	21
Orange juice, fresh	8 oz.	Potassium	496	14
Peaches, dried	5 halves	Potassium	647	18
Potato, baked	1	Potassium	610	17
Prune juice	8 oz.	Potassium	707	20
Pumpkin seeds	1 oz.	Magnesium	152	38
Raisins, golden	½ cup	Potassium	545	15
Skim milk	8 oz.	Calcium	302	30
Soybeans, mature, boiled	½ cup	Magnesium	74	18
Spinach, boiled	½ cup	Magnesium	78	20
Sunflower seeds, dried	1 oz.	Magnesium	101	25
Swiss chard, boiled	½ cup	Magnesium	76	19
Tofu, firm (with calcium)	¼ block	Magnesium	47	12
		Calcium	553	55
Wheat germ, toasted	¼ cup	Magnesium	90	23

Magnesium

From people with diabetes to older women to those already taking anti-hypertensive medicines, magnesium seems to help cool off "hot" high blood pressure readings.

When 28 people with Type II (non-insulin-dependent) diabetes added a magnesium supplement to their diets for six weeks, their systolic blood pressure fell by about seven points. The most dramatic improvement was a reduction from a high reading of 162/82 to a safe 130/66, according to researchers at East Carolina University School of Medicine in Greenville,

North Carolina, and the Center for Health Sciences Research in Primary Care at the Veterans Administration Medical Center in Durham, North Carolina.

The study participants took 384 milligrams of magnesium a day. To get approximately that amount from food sources, you'd have to eat a cup of bran cereal, two tablespoons of pumpkin-seed kernels and a half-cup of boiled wax beans.

When Swedish researchers gave 365 milligrams of magnesium a day to 39 men and women with moderately high blood pressure for eight weeks (following initial treatment with a placebo, or "dummy" pill), they found that systolic blood pressure readings decreased significantly. Patients in this study continued treatment with high blood pressure medication during and after the study.

When 47 middle-aged and elderly women with mild to moderate high blood pressure took 485 milligrams of magnesium daily for six months, their systolic blood pressure fell by 2.7 points and diastolic pressure dropped 3.4 points more than in those who were not taking the magnesium.

The DV for magnesium is 400 milligrams, and Dr. McCarron notes that it seems to take at least this much a day to help tame hypertension. Again, he suggests getting yours from food rather than a supplement, if possible.

Mighty sources of magnesium include 100% Bran, Bran Chex, Bran Buds and All-Bran breakfast cereals, dried pumpkin-seed kernels, wax beans, wheat bran, wheat germ and lima beans.

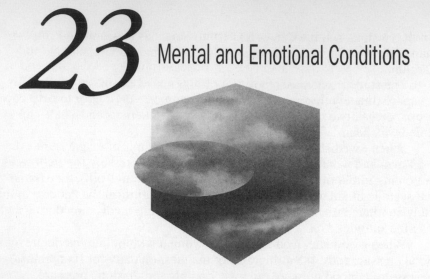

23 Mental and Emotional Conditions

Eating for What's Eating You

Meg Ryan's a pretty unhappy pretty lady throughout most of the hit romantic comedy *Sleepless in Seattle*.

She gets engaged to the wrong man. And eats a bag of potato chips.

She falls head over heels for inaccessible Tom Hanks. And downs a pint of ice cream.

She wallows in her sorrow by watching the classic tear-jerker *An Affair to Remember* while she shovels fistfuls of popcorn into her mouth.

"I love that movie," says nutritionist Elizabeth Somer, R.D., author of *Food and Mood*. "Meg Ryan's doing what we all do—using food for comfort. And she manages to look so cute while she's doing it."

But that's Hollywood. When we try reaching for the Häagen Dazs after a bad day, we end up looking more like Meg Blimp than Meg Ryan. And although sugary treats make us oblivious to the world's woes for a short time, in the long run we're not only a little heavier, we're not much happier, either.

So why do we bury our noses in the fridge instead of a good book when we're feeling blue? Why do we duck into the local Dunkin' Donuts when life pushes us to the brink? Why are some of our precious moments so often punctuated with chocolate?

A lot of it is cultural, concedes Somer. But there's more to it than that. Just as food can help clog or clear your arteries, it can also lift your spirits or bring you down. It can even trigger more serious conditions like depression, says Somer. "You can really change your moods with the right food."

If you're one of those people who rocket through everyday ups and downs, singing the blues as you ride the roller coaster of life, read on. The secret to lifting your mood and smoothing some ups and downs may be as close as your kitchen.

Your Brain Action

As a health-conscious person, you probably know all about eating for a healthier heart and trimmer physique. Now it's time you learned how to feed your brain.

The ten-pound mass of gray matter between your ears is the information center for your life. Every thought, feeling, message and reaction—physical and mental—is channeled through this information superhighway called the nervous system.

At the most basic level, communication flows through your body across billions of minuscule nerve cells called neurons. Unlike other cells in the body, neurons are not round but tree-shaped, complete with roots, a trunk and sprawling branches. The branches get a message and send it down the trunk and into the roots, which are responsible for passing the word on to the next neuron in line. That's tougher than it sounds, because neurons aren't connected. For one neuron to "talk" to another, it has to find a way to fire its message from its roots and across a gap, called a synapse, to the branches of the receiving neuron.

Your Zap Code

Luckily, neurons are equipped with their own fleet of torpedoes that shoot across those gaps and let communication flow. They're nerve chemicals called neurotransmitters. Once the message has been sent, these chemicals either break apart in the synapse or are stored for future use in the receiving neuron.

There are at least 40 different neurotransmitters. Each one is responsible for carrying different messages such as hunger, memory, movement, alertness, sleepiness and so on. A shortage or excess of any of these neurotransmitters means either an overload or a deficit in one of these important signals, which can cause a host of problems, including depression, mania and memory loss.

What does this have to do with whether you ate Froot Loops or cold pizza this morning?

"Some neurotransmitters, such as serotonin, dopamine and norepinephrine, are made directly from components found in food," says Somer. "Changes in your diet can dramatically change the levels of these neurotransmitters and how you feel."

Are You a Carbohydrate Craver?

Sure, a cookie might be just what you need after a bad day. We all seek solace in sweet carbohydrates sometimes. But if you eat the whole box once you've had one, or you can't get through a day without a carbo binge, you may have an imbalance in serotonin levels, says nutritionist Elizabeth Somer, R.D. The imbalance may cause severe carbohydrate cravings and could contribute to weight gain.

To find out if you're a "carbo craver," take this simple quiz from Somer's book, *Food and Mood*, by responding True or False to the following statements.

1. It is difficult to resist sweets and desserts._____
2. I would rather snack on bread, a granola bar, cookies, cakes or other starchy or sweet foods than on peanuts, sliced meats, yogurt or crunchy vegetables._____
3. When I am tired, depressed or irritable, I feel like eating something sweet._____
4. I have a hard time stopping once I start eating sweets, starches or snack-foods._____
5. I am not satisfied after a meal or snack that contains only meat and vegetables._____
6. A breakfast of eggs, bacon and toast is likely to leave me feeling tired and hungry for something sweet by midmorning._____
7. I feel better (more relaxed, more calm or uplifted) after eating something sweet._____

Meeting the Mood Regulators

Of the three neurotransmitters Somer mentions, serotonin is the one that most affects people's moods, she says. "Without enough of it, you can experience symptoms like depression, food cravings and insomnia. How much serotonin you have is often directly related to your diet."

Serotonin is manufactured in the brain from an amino acid called tryptophan, which is found in protein-rich foods like chicken, tuna and tofu. Oddly, however, eating high-protein foods actually *lowers* levels of tryptophan and serotonin in the brain, says Somer.

Why? Because tryptophan isn't the only amino acid found in protein-rich foods. There are more than two dozen of them, and when you eat protein, they all make a beeline for your brain. Tryptophan is the slow horse in this race and ends up getting stuck in the bloodstream.

To get tryptophan into your brain, you have to clear the path of all other amino acids. Your magic wand is composed of carbohydrates. When you eat a carbohydrate-rich meal, your pancreas releases the hormone in

8. After being on a strict diet, I indulge in sweets and starchy foods._____

9. I feel lethargic and irritable when I don't have a midmorning or midafternoon snack._____

10. I would prefer a simple meal with a dessert to a gourmet meal with no dessert._____

11. I feel more energetic after eating a starchy or sweet snack._____

12. I have a craving for something sweet or starchy almost every day._____

13. My cravings for sweets or starchy foods are so strong that I often am unable to resist giving in to them._____

14. The urge to eat sweets or starchy foods is greatest after a meal that contained only meat and vegetables._____

15. I've tried lots of diets but have not had long-lasting success with any of them._____

Scoring: Total the number of statements that are true for you. A score of 5 or less reflects a low probability that you are carbohydrate-sensitive. A score between 6 and 9 suggests that you might be moderately carbohydrate-sensitive, but you can control your cravings. A score of 10 or greater indicates that carbohydrate cravings might be a problem for you.

If you are a carbo craver, Somer recommends eating meals and snacks that include small amounts of complex carbohydrates throughout the day, exercising, drinking plenty of water, eating low-fat foods and finding alternative flavorings like vanilla and cinnamon to satisfy your sweet tooth.

sulin into your blood. Insulin causes other amino acids to be absorbed into the body's cells, leaving a free path for tryptophan to enter the brain and increase serotonin levels.

Once it reaches its destination, tryptophan acts as nature's tranquilizer. If your head is spinning from stress, serotonin is the calming agent that stops the whirl. If you're already calm, serotonin sends you into Dreamland.

Carbohydrates come in two forms—simple, like table sugar and candy bars, and complex, like pasta and whole-grain bread. Simple carbohydrates act like crumpled-up newspapers in your body's furnace. They burn fast and furiously and then, poof, they're gone. Complex carbs are more like logs: They burn a little longer. But from a purely chemical standpoint, it doesn't matter whether the carbohydrate is the simple kind in a Snickers bar or the complex variety in a whole-wheat bagel, says Somer. Both kinds boost serotonin.

Serotonin's counterparts in this brain game are dopamine and norepinephrine, which are also manufactured from an amino acid found in protein-rich foods—tyrosine.

"Low levels of these neurotransmitters also cause depression and poor mental functioning, while high levels stimulate alertness," says Somer. When you're working on a project and your brain starts clicking things into place, you can thank dopamine and norepinephrine.

Unlike tryptophan, tyrosine beats other amino acids in the race for your brain, so eating protein-rich foods raises your levels of tyrosine, dopamine and norepinephrine, she says.

Mind-Meal Manipulation

How much we can manipulate (or are manipulated by) these neurotransmitter levels is a point of contention among researchers.

One camp believes that you can literally switch yourself on or off simply by eating your steak before your potatoes, or vice versa.

They also believe that low levels of neurotransmitters like serotonin are often at the root of common ills such as obesity, because people with low serotonin levels constantly crave (and eat) carbohydrate foods to boost those levels and make themselves feel better.

Others aren't so convinced.

"The tryptophan connection in humans is overblown," argues Larry Christensen, Ph.D., chairman of the Department of Psychology at the University of South Alabama in Mobile. "To get the tryptophan-serotonin effect, you'd have to eat a pure carbohydrate containing no protein at all, like straight sugar," he observes.

Yet there are studies to back both arguments, suggesting that this may be a case where some people are just more sensitive to neurotransmitter effects than others, according to researchers.

So if you're feeling stressed-out or bummed-out or have the winter blahs, give these diet suggestions a try, say the experts. You've got nothing to lose but your blues.

Depression: Good Foods for Blue Moods

You're alone. It's raining. There's nothing on TV. And you're depressed. You open the freezer and reach for the super-deluxe ice cream that seems like your only true friend. You begin to eat. And eat.

If this sounds like something you'd do, you're not alone. Lots of people turn to food to change their mood. All too often, though, all that food indulgence leads to even more "bumming out," say experts.

"It happens all the time," says Dr. Christensen. "You lose your job, you feel depressed, and you start eating. Pretty soon, you're still feeling bad long after the depression about the job has passed. And you're still overeating."

"People who are depressed tend to eat large amounts of refined, processed sweet foods," explains Peter Manu, M.D., director of the Medical Services Department of Psychiatry at Long Island Jewish Medical Center in Glen Oaks, New York, and associate professor of medicine and psychiatry at Albert Einstein College of Medicine of Yeshiva University in the Bronx. "What they don't realize is that by eating all of these foods, they're creating a nutritional deficit. Refined processed flours and sugars have only limited nutritional value," he notes. Not only that, but your body uses up vitamins and minerals in the process of assimilating those substances.

Since carbohydrates increase soothing serotonin levels, it makes sense that you would crave carbohydrates in times of woe. And we all know that a Hershey bar sounds better than a bowl of oatmeal when the weight of the world becomes burdensome. But if you want to rise out of the depression doldrums, it's better to reach for a bagel than a Butterfinger, say experts.

Should You Go Sugarless?

Ever since William Dufty sat down at his typewriter in 1975 and detailed the evils of refined sugar in the book *Sugar Blues*, laymen and experts alike have been debating the health risks of refined sugar.

And while they've been debating, the rest of us have been eating. Sugar consumption continues to rise faster than a bundt cake in a hot oven, with the average American downing over 100 pounds of the sweet stuff a year.

Coffee, Tea or Energy?

We all know people who drag themselves out of bed, growling at everyone in sight until they've had their first shot of the elixir of energy—coffee. Heck, maybe one of those people looks at you from the mirror every morning.

But while most java drinkers associate a steamy cup of Mississippi Mud with increased energy and improved mood, experts say that all that caffeine actually has the reverse effect.

Caffeine depletes the body of B vitamins, which you need for proper brain and nervous system functioning and for converting food to energy, says Michael Murray, N.D., a naturopathic physician in Seattle and author of *Chronic Fatigue Syndrome: Getting Well Naturally.* To make matters worse, it also prevents iron absorption, says Dr. Murray, which can lead to anemia, a condition in which you have too few oxygen-carrying red blood cells and which is a major contributor to fatigue.

"Your body also adapts to the effects of caffeine, so you need more and more coffee for the same effects," says Dr. Murray. "Eventually, you're drinking so much that you develop a medical condition called caffeinism, which causes depression and irritability."

If you can't cut out caffeine completely, experts recommend limiting your consumption to no more than 300 milligrams, or two eight-ounce mugs of coffee, a day.

That's a lot of Tootsie Pops. And although licking all those lollies seems to have made us jubilant youths, dumping all that sugar into our systems through processed foods and baked goods is making us pretty miserable adults, say researchers.

"Sweets will raise serotonin levels and make you feel better temporarily, but in the long run they add to your depression problem rather than solve it," says Somer. "You feel better for an hour, maybe even two, but once your blood sugar levels start to drop, you crash, feel awful and want more sugar."

"Some cases of depression clear up completely just by eliminating sugar from the diet," says Dr. Christensen, who has studied the food-mood connection for more than a decade.

He acknowledges, however, that shaking the sugar habit isn't a panacea for depression. Some people are more sensitive than others. Some aren't affected at all. But for those who are, a sugar-free diet is a lifesaver, and not the edible kind.

If sweet treats can give us a quick "up," how can they bring us down so far? Researchers aren't sure, but they believe that too much dietary sugar probably triggers temporary oversecretion of feel-good hormones such as the morphine-like compounds called endorphins. This short-lived high is followed by a serious crash, resulting in wild fluctuations in blood sugar, energy and mood.

Needing the Bs

Besides sending our bodies into overdrive, too much sugar also saps our vitamin and mineral stores, say the experts. Sugary foods not only have a tendency to replace nutritious foods in the diet, says Dr. Manu, they also use up valuable vitamins and minerals as your body processes these nutritionally deficient foods. As that happens, you may end up feeling worn out and depressed, especially if what you're lacking is B vitamins, say the experts.

B-complex vitamins, particularly vitamin B_6, folic acid and vitamin B_{12}, are crucial for sound mental health, says Somer. "And you don't have to be deficient in these vitamins to feel the effects," she says. "Just being on the borderline can cause depressive symptoms."

This makes a lot of sense, say experts, when you consider that overt deficiencies of B vitamins may cause serious psychiatric problems like dementia and paranoia. It doesn't happen that you're fine one day and have dementia the next, says Somer. Your mood gradually falls along the way.

"Women in particular tend not to get enough B vitamins like vitamins B_6 and B_{12}, because they don't eat enough foods that are rich in these nutrients, like meat," says Somer. "Folic acid may be our nation's most common vitamin deficiency. And surveys show that many women consume less than the two milligrams of vitamin B_6 they need each day. Women are also the most frequent victims of depression."

Nutrients for Your Noggin

If neurotransmitters are the carrier pigeons that transmit messages throughout your nervous system, then vitamins and minerals are birdseed. Without the proper nutrients, neurotransmitters can't operate, say experts. They recommend the following nutrients for optimal neurotransmitter functioning.

Nutrient	Daily Value	Food Sources
Thiamin	1.5 milligrams	Wheat germ and sunflower seeds
Riboflavin	1.7 milligrams	Mackerel and yogurt
Vitamin B_6	2 milligrams	Banana and baked potato
Vitamin B_{12}	6 micrograms	Herring and tuna
Folic acid	400 micrograms	Lentils and pinto beans
Vitamin C	60 milligrams	Oranges and broccoli
Iron	18 milligrams	Cream of Wheat cereal and tofu
Magnesium	400 milligrams	Tofu and sunflower seeds
Selenium	70 micrograms	Tortilla chips and tuna

To put more of these essential B vitamins in your diet, fill up on lentils, pinto beans and spinach for folate (the naturally occurring form of folic acid) and baked potatoes, bananas and chick-peas for vitamin B_6. Clams and oysters are among the top sources of vitamin B_{12}.

Obviously, not all of these foods are high on everyone's list of top favorites. "I also recommend taking a good multivitamin/mineral supplement," says Somer. "Many people just don't get everything they need through diet."

But note: This advice is for the occasional bout with the blues only, not for the kind of depression that requires medical treatment. If you're so down that normal activities seem impossible, you have no interest in friends or hobbies, you have suicidal thoughts and problems concentrating or you are sleeping a lot more or less than usual, you need to see a medical doctor.

Stress: Eating under Pressure

One thing is certain, from the times when Tyrannosaurus Rex chased us down as an appetizer to these enlightened times when rush hour traffic chases us down the freeway, every person alive has had to deal with tension. Stress was, is and always will be an inevitable part of life. But how you deal with it is not so inevitable. In fact, you have quite a range of choices—among them, the choice of foods you eat.

While experts shy away from making universal dietary recommendations for staying in tip-top health during stressful times, they agree that

Love Is like a Box of Chocolates

Love is like a red, cellophane-wrapped, heart-shaped box of chocolates. Not quite the way *you* think of that sweet emotion? Well, maybe not, but sweets for the sweet is the rule for millions of Americans. Why else would we plunk down more than $580 million for chocolate for Valentine's Day?

"Chocolate is the number one most-craved food, especially among women, and *especially* among women with premenstrual syndrome!" says nutritionist Elizabeth Somer, R.D., author of *Food and Mood.* "And nothing satisfies that craving except chocolate. It's a definite mood elevator."

No one really knows what the magical ingredient in chocolate is, but scientists have been guessing. Over the years, they've attributed our passion for chocolate to as many different factors as there are kisses in the city of Hershey.

Some experts say that chocolate simulates the feelings of being in love by elevating endorphins, the same brain chemicals that give exercisers a "runner's high." Others say it fills in for a magnesium deficit. Still others say that it simply raises our levels of the soothing brain chemical serotonin. All of these theories may be true, say experts. But lots of foods do the same thing, don't they? So we still don't know the answer to the burning question: Why chocolate?

Somer has a less technical answer. "It's probably a learned response," she says. "Nothing melts in your mouth quite like chocolate."

That doesn't mean that chocoholics should throw resolve to the wind. But neither does it mean that you have to suffer cold turkey, says Somer. "Just plan your chocolate splurges. One of the best, lowest-fat treats you can give yourself is a 'cold fondue' of two cups of cut fresh fruit and a quarter-cup of chocolate syrup. Dip away and enjoy."

---

stress tends to breed bad eating habits and that stressed-out people often eat excessively to make themselves feel better.

It's understandable, when you think about how sick stress can make you feel. Just for starters, your stressed-out body is likely to respond with a powerful fight-or-flight reaction.

To get the picture of the fight-or-flight jump-start, imagine what would happen if you were strolling down the sidewalk, minding your own business, when an unleashed pit bull came snarling around the corner, hurtling at you with fangs bared and jowls dripping.

The blood is sucked from your stomach. A tidal wave of blood cells shoots into your arms and legs, giving you the oomph to either clobber that raging pit bull or hightail it in the other direction. While your brain overloads at lightning speed, computing all possible options, your adrenal glands pump you full of the body-boosting hormone adrenaline to make sure you have the energy for your fight or flight.

It's a dandy mechanism. The trouble is, it doesn't take anything as potentially dangerous as the onslaught of a frothing dog to touch off this punch-or-sprint reaction. You can feel the same degree of fight-or-flight stress if an iron-fisted boss bursts into your office, railing at you for a botched assignment. Now what do you do? Unless you bolt out the door or bop him in the mouth, all of those hormones and blood cells that are coursing through your body only serve to disrupt your digestion and upset your stomach.

Over the long term, stress can also increase the risk of a host of all-too-common ills, including eating disorders, heart disease and even some cancers, say experts.

How Sweet It Isn't

The primary dietary advice that experts give for controlling stress concerns simple and complex carbohydrates: Dump the former and load up on the latter.

We've already mentioned that too much sugar, a simple carbohydrate, robs your body of vital nutrients, especially B vitamins. This in itself causes nervous tension and anxiety. But in addition, sugary foods also fuel the fight-or-flight response, which overworks your adrenal glands and triggers vasoconstriction, or narrowing of the blood vessels. And when your blood vessels constrict, that further contributes to your body's stress, say experts.

Our blood sugar naturally increases when we're under stress, and we don't need to add to it, says Harold Bays, M.D., director of the Lipid Center at the Columbia Audubon Regional Medical Center in Louisville, Kentucky. "Stress-related rises in blood sugar are especially a problem for someone who either has diabetes or has borderline diabetes," he says.

"I had a woman come to see me who had had diabetes for years, but her blood sugar was under control," recalls Dr. Bays. "Suddenly, her blood sugar was in the 300 to 400 range, which is very high. I couldn't find any physical cause for it. As it turned out, she was extremely upset that her nephew was going to Operation Desert Storm in the Persian Gulf War, and it was driving her blood sugar up through the roof."

We probably crave sugary, sweet foods when we're under pressure because stress breaks down brain neurotransmitters, including calm-inducing serotonin, leaving us feeling down and irritable. And that's when we go searching for a quick chocolate-covered fix, says Somer.

Following the Beans-and-Rice Road

For a healthier and longer-lasting serotonin boost, experts recommend reaching for carbohydrates. Somer suggests sticking to the following dietary guidelines to keep your body healthy, trim and stress-free.

- Eat a variety of vegetables, fruits, grain products and complex carbohydrates every day.
- Don't overeat. Spread meals and snacks evenly throughout the day.
- Limit your intake of refined sugar, salt and alcohol.
- Avoid foods high in total fat and cholesterol.
- Drink eight glasses (eight ounces each) of water a day.
- Make sure you're getting all of your essential vitamins and minerals.

Shining like Lady Liberty

Hans Selye, the late Canadian scientist who coined the term *stress*, described the phenomenon as "the rate of wear and tear on the body." Scientists today know that wear and tear occurs partially because stress accelerates our body's production of tissue-damaging molecules known as free radicals.

Free radicals are the product of a process of oxygen breakdown known as oxidation, the organic form of the process that makes iron rust and silver tarnish. It's what made the Statue of Liberty show her age, before she got her million-dollar face-lift.

There are ways to help prevent stress-induced free radicals from wearing down your immunity and contributing to such life-threatening conditions as heart disease and even some cancers. To fend off this process, experts recommend arming yourself with free radical–fighting nutrients appropriately called antioxidants.

Antioxidants step between free radicals and your body's cells, attaching themselves to the potent run-amok free radical molecules and rendering them harmless. Some of the best antioxidants are beta-carotene, vitamin C and vitamin E. If stress has you in its grip, get a grip on foods full of these nutrients as well as an antioxidant-rich multivitamin/mineral supplement, advises Somer.

For optimal stress resistance, experts recommend getting 10,000 international units of beta-carotene, at least 500 milligrams of vitamin C and up to 400 international units of vitamin E daily through a combination of food and supplementation.

Good food sources of vitamin C include citrus fruits, tomatoes and red bell peppers. Wheat germ, almonds and vegetable oils are rich in vitamin E, and carrots, broccoli and sweet potatoes are beta-carotene boosters.

Putting the Stops on PMS

Women's menstrual cycles have been called a lot of unflattering names—the nuisance, the plague, the curse. But any woman who's ever endured the bloating, cramping and mood swings that assail her during the week to ten days before menstruation knows what the real curse is.

The physical and emotional upheaval that precedes your period—

known as premenstrual syndrome—can be the most trying of times, says Somer. "On top of all the other symptoms they're experiencing, a lot of women also have intense food cravings with PMS," she says. "They especially crave sweet foods, like chocolate. Sugar consumption can go up to 20 teaspoons a day for some women!"

The key to taming the premenstrual beast is understanding why your body is screaming for chocolate-covered pretzels and then making the right dietary changes to soothe it, says Somer.

The crux of your cravings, says Somer, is probably our good friend serotonin again. "Serotonin levels drop in response to female hormones, which causes us to feel anxious and depressed. So it's natural that we'd look to sweet carbohydrates for a pick-me-up."

Another reason that we reach for sweets during "that time of the month" is that we have a shortage of endorphins, according to Somer. "Studies show that women who have PMS have lower levels of pleasure-producing brain chemicals called endorphins during the two weeks before menstruation than at any other time," she says. "This could also cause them to want more sugar."

The simple dietary solution is to maximize your serotonin levels and avoid the sharp ups and downs of the sugar roller coaster. Choose snacks that are high in complex carbohydrates, suggests Somer. That means eating healthful foods like pasta, bagels or even low-fat, lower-sugar treats like unfrosted angel food cake topped with blueberries, she says.

Women's health experts also recommend that women with PMS eliminate as much caffeine as possible from their diets and cut their alcohol consumption to no more than five drinks a week.

Smiling through SADness

It's dark when you get up in the morning. It's dark when you come home from work. It's dark everywhere. Except in the fridge, where all that food awaits, promising to help you make it through those l-o-o-o-n-g winter months.

This is a thumbnail sketch of people with seasonal affective disorder, or SAD, a form of depression that descends with the shortening of the days and lifts with the blooming of the daffodils. People who experience it tend to lose interest in all activities except two: sleeping and eating.

"The further away you are from the equator, the more likely you'll suffer from SAD," says Dr. Manu. "In New York, beginning about the end of October and going until March, people with SAD experience intense carbohydrate cravings and weight gain."

Studies have shown that people with SAD don't have different levels of the soothing brain chemicals tryptophan and serotonin. They do, however, have higher levels of the stimulating amino acid tyrosine. Scientists believe that this jazz-you-up chemical could be blocking out the calming chemicals and contributing to depression and carbohydrate cravings.

Most of these seasonal carbohydrate cravers aren't satisfying their cravings with brown rice and sweet potatoes, say experts. Instead, they're going for Twinkies and cheesecake. Although both help raise serotonin temporarily, in the long run the junk food only deepens your funk, says Dr. Manu.

"Refined, processed foods made with flour and sugar don't provide the body with essential vitamins and minerals," he explains. "Because the body has to use nutrients to process these foods, a steady diet of them actually creates a nutritional deficit."

For people experiencing SAD, Somer recommends two things: light therapy and complex carbohydrates.

"This is a case where diet probably can't do it all alone," she says. For serious cases of SAD, she notes, people need regular exposure to special high-intensity lights—called SAD lights—throughout the day. "And you need to work good nutritional complex carbohydrates into every meal and every snack," says Somer.

24 Migraines

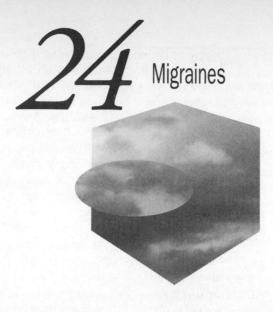

Feeding Your Aching Head

"It starts as a hot pain behind your eye and builds to a crescendo until you can't stand light, noise or even the slightest touch. You just want to die for a while," says Jane Yeager, a Pennsylvania woman in her fifties. When a migraine hits, she utters her silent wish for temporary death while lying in a pitch-black room with cool washcloths over her eyes.

Migraine headaches are a whole dimension beyond regular headaches, which are content to do their dirty work above your neck. Migraines start in your head, but a blistering attack wages war on your whole body, causing severe throbbing head pain, nausea, vomiting, dizziness, cold hands, tremors and sensitivity to light and sound. They can hang on for a few hours but often last more than a day.

Like a nuclear missile, some migraine headaches send out a "red alert" warning signal before they launch their attack. It's called an aura. Some experience this aura as flashing lights, multiple small dots, zigzagging lines or areas of total darkness and tingling or numbness in an arm or leg. Other symptoms include strange odors, restlessness, hallucinations, confusion and speech impairment.

Searching for Causes

Migraines are largely hereditary, so you're more susceptible if your mom or dad had them. And you're also more likely to get them if you're a woman, since women are three times more susceptible than men.

In Good Company

It's small consolation, we know. But if you suffer from migraines, you've got plenty of companions. Nearly 18 million Americans endure migraines, and more than 157 million workdays are lost each year because of them, according to the National Headache Foundation in Chicago.

While migraines may slow you down, they could also be a mark of distinction. Among the famous historical figures who were known to be migraineurs are Julius Caesar, Ulysses S. Grant, Edgar Allan Poe, Karl Marx, Saint Paul, Thomas Jefferson, Frederic Chopin, Charles Darwin, Leo Tolstoy and Sigmund Freud.

For the migraine-prone, lots of things can set off an attack— changing hormone levels prior to menstruation or during ovulation, poor eating or sleeping habits, stress, chemicals in food (including additives and preservatives) or low blood sugar. Even changes in the weather or moving to a higher altitude can prompt the onset of migraine.

What's going on behind your eyes during a bout with migraine is almost as puzzling as the world Alice saw behind the famed Looking Glass. Scientists believe that these mind-boggling headaches are triggered by a chain of events that begins with an electrical spasm in the back of the brain. The spasm causes blood vessels in this area to constrict, while the vessels at the top of the brain dilate. Blood gushes into the arteries around your temples, causing throbbing pain and inflammation in the covering of your brain.

What causes that initial spasm is still a mystery, but the reaction seems to be related to a brain chemical. "We know that the neurotransmitter serotonin plays a large role in triggering migraines," says Alan Rapoport, M.D., co-founder and co-director of the New England Center for Headache in Stamford, Connecticut, and assistant clinical professor of neurology at Yale University School of Medicine. "In fact, most of the newer migraine medications work primarily by stimulating the brain's serotonin receptors."

Keeping Your Fingers Off the Triggers

Although people who experience frequent attacks may have to take preventive medications, others can waylay migraine attacks by making lifestyle changes, especially in their diet, say experts. To head off migraines, you should fill up on whole, natural, unprocessed foods, especially vegetables and grains, say experts.

"You can prevent migraine headaches at least 40 percent of the time just by making dietary changes," says Frederick Freitag, D.O., associate director of the Diamond Headache Clinic in Chicago. But to do that, you have to avoid food triggers as well as eat healthfully. Some foods that are known to trigger migraines are wine, cheese, onions, tomatoes and nuts.

While it's not known why some of these foods trigger migraines in some people, chemical culprits have been found in others. Among the chief troublemakers are substances called vasoactive amines.

Avoiding Amines

For some, a hot fudge sundae studded with walnuts is a midsummer night's dream. For migraine sufferers, however, this mouthwatering treat can be a nightmare. Chocolate, along with many other common foods, contains an amine called phenylethylamine, which can cause your blood vessels to constrict, then dilate, triggering a headache.

Scientists believe that the worst of the amines is tyramine, an amino acid found predominantly in strong, aged cheeses and foods like pickled herring and liver. If you get migraines, you'll also have to watch out for homemade yeast breads and alcoholic beverages like wine and beer, say headache experts. All of these foods—as well as the pods of lima beans and snow peas—contain the dreaded amines.

"Alcohol is actually at the very top of the list of food factors that affect the most people with migraine," says Dr. Rapoport. "It is a vasodilator, meaning that it expands blood vessels, which can trigger migraine. Chocolate may be the second biggest offender."

Surprisingly, even citrus fruits and juices can trigger migraines in people who are particularly sensitive to a food factor in citrus known as synephrine, say experts.

Nixing the Nasty Nitrites

Many cured meats contain nitrites, chemicals that are added to salt when curing meats. Unfortunately, nitrites also cause your blood vessels to

---

Regular or Diet?

When it comes to knocking a couple of hundred calories from a cola, nothing does the job quite like aspartame, commercially known as Nutra-Sweet. Unfortunately for some who are prone to migraines, nothing else triggers quite the headache, either. At least that's the word from headache specialists.

"It's a controversial area, and the research has not been conclusive," says Alan Rapoport, M.D., co-founder and co-director of the New England Center for Headache in Stamford, Connecticut, assistant clinical professor of neurology at Yale University School of Medicine and co-author of *Headache Relief for Women*. "But a large percentage of the people who are prone to migraines get more headaches if they consume beverages and foods containing this chemical."

dilate, setting the stage for a migraine.

Head pounders caused by nitrites are commonly called hot dog headaches, because the worst offenders are meat and meat products like hot dogs, bacon, ham and salami. But remember, these head-thumping chemicals are found in many other preserved meats as well. If you want to lower your risk of an onslaught of migraine, doctors agree that you should go for fresh meat instead of preserved products.

Brew Some Relief

Ah, Saturday! A day to thumb your nose at the alarm clock, curl up, sleep in and awaken with an eye-popping headache! At least, that seems to be the story for many of the people who are prone to migraines.

Noticing that a certain segment of such people got most of their attacks on their days off, researchers investigated their caffeine-drinking habits. Sure enough, they found that those who had headaches on their days off consumed more than twice as much caffeine daily and slept in later on weekends than those who didn't have weekend headaches.

By sleeping in, the migraine group delayed their first caffeine fix of the day by a couple of hours. But that delay alone was enough to trigger a withdrawal headache. "If it isn't a migraine, it acts and feels just like one," says Dr. Freitag.

Actually, caffeine has different effects on migraine, depending upon how much you're used to: Excessive caffeine—more than one or two cups a day for those who get migraines—can trigger headaches. But if you're not a regular caffeine consumer, one cup can go a long way toward providing migraine relief.

"Caffeine constricts the dilated blood vessels around your temples," says Dr. Rapoport. "It also increases the efficacy of pain medication. That's why it's in most headache medications."

An Ache from MSG

Monosodium glutamate (MSG) may bring out all those wonderful subtle and spicy flavors in wonton soup, but if you're one of the many people who are sensitive to this flavor enhancer, it might also bring on a whopping headache.

Like other headache triggers, MSG launches its attack by dilating blood vessels and exciting certain nerves in the brain. Often people who get headaches from MSG have other symptoms as well, such as feelings of pressure in the neck and face, sweating, tingling in the fingers and abdominal cramps. These symptoms are so common that they've been dubbed Chinese restaurant syndrome. If you get headaches and other symptoms from this aggravating additive, ask for your food to be prepared without MSG or seasoning salt (which contains MSG) the next time you're ordering Chinese.

Although it can cause headache in anyone, MSG also can trigger migraine, says Dr. Rapoport. "We think MSG is toxic to the brain and actually triggers the electrical dysfunction in the brain that starts the migraine process."

Resources for Healing

Organization

National Headache Foundation
428 West St. James Place, 2nd Floor
Chicago, IL 60614

Books

Headache and Diet: Tyramine-Free Recipes
Seymour Diamond, M.D.
International Universities Press

Headache Relief for Women
Alan M. Rapoport, M.D., and Fred D. Sheftell, M.D.
Little, Brown

Migraine: The Complete Guide
The American Council for Headache Education Staff, Lynne M. Constantine and Suzanne Scott
Dell

25 Multiple Sclerosis

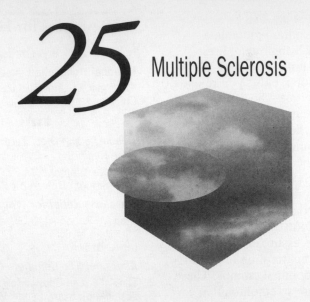

A Healing Diet?

Five years after learning she had multiple sclerosis (MS), a New York City–area massage therapist is able to rock-climb, downhill ski and even enjoy belly-dancing classes.

"I am no worse than anyone else in these classes," she notes, "which does amaze me, considering the fact that I used to fall and have trouble balancing on a bicycle."

What reversed her MS? She credits a low-fat diet devised by Oregon neurologist Roy L. Swank, M.D., Ph.D.—a diet that Dr. Swank claims can halt the progressive nerve damage responsible for MS symptoms such as loss of balance, reduced muscle coordination, fatigue, blurry vision and even paralysis.

It's a claim that's discounted by conservative MS experts and groups like the National Multiple Sclerosis Society. But Dr. Swank's eating strategy is by no means the first to be proposed for this chronic and incurable disease. People with MS have long sought relief through food, trying schemes as varied as a sucrose-free eating plan, low-calorie liquid diets, raw food regimens and programs that restrict wheat, fruit or meat.

"No diet has ever been demonstrated in a scientific fashion to be especially beneficial for halting or reversing MS," says Aaron Miller, M.D., director of the Division of Neurology at Maimonides Medical Center in Brooklyn and a member of the National Multiple Sclerosis Society medical advisory board. But Dr. Miller notes that while no diet will stop the disease,

The Food Allergy Connection

Could what they had for lunch trigger a new cycle of nerve damage for people with multiple sclerosis (MS)? Food sensitivities may be an overlooked cause of recurring MS degeneration, according to William J. Rea, M.D., director of the Environmental Health Center in Dallas.

"A food sensitivity probably would not cause multiple sclerosis, but it could make it worse once someone has MS," Dr. Rea says. Although food triggers can be highly individual, common problem foods for people with MS include wheat, sugar, corn, beef and milk, he says.

You're more likely to be food-sensitive if you're also sensitive to odors, he says. "If perfume, gasoline, cigarette smoke and even things like new carpeting and new clothing bother you or give you a headache, sensitivity is possible."

How can you track down food sensitivities that might make MS flare?

Keep a food diary, suggests Dr. Rea, and note what you eat and how you feel afterward. "See if you feel worse an hour or so after you eat. People may feel tired, weak and fatigued and perhaps have headaches or notice their thinking is fuzzy," he says. "Then try leaving those foods out of your diet."

One caution: You may need a doctor's help in striking a new nutritional balance if many foods seem to be culprits. If you're excluding important food groups like dairy products or meats, your doctor will want to recommend supplements to make up for lost nutrients.

---

eating less fat and getting more fiber can improve the quality of life for people with MS.

What's the Connection?

Fiber, found in abundance in fruits, vegetables and whole grains, can help prevent constipation—a particular problem with MS because the disease can make the bowels sluggish, according to Dr. Miller. And a low-fat eating plan can help prevent weight gain. "Flexibility, mobility and balance are already difficult for many people with MS," Dr. Miller says. "Gaining weight makes them even more difficult."

But Dr. Swank says such a diet can do more.

"When I did a study in Norway, I found the incidence of multiple sclerosis was lowest along the coast, where intake of saturated fat was very low. But inland, in farming areas where people eat more cheese and meat, the incidence was higher. And in mountainous areas, where people really live on animal products, there was eight times more MS than along the coast."

As a result, in the late 1940s, Dr. Swank began to prescribe a diet for people with MS that contains less than 20 grams of saturated fat a day. That's about the amount of fat in three to four one-ounce slices of American cheese or the combined total from two Italian sausage links and two teaspoons of salted butter.

He kept track of 144 low-fat eaters for 35 years and found that those who started the program soon after MS was diagnosed and followed it carefully had only mild symptoms. Most were still able to walk and hold jobs, although they felt tired and had some memory problems. Those who veered away from the low-fat plan experienced more severe symptoms: They were often bedridden or confined to a wheelchair.

Dr. Swank says he cannot explain how the diet might work to halt the progression of MS. "I think it allows for improved circulation in the brain, which prevents new nerve damage from happening," he says. "The important thing is starting the diet early. If you already have disabilities caused by MS, it cannot reverse them."

Dr. Swank's Lean Cuisine

Critics say that it's impossible to know whether or not diet is truly responsible for the differences found in Dr. Swank's study. But they also say the Swank diet is not dangerous.

"It's very close to the low-fat diet the American Heart Association recommends that all Americans follow to prevent heart disease," notes Dr. Miller. "If my patients wanted to try it, I would just make sure that they didn't stop taking the newer medications we now have that are scientifically known to help. Beyond that, cutting back on fat is a healthy thing to do."

Here are the basics of the Swank plan.

Keep it lean. These days, Dr. Swank suggests that people with MS keep saturated fat intake to 15 grams a day. You can do this by reading food labels and by eliminating red meat, full-fat dairy products such as whole milk and cheese, and palm and coconut oils from your diet.

"For animal protein, have white-meat chicken, turkey and fish," he says. "If you really miss red meat, a three-ounce portion of a lean meat once in a while is okay. So is the occasional egg."

Add some vegetable oil. Fit in about 1½ tablespoons of vegetable oil a day, Dr. Swank suggests. To get that much, splash olive oil on your salad, sauté your chicken or fish in a little sesame oil or bake with canola oil in place of butter. "I've found the oil helps people feel satisfied, even when they're not eating much saturated fat," Dr. Swank says.

Don't forget the fish oil. Swallow a teaspoon of fish oil every day, Dr. Swank suggests. "My feeling is that there are nutrients in animal protein that may be missing because people are not eating red meat," he says. "So the fish oil is for general nutritional balance."

Feast in the produce aisle. Eat a variety of fruits and vegetables. "The bigger the variety, the more varied the nutrients you'll be getting," Dr. Swank notes.

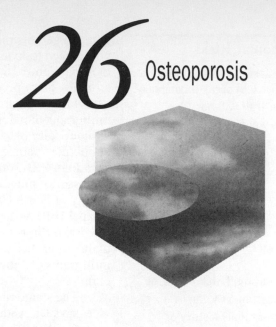

26 Osteoporosis

Winning the Battle of the Bone

A generation ago, almost no one outside the medical profession had heard of osteoporosis, the brittle-bone disease that affects more than 25 million Americans annually, most of them women. Today health-conscious people, especially women, know that we have to take care of our bones.

If you're chugging milk, swallowing calcium supplements or getting hormone replacement therapy, you probably think that you're doing everything you can to keep your bones strong. But many experts outside the mainstream of the Western medical profession say that there's more to preventing osteoporosis than loading up on calcium. Maybe we have a lot more control over how our bones age than most of us realize.

The Roots of the Calcium Crusade

Ask the average family doctor how you can prevent osteoporosis, and the first word out of her mouth will probably be "calcium."

Organizations like the National Institutes of Health in Bethesda, Maryland, and the National Osteoporosis Foundation say that most of us simply aren't getting enough calcium. Usually such organizations favor a "supply-side" approach, urging women under 50 to get 1,000 milligrams of calcium daily and recommending a whopping 1,500 milligrams a day for older women.

To get this much calcium, you'd need to load up on the most calcium-rich foods around—dairy products. "It would be very hard to get 1,000 milligrams of calcium a day without dairy products, and I doubt most people could do it," says John J. B. Anderson, Ph.D., professor of nutrition at the University of North Carolina at Chapel Hill. A glass of skim milk has 300 milligrams, and a cup of plain yogurt has as much as 400 milligrams of easy-to-absorb calcium.

The standard medical advice, says Dr. Anderson, also specifies that you should stay away from cigarettes and avoid excessive alcohol consumption. Along with that, he says, you should follow a regular exercise program. And if you take all of these recommendations to heart, research has shown that you have a much better chance of keeping your bones strong and healthy.

A Balancing Act

That said, a number of physicians outside the medical mainstream raise some questions as to whether this supply-side approach is really the answer to osteoporosis.

"Loads and loads of people have added calcium to their diets, but this has had a minimal effect on osteoporosis in this country," says Andrew Nicholson, M.D., of the Physicians' Committee for Responsible Medicine, a national organization of doctors that advocates preventive health care. "The rates of hip fracture remain astronomical."

The problem isn't how much calcium we're getting, he believes—it's how much calcium we're *losing*.

"The key to preventing osteoporosis is having a positive calcium balance," he explains. "There are two factors that determine how much calcium you have in your body—how much you consume and how much you lose in your urine."

Instead of loading up on calcium, the alternative approach focuses on diet and lifestyle changes that can help your bones hang on to the calcium they've already got.

The Price of Protein

Experts like Dr. Nicholson believe that when it comes to calcium loss, the main culprit is animal protein. Most Americans eat an excess of animal protein—often more than 100 grams per day—in the form of meat, eggs and dairy products. In fact, says Dr. Nicholson, many of us would feel much better if these protein sources were eliminated from our diets.

When scientists at Yale University compared the rates of hip fracture in 16 countries, they found that fractures were most common in populations that ate the most animal protein, including Americans, Britons and Scandinavians. By contrast, countries where the traditional diet contained little or no animal protein had the lowest rates of hip fracture, even though their diets were much lower in calcium.

Amazingly enough, there didn't seem to be any connection between an increased amount of calcium in the diet and a reduced rate of hip fractures. In fact, the countries where fractures were most common actually had the *highest* average intakes of calcium.

"Of course, that doesn't mean that calcium causes hip fractures," says Dr. Nicholson. "It's probably because the high-calcium diets were also very high in animal protein."

How does our meaty, cheesy, creamy Western diet put our bones in jeopardy? Researchers believe it's because meat, eggs and dairy are very high in sulfur, which your body converts into sulfuric acid. A regular diet of these foods actually makes your blood slightly acidic, which, studies show, increases the amount of calcium you excrete in your urine.

On the other hand, the protein-rich beans, peas and whole grains favored by vegetarians contain much less sulfur than animal products, so they don't have the same calcium-depleting effect.

Making the Change

Proponents of the alternative view believe that if you eliminate animal protein from your diet completely, you can gain the upper hand in the battle to maintain healthy bones—regardless of your age.

"It's never too late," according to Dr. Nicholson. "If you are living a typical American lifestyle, you will continue to lose calcium every day unless you do something to stop it. But if you change your

Resource for Healing

Organization

National Osteoporosis Foundation
1150 17th Street, NW, Suite 500
Washington, DC 20036.

A Bone-Building Lifestyle

When it comes to preventing osteoporosis, nutrition is only one bone pre-server. Here are some other ways you can help prevent bone loss.

Shake your skeleton. Physical activity is probably at least as important as diet for maintaining bone health, says John J. B. Anderson, Ph.D., professor of nutrition at the University of North Carolina at Chapel Hill.

Weight-bearing activities like walking or jogging help build bone in the lower spine and hip, where some of the most serious osteoporosis-induced fractures occur. To reap the benefits, you'll need to exercise for at least 20 minutes three times a week.

You're also likely to have healthier bones if you do some resistance training, like lifting light weights or exercising with resistance bands. In a study at Tufts University in Boston, postmenopausal women who lifted weights twice a week for 45 minutes at a time had significantly denser bones than women who did no resis-tance training.

Keep salt out. Some studies suggest that a salty diet can increase the amount of calcium you lose in your urine, leading to a shortage of calcium in the blood-stream. To make up the difference, your body dips into your bones' calcium re-serves, which is bad news for anyone who's concerned about osteoporosis.

The good news: By cutting back on your sodium intake, you may be able to make a real difference in your bones' density. One Australian study found that cut-ting sodium intake in half was as beneficial for bones as getting an extra 891 mil-ligrams of calcium a day. (For tips on cutting your sodium intake, see chapters 8 and 22.)

Clear out caffeine. If you drink coffee from dawn till dusk—or guzzle several diet colas a day—you aren't doing your bones any favors. When researchers ques-tioned 980 women about their coffee-drinking habits, they found a clear relation-ship between low bone density and a high caffeine intake combined with a low-calcium diet.

How much caffeine is too much? If your diet is low in calcium to begin with,

---

eating habits today, by tomorrow, for most people, there will be a measur-able difference in urinary calcium loss. Even if you're 60 and already have some degree of osteoporosis, you can still keep it from progressing."

Another Culprit

Protein, however, isn't the only dietary factor that can contribute to a calcium deficit. Some intriguing new research shows that consuming too much of the mineral phosphorus can also rob your body of calcium.

as few as two cups of caffeinated coffee a day may take a toll. Scientists still have a lot to learn about caffeine and osteoporosis, but in the meantime, cutting back on caffeinated coffee, tea and sodas makes sense.

Ban the bar habits. Two of the worst health habits around—smoking cigarettes and drinking to excess—are as bad for your bones as they are for the rest of you.

Researchers have known for a long time that smokers run a greater-than-average risk of breaking a hip or wrist. Studies of postmenopausal twin sisters reveal that smokers have significantly lower bone density than their nonsmoking sisters. Smoking seems to upset the balance of hormones that control the body's calcium balance. And drinking too much alcohol—more than one or two drinks a day—seems to interfere with the body's ability to hold on to calcium. Both habits add up to weaker bones and more fractures.

Get fortified. Vitamin D, which is necessary to help the body use calcium efficiently, is produced by your skin when it's exposed to sunlight. "Many older women don't get adequate vitamin D, especially if they avoid the sun or wear sunblock all the time," says Dr. Anderson.

If you avoid the sun, or if you live in a northern climate with long, sunless winters, the easiest way to get vitamin D is through fortified foods, including milk and some cereals. Two glasses of milk will give you the Daily Value of 400 international units. But while this amount is enough to prevent a deficiency, research shows that it might not be enough to keep your bones in top shape. A study at Tufts University found that after a year of getting 800 international units of vitamin D a day, 247 postmenopausal women living in the Boston area—not noted for sunny winters—had less bone loss than women who didn't get the extra D. The vitamin was especially beneficial during the winter and spring.

Vitamin D can be toxic when taken in large doses, so it's important not to overdo it. If you want to try some extra D, make sure that your daily intake from supplements doesn't exceed 600 international units, and you shouldn't get more than 800 international units from a combination of food and supplements.

A certain amount of phosphorus—found in most foods, but especially in some sodas and processed foods—is necessary for good nutrition. "The ideal diet would have roughly equal amounts of phosphorus and calcium," says Mona S. Calvo, Ph.D., a member of the Clinical Research and Review staff in the Office of Special Nutritionals at the Food and Drug Administration in Washington, D.C. "What we're seeing today is an increase in the proportion of phosphorus in the American diet. Due to changes in our food choices, our calcium intake has stayed the same or even decreased, while phosphorus consumption has gone up."

Rather than phosphorus intake being the main concern, it's this imbalance between phosphorus and calcium that seems to put bones in jeopardy, says Dr. Calvo. A number of studies have shown that a low-calcium, high-phosphorus diet produces severe osteoporosis in animals. We don't have all the answers yet, but some studies show that a high-phosphorus diet combined with low calcium intake may cause the body to produce too much parathyroid hormone, a compound that regulates the body's use of calcium. And research has shown that this condition, known as secondary hyperparathyroidism, can lead to osteoporosis.

Dr. Calvo believes that the increasingly low-calcium, high-phosphorus American diet most commonly seen among young people sets the stage for future risk of osteoporosis. The problem starts when we replace naturally calcium-rich foods with foods higher in phosphorus that are also deficient in calcium. If we drink soda instead of skim milk and eat processed lunch meat instead of lean, fresh meat, we're getting more phosphorus without making up the lost calcium. "Fifty years ago we didn't have readily available food choices like instant potato dishes, instant pudding, refrigerator biscuits and restructured meats such as chicken nuggets—many of which are very high in phosphorus," Dr. Calvo says. She explains that phosphate additives serve a useful purpose in modern foods by adding smooth texture or spreadable consistency, but she emphasizes that a healthy diet shouldn't focus on processed foods alone. "Many people today eat a diet based on convenience foods, supplying two or three times the Recommended Dietary Allowance of phosphorus, without a corresponding increase in their calcium consumption."

If you're concerned about your phosphorus intake, Dr. Calvo recommends first scanning food labels to be sure you're getting enough calcium in your diet. Since phosphorus isn't always mentioned on the label as a nutrient, check the ingredient list for phosphorus-containing food additives. You can recognize these additives by spotting the term *phosphate*.

Calcium without the Moo

As you're cutting back on animal protein and phosphorus, you still need to make sure you're getting enough calcium. Proponents of the alternative view do agree that calcium is important. But unlike mainstream doctors and nutritionists, they don't think dairy products are necessarily the best sources.

"Studies consistently show that countries where people eat the most dairy products also have the highest rates of osteoporosis," says T. Colin Campbell, Ph.D., professor of nutritional biochemistry at Cornell University in Ithaca, New York, and one of the architects of the China Project on Nutrition, Health and Environment, a long-term study of the relationship between diet and health. "The more dairy products a population eats, the more osteoporosis there is."

A Dairy-Free Way

Dairy products aren't the only good sources of calcium, says Andrew Nicholson, M.D., of the Physicians' Committee for Responsible Medicine, a national organization of doctors that advocates preventive health care. Here are some sources of calcium that include vegetables, cereals, legumes and fortified orange juice—everything but meat and dairy.

Food	Portion	Calcium (mg.)
Bread, calcium-fortified	1 slice	300
Orange juice, calcium-fortified	8 oz.	300
Rice Dream enriched rice beverage	8 oz.	300
Soy milk, calcium-fortified	8 oz.	300
Total cereal	1 serving	300
Bok choy, cooked	1 cup	200
Tofu, low-fat	1 cup	200
Turnip greens, cooked	1 cup	200
Broccoli, cooked	1 cup	100
Kale, cooked	1 cup	100
Kidney beans, canned	1 cup	100
Oatmeal, instant	1 packet	100
Pinto beans, canned	1 cup	100

The problem with dairy products, experts say, is that they're high in animal protein—the same stuff that's been shown to increase calcium excretion. "Much of the calcium you get is probably counterbalanced by the protein that pulls it into the urine," says Dr. Nicholson. "If you get most of your calcium from dairy, you're already at a disadvantage compared to someone who gets less calcium but gets it from plant sources."

But if you cut back on dairy products—or eliminate them entirely—how can you get enough calcium in your diet? Michael Klaper, M.D., a nutritional medicine specialist in private practice, says, "In America there's a perception that dairy products are the only good sources of calcium. But most people in Africa, Asia and South America maintain healthy bones while drinking very little milk—or none at all."

Get Greens for Calcium

Both Dr. Nicholson and Dr. Klaper suggest that women get most of their calcium from beans, green vegetables, nuts and seeds (including sesame seeds and tahini butter made from sesame) as well as from calcium-fortified foods such as orange juice, soy milk, rice milk and cereals. While the plant sources are not as loaded with calcium as milk or yogurt, all of these foods provide significant amounts of the mineral.

Proponents admit that it would be pretty hard to get the recommended 1,000 to 1,500 milligrams a day of calcium on a dairy-free diet. But they're convinced that with the right lifestyle and a diet low in animal protein, people don't have to get daily doses that are this high.

"If a woman isn't doing things that make her lose calcium, such as following a high-protein diet, getting excessive amounts of sugar, salt, caffeine or phosphorus, smoking cigarettes or drinking alcohol—and if she exercises regularly—then she probably doesn't need 1,500 milligrams of calcium a day," says Dr. Klaper. "That recommendation was made because the average American woman is in a high state of calcium loss due to a sedentary lifestyle, a high-protein diet and other factors that result in excessive calcium loss through the urine."

Just how much calcium do you need on a plant-based diet? Provided you're active, don't smoke or drink, don't consume the other calcium thieves already mentioned and eat little or no animal protein, Dr. Klaper believes that approximately 800 milligrams a day should cover it for most people. In practical terms, that's a cup of soy milk on your calcium-fortified breakfast cereal, a half-cup of beans in your lunchtime chili and a half-cup each of broccoli and bok choy in your Chinese stir-fry. Sneak in a glass of calcium-fortified orange juice sometime during the day, and you're more than covered.

An important exception, notes Dr. Klaper, is the elderly. Homebound elderly people may have higher calcium needs since their levels of exercise and vitamin D intake—from exposure to sunlight—are often minimal. According to Dr. Klaper, an especially generous intake of calcium and vitamin D may help the elderly avoid or reverse osteoporosis.

"I feel that older people who are at greater risk for osteoporosis are wise to consume an additional 500 to 700 milligrams of calcium per day, for a total of 1,200 to 1,500 milligrams daily," recommends Dr. Klaper. "Calcium supplements and fortified beverages can help to supply this extra amount."

Some experts caution that the calcium in beans and vegetables is a little harder for the body to absorb than that found in dairy products, so if you're depending on plant sources, it's important to make sure you get as much calcium from your food as possible. "To get to the calcium, you have to break down the cell walls of the plant, which contain fiber," says Dr. Anderson. "Cooking—even steaming lightly—will help, and it's important to chew very well so you get as much of the calcium as possible."

Finally, if you're concerned about getting enough calcium on a plant-based diet, calcium-fortified foods are an easy way to get some extra insurance, says Dr. Klaper. Glass for glass, fortified orange juice or soy milk provides as much calcium as cow's milk. Fortified breads and cereals also give you a boost; just read the labels to find out how much. And if you want an extra boost from nonfood sources, calcium supplements are also an option.

Part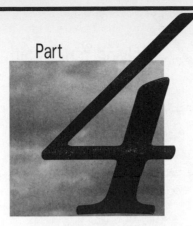

**Your Guide to Healing
with Alternative Nutrition**

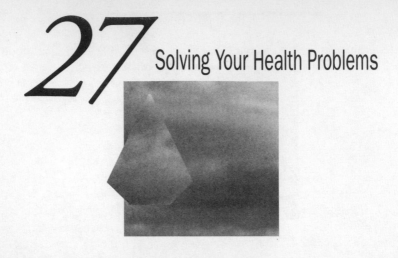

27 Solving Your Health Problems

How to Choose Your Healing Diet

Well, the secret's out.

Not only is there more than one way to skin a cat, there's more than one way to help solve health problems and fight disease.

In this book, we've described a number of diets that will help fight a cold. And we've noted numerous diets, herbs and supplements that will help prevent arthritis, lower your risk of cancer or ease constipation. Whether you want to dodge diabetes, avoid heart disease, lower high blood presure or guard against bone-wasting osteoporosis, somewhere in this book there's an alternative diet that you can enlist in your ongoing crusade for good health.

The following chart will help guide you. In the left-hand column you'll find the diseases and health conditions that are described in the chapters of this book, arranged alphabetically from acne to yeast infections. All of the diets described —from the additive-free diet to the yeast-free diet— are listed alphabetically across the top of the chart.

You can use the chart in two ways. If you're about to try one of the alternative diets mentioned in this book, you can read down to find out what it will do to improve your health and help stop disease. Or if you already have a health problem that you'd like to remedy, you can find it in the left-hand column, then read across the top to find out which diets might be effective.

In addition, the chart includes a rating system. While medical doctors and alternative medicine practitioners agree about the effectiveness of some diets, there is debate about others. The rating system has four categories, each indicated by a symbol. Here's how the ratings were determined by our researchers.

■ indicates that there's strong scientific evidence—supported by scientific studies—that the diet can help prevent or cure a specific health problem.

▬ indicates that there's evidence supported by some studies, but it's contradicted or not supported by others.

☰ indicates that the evidence is based on stories of patients who say that they have been treated or cured—in other words, it's anecdotal.

▤ indicates that there's little or no evidence that the diet helps, but some practitioners or doctors speculate that it should or does.

Keep in mind that this chart is only a guide. You can try any of the diets in this book—following the guidelines in each chapter—and you may find additional benefits to your overall health.

Health Problems and Diseases

Health Problems and Diseases	Additive-Free Diet	Alternative Supplements	American Diabetes Association Diet	Ancestral Nutrition	Ayurveda	Chinese Nutrition	Clear Liquid Diet	Elimination Diet	Fasting	Fish/Fish Oil Diet	Fruit- and Vegetable-Rich Diet	Gluten-Free Diet	Herbal Nutrition	High-Carbohydrate, High-Fiber Diet	High-Fiber Diet
Acne					Some	Some			Some						
Addiction		Some							Some						
Aging		Some							Some						
AIDS*		Some			Some										
Allergies/Hay Fever		Some			Some				Some						
Alzheimer's Disease		Some			Some										
Amenorrhea					Some										
Anxiety					Some								Some		
Arthritis		Some			Some	Some		Some	Some	Some					
Asthma	Some	Some			Some	Some			Some						
Bladder Infections (chronic)						Some									
Boils					Some										
Cancer Prevention		Some									Strong		Some	Strong	
Cataract Prevention											Some				
Chronic Fatigue Syndrome	Some	Some			Some	Some			Some						
Cold Prevention/Treatment					Some	Some							Some		
Cold Sores		Some													
Colitis		Some							Some						
Constipation		Some			Some	Some	Some				Strong		Some	Some	
Crohn's Disease/IBD					Some	Some									
Depression	Some	Some			Some								Some		

KEY: ■ Strong evidence   ▬ Some evidence

416   *Remedies may slow progression

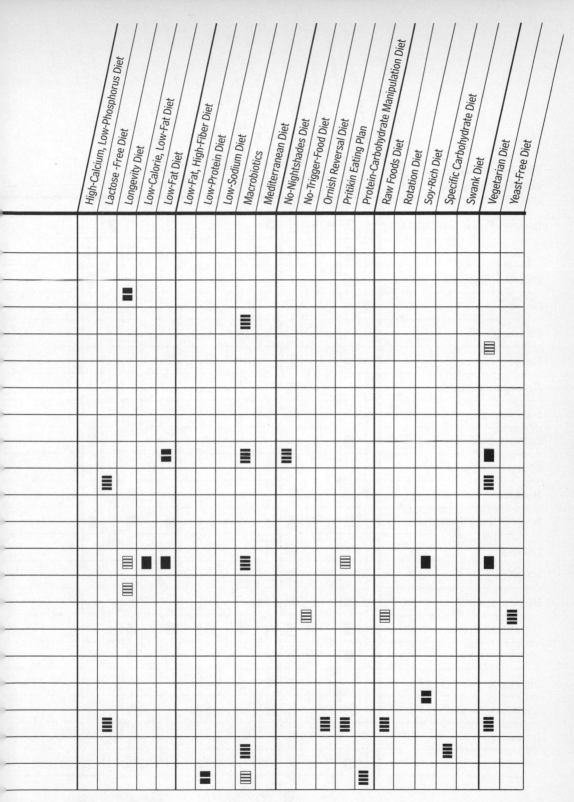

■ Anecdotal evidence   ☰ Possible benefits

Health Problems and Diseases — Diets, Herbs and Supplements

Health Problems and Diseases	Additive-Free Diet	Alternative Supplements	American Diabetes Association Diet	Ancestral Nutrition	Ayurveda	Chinese Nutrition	Clear Liquid Diet	Elimination Diet	Fasting	Fish/Fish Oil Diet	Fruit- and Vegetable-Rich Diet	Gluten-Free Diet	Herbal Nutrition	High-Carbohydrate, High-Fiber Diet	High-Fiber Diet
Diabetes Prevention/Control		▦	■	▦	▦	▦			▦*				■		
Diarrhea		▦			▦	▦	▦						▦		▦
Digestive Problems		▦											▦		▦
Eczema	▦	▦			▦			▦							
Endometriosis					▦										
Fatigue		▦			▦			▦			▦				
Fibrocystic Breasts					▦										
Food Allergies	▦				▦										
Gallstones		▦						▦							▦
Gluten Intolerance												▦			
Headache	▦	▦			▦			▦					▦		
Heart Disease Prevention		▦		▦	▦	▦		▦		■			▦	■	
Hemorrhoids					▦	▦									
Hepatitis					▦										
Herpes (genital)		▦			▦										
High Blood Pressure		▦		▦	▦	▦		▦		■			▦		
High Cholesterol		▦		▦	▦								■	■	
Impotence					▦	▦									
Infections (chronic)		▦				▦		▦					■		
Infertility					▦										
Insomnia		▦			▦								▦		

KEY: ■ Strong evidence   ▦ Some evidence

*People with Type I (insulin-dependent) diabetes should not fast

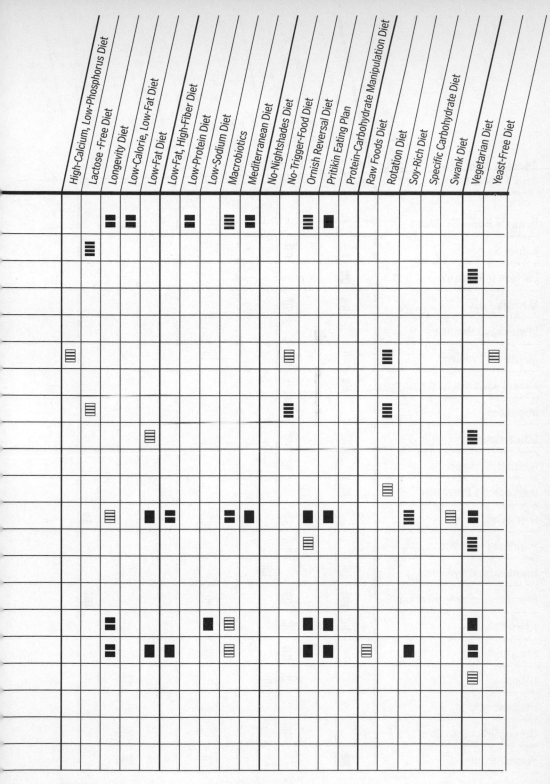

High-Calcium, Low-Phosphorus Diet · Lactose-Free Diet · Longevity Diet · Low-Calorie, Low-Fat Diet · Low-Fat Diet · Low-Fat, High-Fiber Diet · Low-Protein Diet · Low-Sodium Diet · Macrobiotics · Mediterranean Diet · No-Nightshades Diet · No-Trigger-Food Diet · Ornish Reversal Diet · Pritikin Eating Plan · Protein-Carbohydrate Manipulation Diet · Raw Foods Diet · Rotation Diet · Soy-Rich Diet · Specific Carbohydrate Diet · Swank Diet · Vegetarian Diet · Yeast-Free Diet

▤ Anecdotal evidence   ▤ Possible benefits

(continued)

Health Problems and Diseases	Additive-Free Diet	Alternative Supplements	American Diabetes Association Diet	Ancestral Nutrition	Ayurveda	Chinese Nutrition	Clear Liquid Diet	Elimination Diet	Fasting	Fish/Fish Oil Diet	Fruit- and Vegetable-Rich Diet	Gluten-Free Diet	Herbal Nutrition	High-Carbohydrate, High-Fiber Diet	High-Fiber Diet
Irritable Bowel Syndrome															
Kidney Stones					▦										
Lactose Intolerance	▦														
Memory Loss	▦				▦										
Menopausal Problems															
Menstrual Problems					▦								▦		
Mental and Emotional Problems	▦				▦										
Migraines											▦				
Miscarriage					▦										
Multiple Sclerosis					▦										
Osteoporosis Prevention	▦		▦								▦				
Overweight					▦				▦					▦	▦
Parkinson's Disease					▦										
Premenstrual Syndrome	▦			▦									▦		
Prostate Cancer Prevention	▦				▦					▦	▦			▦	
Psoriasis	▦				▦										
Sinusitis					▦				▦						
Ulcers					▦	▦							▦		
Underweight					▦										
Urinary Tract Infections					▦								▦		
Yeast Infections	■								▦				▦		

KEY: ■ Strong evidence   ▦ Some evidence

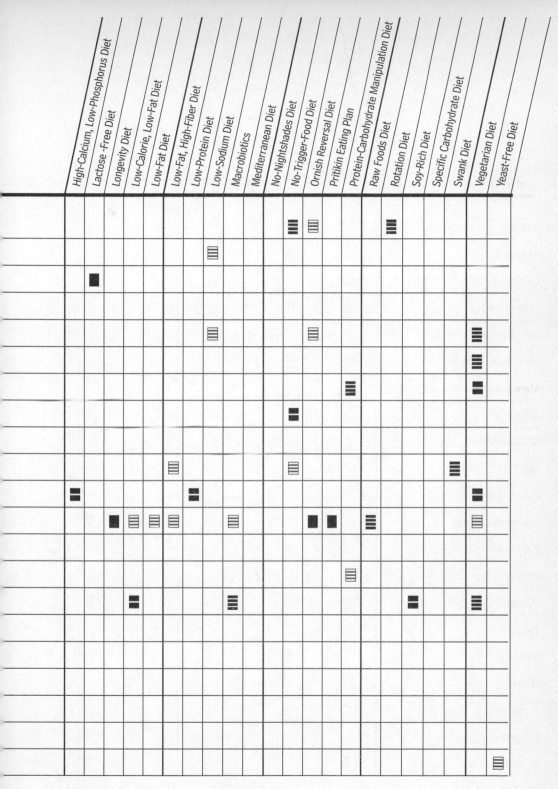

	High-Calcium, Low-Phosphorus Diet	Lactose-Free Diet	Longevity Diet	Low-Calorie, Low-Fat Diet	Low-Fat Diet	Low-Fat, High-Fiber Diet	Low-Protein Diet	Low-Sodium Diet	Macrobiotics	Mediterranean Diet	No-Nightshades Diet	No-Trigger-Food Diet	Ornish Reversal Diet	Pritikin Eating Plan	Protein-Carbohydrate Manipulation Diet	Raw Foods Diet	Rotation Diet	Soy-Rich Diet	Specific Carbohydrate Diet	Swank Diet	Vegetarian Diet	Yeast-Free Diet

■ Anecdotal evidence   ▤ Possible benefits

Credits

The menu in "Try It for a Week" on pages 62–63 is reprinted by permission of SevenStar Communications from *The Tao of Nutrition* by Maoshing Ni, Ph.D., C.A., with Cathy McNease, B.S., M.H. Copyright © 1993 by Maoshing Ni and Cathy McNease.

The recipe for Tofu and Spinach Soup on page 63 is reprinted by permission of Tao Publishing from *The Tao of Balanced Diet: Secrets of a Thin and Healthy Body* by Dr. Stephen T. Chang. Copyright © 1987 by Stephen T. Chang.

"What's Your Dominant Dosha?" (originally titled "Determining Your Body-Mind Constitution") on pages 84–85 is reprinted by permission of the Putnam Publishing Group/Jeremy P. Tarcher, Inc., from *A Woman's Best Medicine: Health, Happiness, and Long Life through Ayur-Veda* by Melanie Brown, Ph.D., Veronica Butler, M.D., and Nancy Lonsdorf, M.D. Copyright © 1993 by Melanie Brown, Veronica Butler and Nancy Lonsdorf.

The food guidelines in "Do's and Don'ts to Balance Dosha" on pages 90–91 are reprinted by permission of Lotus Press from *Ayurveda: The Science of Self-Healing* by Vasant Lad, B.A.M.S., M.A.Sc. Copyright © 1984 by Vasant Lad.

The menu in "Try It for a Week" on pages 100–101 is reprinted by permission of the Kushi Institute, Becket, Massachusetts.

The recipes for Hot Korean Vegetables and Noodles and Mint Tulip on page 104, Scrambled Tofu and Fresh Dilled Eggplant on page 106 and Avocado Spread on page 107 are reprinted by permission of Lotus Press from *The Ayurvedic Cookbook: A Personalized Guide to Good Nutrition and Health* by Amadea Morningstar with Urmila Desai. Copyright © 1990 by Amadea Morningstar and Urmila Desai.

The recipes for Vegetarian Stroganoff and Light Basil Sauce on page 103, Pasta Primavera and Pesto Sauce on page 105 and Nice Burgers on page 107 are reprinted by permission of Lotus Press from *Ayurvedic Cooking for Westerners: Familiar Western Food Prepared with Ayurvedic Principles* by Amadea Morningstar. Copyright © 1995 by Amadea Morningstar.

The menu in "Try a Low-Cal Day" (originally titled "Third Day Menu") on page 166 and the recipes for Tropical Dream Bars on page 166 and Stuffed Peppers on page 167 are reprinted by permission of Four Walls Eight Windows from *The Anti-Aging Plan: Strategies and Recipes for Extending Your Healthy Years* by Roy L. Walford, M.D., and Lisa Walford. Copyright © 1994 by Roy L. Walford and Lisa Walford.

"Are You a Carbohydrate Craver?" on pages 386–87 is adapted from *Food and Mood: The Complete Guide to Eating Well and Feeling Your Best* by Elizabeth Somer, M.A., R.D. Copyright © 1995 by Elizabeth Somer. Reprinted by permission of Henry Holt and Co., Inc.

"Are You at Risk?" (originally titled "Osteoporosis: Can It Happen to You?") on page 406 is reprinted by permission of the National Osteoporosis Foundation, Washington, D.C.

Index

Note: <u>Underscored</u> page references indicate boxed text. **Boldface** page references indicate tables.

A

Acetaminophen, fasting and, <u>182</u>
Acetylcholine, lecithin and, 221
Acidophilus, health claims for, 219–20
Acidosis, kombucha and, 227
Acid reflux, preventing, <u>315</u>
Acne
  Ayurveda for, 96
  Chinese nutrition for, 66
  dietary remedies for, **416**
Acupuncture, Chinese medicine and, 65–66
Addictions
  amino acid supplements for, 197
  fasting and, 183
  dietary remedies for, **416**
  to foods causing allergies, 349
Additive-free diet, for food allergies and
    sensitivities, 347–48, **416, 418, 420**
Additives, food allergies and, 344–48
Adolescents, Longevity Diet and, <u>165</u>
Adzuki beans, in macrobiotic diet, <u>39</u>
Aflatoxin B$_1$, cancer and, 238, 239
Aging
  DHEA and, <u>206</u>
  dietary remedies for, **416–17**
  fasting and, 183
  melatonin and, 222
  royal jelly and, 230–31
AHA, 361, 363
AIDS
  Ayurveda for, 98
  dietary remedies for, **415, 416, 417**
  mushroom extracts for, 225
Alcohol consumption
  cancer and, 269, 277
  chronic fatigue syndrome and, 286

diabetes and, 302
fatigue and, 335–36
food allergies and, 344
heart disease and, 132–33
migraines and, 399
Ornish program and, 132–33
reducing, benefits for
  blood pressure control, 378
  diarrhea control, 314
  ulcer relief, <u>321</u>
vegetarians and, 9, 11
Alcoholism, amino acids and, 197
Allergens, hidden, in food, 343
Allergies
  Ayurveda for, 95
  bee pollen for, 200
  dietary remedies for, **416**
  food (*see* Food allergies)
Almonds, sprouting method for, **174**
Alpha-galactosidase. *See* Beano
Alpha-interferon, echinacea and, 241
Alternative supplements
  amino acids, 195–98 (*see also* Amino
    acids)
  aspirin, 198–99, 372
  bee pollen, 199–200
  brewer's yeast, 201–2, 207
  coenzyme Q$_{10}$, 204–5, 289–90
  conditions helped by, **416, 418, 420**
  DNA/RNA, 205–7
  enzymes, 171, 207–8 (*see also specific*
    enzymes)
  evening primrose oil, 208–10
  fiber, 210–12 (*see also* Fiber, dietary)
  fish oil, 213–16 (*see also* Fish oil)
  foods vs., <u>226</u>
  ginkgo, 216–18

Cholesterol (*continued*)
elevated, heart disease risk and, <u>136</u>
family history and, 357
game meat consumption and, 25
heart disease and, 137
high blood pressure and, <u>379</u>
high-density lipoprotein (*see* High-density lipoproteins)
hunter-gatherer diet and, 33
Longevity Diet and, 160
low-density lipoprotein (*see* Low-density
lipoproteins)
lowering
dietary strategies for, 356, 357,
418–19
fiber and, 367–69
garlic for, 212, 243, 245–46, 374
green tea for, 246
herbs for, 245–46
lecithin for, 221–22
lifestyle changes for, 357
macrobiotics and, 46–47
mushroom extracts for, 224, 225
soluble fiber for, 211, 305
soy products and, 372–73
vegetarian diet for, 8, 13
meat eating and, 47, 120
royal jelly and, 231
sugar and, 130
Choline, health claims for, 221–22
Christianity, dietary practices in, 71–74
Chromium, in brewer's yeast, 201
Chronic diseases, Ayurveda for, 97–99
Chronic fatigue syndrome (CFS)
dairy products and, 286–87
dietary remedies for, **416–17**
elimination of artificial ingredients for,
284
theories about, 281, 283–84
food sensitivities and, 285–86
prevalence of, 282–83
symptoms of, 281, <u>282</u>
vitamin/mineral supplements for,
287–90
yeast-free diet for, 285
Cinnamon, for ulcers, 250
Circulatory system disorders, Ayurveda for,
89
Claudication, intermittent, Pritikin Eating
Plan and, 142
Clear liquid diet, for bowel problems, 311,
416, 418
Cloves, for heart disease prevention, 244
Coconuts, fat content of, 128

Coenzyme Q$_{10}$, health claims for, 204–5,
289–90
Coffee. *See also* Caffeine
decaffeinated, 132, <u>321</u>
eliminating
for diarrhea control, 314
in Ornish program, 132
inositol supplements and, 219
Colds
Ayurveda for, 95
Chinese nutrition for, 67
dietary remedies for, **416**
herbal remedies for, 240–41
Cold sores, 197, 225, **416**
Colitis, ulcerative
dietary remedies for, **416**
evening primrose oil for, 209–10
fasting for, 187–88
Collard greens, in macrobiotic diet, <u>38</u>
College of Maharishi Ayur-Veda Health
Center, <u>99</u>
Colon cancer
aspirin for, 199
calcium and, 267
fiber and, 9, 211, 268–69
folate and, 267
garlic for, 236
low-fat diet for, 269
preventing, dietary strategies for, 266,
<u>270</u>
Reversal Diet and, 122
sugar and, 272–73
Colorings, food, adverse effects of, 20, <u>346</u>
Congestive heart failure, macrobiotics and,
45
Constipation
Ayurveda for, 89, 92
Chinese nutrition for, 67
dietary remedies for, **416**
with irritable bowel syndrome, 318–19
molasses for, 303
in multiple sclerosis, 403
prunes for, <u>306</u>
vegetarian diet for, 13
wheat bran for, <u>304</u>
Constitution, physical
Ayurvedic concept of, 81–82
yin/yang concept of, 58, **59**, 61
Cooking methods
calcium and, 412
for cancer prevention, 270–71
for defatting meat, <u>366</u>
for diabetes control, 300
low-fat, <u>118</u>

macrobiotic diet and, 41–43
vegetarianism and, 20
Cooking utensils and tools, for macrobiotic
  diet, 54–55
Coriander, digestion and, 92
Corn, sprouting method for, **174**
Cornbread
  Dorothy Hulsey's Healthy Cornbread, 141
Coronary artery disease
  Ayurveda for, 89
  Chinese nutrition for, 67
  macrobiotic diet for, 45
  Pritikin Eating Plan for, 135
Coughs
  Ayurveda for, 95
  herbal remedies for, 241–42
Couscous, in Chinese nutrition, 61
Cow worship, 78
Cranberry tea, for urinary tract infections,
  251
Crash dieting, gallstones and, 323
Crohn's disease
  Ayurveda for, 98
  Chinese nutrition for, 57, 67
  dietary remedies for, **416–17**
  macrobiotic diet for, 52
  Specific Carbohydrate Diet for, 324
Cumin, digestion and, 92
Curcumin, as antioxidant, 239

D

DADS, cancer-fighting potential of, 236–37
Daikon, in macrobiotic diet, 38
Dairy Ease, for lactose intolerance, 208, 313
Dairy products. *See also specific products*
  in ancestral nutrition, 24
  cancer prevention and, 277
  chronic fatigue syndrome and, 286–87
  irritable bowel syndrome and, 320
  lactose intolerance and, 208
  low-fat, Reversal Diet and, 123, 126
  osteoporosis and, 11–12, 410–11
  in Pritikin Eating Plan, 147
  religious laws and, 75, 77
Dandelion leaf tea, for premenstrual
  syndrome, 250
Dandelion root, for indigestion, 247
D-carnitine, vs. L-carnitine, 196–97
Decaffeinated beverages
  avoiding, for ulcer prevention, 321
  in Ornish program, 132

Dehydration, from diarrhea, 311
Dehydroepiandrosterone (DHEA), for age-
  related diseases, 206
Depression
  amino acid supplements for, 197
  Ayurveda for, 93–94
  B-complex vitamins and, 390–91
  carbohydrate cravings and, 388–99
  dietary remedies for, **418–19**
  macrobiotics for, 53
  neurotransmitters and, 388
  in seasonal affective disorder, 395–96
  sugar consumption and, 389–90
Detoxification, fasting for, 73–74, 181
DGLA, heart disease and, 209
DHA, in fish oil, 213
DHEA, for age-related diseases, 206
Diabetes
  alcohol consumption and, 302
  American Diabetes Association diet for,
    294–96
  bee products and, 201
  brewer's yeast for, 201
  Chinese nutrition for, 67–68
  dietary remedies for, 291–92, **418–19**
  "eating smart, eating easy" plan for,
    299–302
  evening primrose oil for, 209–10
  exercise for, 300
  fiber for, 301, 302
  fish oil and, 216
  heart disease risk and, 136
  high-carbohydrate, high-fiber diet for,
    296–97
  high blood pressure and, 377, 379
  individuality of food plans and, 293–94
  inositol supplements for, 218
  Longevity Diet and, 160–61, 165
  long-term complications of, 292
  low-density lipoproteins in, 293
  macrobiotics and, 52
  Mediterranean plan for, 297–99
  overweight and, 293, 299
  Pritikin Eating Plan and, 135, 144–45
  Type I (insulin-dependent), 257, 292, 297
  Type II (non-insulin-dependent), 292,
    297
    fasting and, 187
    hunter-gatherer diet and, 28–29
    Pritikin Eating Plan and, 144–45
Diabetic retinopathy, shark cartilage for,
  203–4
Diallyl disulfide (DADS), cancer-fighting
  potential of, 236–37

Diarrhea
  Ayurveda for, 92
  brewer's yeast for, 202
  causes of, 311
  dietary remedies for, 311, 314, **418–19**
  with inflammatory bowel disease, 325
  milk and, 303
  prevalence of, 311
Digestion, Pritikin Eating Plan and, 146, 148
Digestive problems. *See also specific problems*
  Ayurveda for, 89, 92
  dietary remedies for, **418–19**
  fiber and, 211
  food alternatives for, 303, 305
Dihomogamma-linolenic acid (DGLA), heart disease and, 209
Dill
  cancer-fighting potential of, 240
  Fresh Dilled Eggplant, 106
Dimenhydrinate, for nausea, 249
Discharging of disease, macrobiotic diet for, 53
Diuretics, for blood pressure control, 131
Diverticulitis
  fiber supplements for, 211
  vegetarian diet for, 13
Diverticulosis, vegetarian diet for, 13
Dizziness
  fasting for, 189
  ginkgo for, 217
DNA damage, preventing, 162, 222–23
DNA/RNA supplements, health claims for, 205–7
Docosahexaenoic acid (DHA), in fish oil, 213
Dopamine, energy levels and, 334, 385, 387
Doshas. *See* Ayurveda, doshas
Dramamine, for nausea, 249
Drug addiction, amino acid supplements for, 197
Dulse, in macrobiotic diet, 39
Dyes, food, adverse effects of, 346

E

Eating
  lying down after, heartburn and, 315
  scheduling, benefits for
    diabetes control, 300–301
    gallstone prevention, 323

  heartburn and, 315
  irritable bowel syndrome, 316
  ulcer relief, 321
  speed of, reducing, 309, 316
Echinacea, for colds and flu, 240–41
Eczema
  Ayurveda for, 96
  dietary remedies for, **418**
  evening primrose oil for, 210
  fasting for, 189
Egg-free diet, for food allergies and sensitivities, 343
Eggplant
  Fresh Dilled Eggplant, 106
Eggs
  in low-fat diet, 363
  Reversal Diet and, 123, 126
Eicosapentaenoic acid (EPA), in fish oil, 213
Elimination diet, for food allergies, 257–59, 259, **416**
Emotional and mental problems. *See also* Depression; Stress
  Ayurveda for, 93–94
  B-complex vitamins for, 390–91
  dietary remedies for, **420–21**
  ginkgo for, 217–18
  Protein-Carbohydrate Manipulation Diet for, 389–91
  vegetarian diet for, 12, **421**
Endometrial cancer, dietary fat and, 266, 269
Endometriosis, Ayurveda for, 94, **418**
Endorphins, chocolate and, 392
Energy
  caffeine and, 389
  lack of (*see* Chronic fatigue syndrome; Fatigue)
  levels, hunter-gatherer diet and, 32–34
  nutrients for, 336–37
  production, during fasting, 179–80
Environmental toxins, eliminating by fasting, 189
Enzymes. *See also specific enzymes*
  in fruits and vegetables, 171, 207–8
  health claims for, 207–8
Eosinophilia-myalgia syndrome, tryptophan and, 196
EPA, in fish oil, 213
Epilepsy, fasting and, 257
Epinephrine, for anaphylactic shock, 344
Epstein-Barr virus
  chronic fatigue syndrome and, 281
  fasting and, 186

Esophageal cancer
   black tea and, 238
   foods associated with, 269
   green tea and, 237
   low-fat diet for, 269
Esophagus irritation, foods causing, 315
Essene religious order, fasting and, 73–74
Essential hypertension, excess salt
      consumption and, 150
Estrogen, soy products and, 278
Ethnic restaurants, choices for Pritikin
      Eating Plan, 155
Eucalyptus, for coughs, 241–42
Eugenol, for heart disease prevention, 244
Evening primrose oil, health claims for,
      209–10
Exercise
   for diabetes control, 300
   food allergies and, 344
   in Ornish program, 109
Exhaustion syndrome, diabetes and, 67

F

Faith, health and, 71
Family history
   cholesterol levels and, 357
   heart disease risk and, 136
FAN, 343, 348
Fast-food lunch, vs. Pritikin lunch, **145**
Fasting
   advocates of, 187
   autolyzation and, 179
   benefits for
      addiction, 183
      aging, 183
      asthma, 184
      benign tumors, 185
      cardiovascular disease, 185–86
      chronic infections, 186–87
      diabetes, 187
      headaches, 188
      high blood pressure, 188, 376
      prostate enlargement, 189
      rheumatoid arthritis, 183–84, 256–57
      ulcerative colitis, 187–88
      weight loss, 189
   conditions helped by, **416, 418, 420**
   contraindications for, 181, 257
   energy production during, 179–80
   Essene religious order and, 73–74
   experts on, 179

healing aspects of, 177–78, 183, 189
historical aspects of, 186
hunger and, 180–81
information resources for, 190
liver function in, 178–79
longest, record for, 191
planning for, 190
purpose of, 176
return from, 190–91
vs. starvation diet, 178
tips for, 182
types of, 180
Fatigue
   alcohol and, 335–36
   Ayurveda for, 98
   causes of, 331–32
   chronic (*see* Chronic fatigue syndrome)
   dietary remedies for, **418–19**
   fasting for, 189
   fats and, 335
   from food allergies, 336–38
   information resources for, 338
   iron deficiency and, 332–33
   sugar and, 334–35
   weight-loss diets and, 115
Fat(s), dietary. *See also* Low-fat diet
   arthritis and, 260
   butter vs. margarine, 362
   cancer and, 8, 145–46, 269, 280
   chronic fatigue syndrome and, 286
   consumption, reducing
      for diabetes control, 294, 295
      for gallstone prevention, 323
      menus, sample, 364–65
   fatigue and, 335
   heart disease and, 137–38
   insulin and, 296
   intake, healthy range for, 274
   irritable bowel syndrome and, 320–21
   monounsaturated, 275, 297
   polyunsaturated, 275, 277
   recommended percentages of, 273–74,
      361–62 (*see also* Ornish program;
      Pritikin Eating Plan)
   removal from meat, 366
   saturated
      eliminating, for diabetes control,
         299–300
      low-density lipoproteins and, 359–60
      ovarian cancer and, 273
   in tofu, 279
   unsaturated, 123
FD&C Yellow No. 5, adverse effects of, 346
Fennel, digestion and, 92

Gluten intolerance (*continued*)
  symptoms of, 326
  wheat-free diet for, <u>328</u>, 328–29
Glycyrrhizin, for ulcers, 251
Gout, uric acid and, 255, <u>256</u>
Grains. *See also* Macrobiotic diet; *specific grains*
  in ancestral nutrition, <u>24</u>
  in Chinese nutrition, <u>60–61</u>, 64
  in macrobiotic diet, <u>38</u>
  Nice Burgers, <u>107</u>
  in Reversal Diet, <u>127</u>, 128
  sensitivity to, 24
  whole, 30
    for constipation, <u>304</u>
    fiber content of, 308
    for heart disease prevention, <u>371</u>
Grapefruit, in macrobiotic diet, 40
Grape juice, for heart disease prevention, <u>370</u>, 371–72
Grating, for raw foods diet, 175
Green peas, sprouting method for, **174**
Green tea, benefits for
  cancer prevention, 237–38
  lowering cholesterol, 246
Grilling
  cancer and, 269
  as low-fat cooking method, <u>118</u>
Group support, in Ornish program, <u>109</u>
Growth hormone, L-arginine and, 195

H

Hamburger(s)
  defatting method for, <u>366</u>
  vs. veggie burger, 2, <u>3</u>
HAs, cancer and, 8–9
Hay fever, Ayurveda for, 95, **416**
HDL. *See* High-density lipoproteins
Headaches
  Ayurveda for, 94
  dietary remedies for, **418–19**
  fasting for, 188
  migraine (*see* Migraines)
Hearing loss, ginkgo for, 217
Heart attack prevention
  aspirin for, 198
  fish oil and, 214
Heartburn, preventing, 303, <u>315</u>
Heart disease
  alcohol consumption and, 132–33
  coronary artery, 45, 67, 89, 135

deaths from, 112
  preventing
    ancestral diet and, 24–25
    coenzyme Q_{10} and, 204–5
    dietary strategies for, **418–19**
    evening primrose oil for, 209–10
    food choices for, <u>370–71</u>
    garlic for, 374
    herbs for, 242–45
    Longevity Diet and, 160
    low-fat diet for, 119, 354–55
    macrobiotics and, 35, 37, 45–47
    religion-based diets and, 71
    restaurant selections for, <u>368</u>
    soy and soy products for, 372–73
  risk factors for, <u>136</u>
  symptoms, lifestyle changes and, 112–13
  vegetarianism and, 6–8
Heart failure, coenzyme Q_{10} and, 204
Helicobacter pylori, ulcers and, <u>320</u>
Hemorrhoids
  Ayurveda for, 93
  Chinese nutrition for, 68
  dietary remedies for, **418**, **419**
Hepatitis, Ayurveda for, 93, **418**
Herbs. *See also specific herbs*
  for Ayurveda, <u>92</u>
  benefits for
    blood pressure reduction, 245
    cancer prevention, 236–40
    colds, 240–41
    coughs, 241–42
    diarrhea, 242
    flu, 240–41
    heart disease prevention, 242–45
    indigestion, 247–48
    insomnia, 248–49
    menstrual cramps, 249
    nausea, 249–50
    premenstrual syndrome, 250
    ulcer prevention, 250–51
    urinary tract infections, 251
  conditions helped by, **416**, **418**, **420**
  healing aspects of, 234–35
  information resources for, <u>252</u>
Herpes, genital, Ayureveda for, 94–95, **418**
Heterocyclic amines (HAs), cancer and, 8–9
High blood pressure. *See also* Hypertension
  alcohol consumption and, 378
  deaths from, 375
  diagnosing, 377
  dietary remedies for, **418–19**
  heart disease risk and, <u>136</u>
  pregnancy-induced, fish oil and, 216

reducing
  Ayurveda for, 89
  Chinese nutrition for, 68
  coenzyme Q_{10} and, 205
  fasting for, 188, 376
  fish oil and, 213
  foods for, **382**
  herbs for, 245
  hunter-gatherer diet and, 27
  lecithin for, 222
  Longevity Diet and, 160
  macrobiotics and, 46–47
  minerals for, 380–83
  mushroom extracts for, 225
  salt consumption and, 378–80
  vegetarian diet for, 7, 13, 377–78
  weight loss and, 378
  risk factors for, 377
High-calcium, low-phosphorus diet, 410, **417, 419, 421**
High-carbohydrate, high-fiber diet, 296–97, 302, **416, 418, 420**
High-density lipoproteins (HDL)
  fish oil and, 26
  garlic and, 246
  monounsaturated oils and, 360
  preserving, 356, 360–61
  trans-fatty acids and, 362
  vitamin C and, 172
High-fiber diet
  conditions helped by, **416, 418, 420**
  menu, sample, 302
High-protein diet, 11, 127
Hinduism, dietary practices in, 70, 78–79
Hing, digestion and, 92
Histamine, food sensitivity and, 345–46
HIV. *See* AIDS
Hiziki, in macrobiotic diet, 39
Hormone-responsive cancer, macrobiotics and, 50
Hormones. *See specific hormones*
Hot dog headaches, 400
Hot pepper, for ulcers, 251
Hunger
  Essene religious order and, 73–74
  in fasting, 180–81
  Longevity Diet and, 168–69
  Muslims and, 77
Hunter-gatherer diet
  benefits of, 32–34
  blood pressure and, 27
  conditions helped by, **418, 420**
  fiber in, 26–28
  heart disease and, 24–25

mail-order food sources, 31
menus, sample, 32–33
nutrients in, 22–23
osteoporosis and, 29–30
transition to, 23, 30–32
Type II diabetes and, 28–29
Hypertension. *See* also High blood pressure
  essential, 150
  malignant, 89
  transient, 89

I

IBD. *See* Inflammatory bowel disease
IBS. *See* Irritable bowel syndrome
Immune system
  echinacea and, 240–41
  fasting and, 186–87
  food allergies and, 341
Impotence
  Ayurveda for, 95
  Chinese nutrition for, 68
  dietary remedies for, **418, 419**
  vegetarian diet for, 13
Indigestion, herbal remedies for, 247–48
Indoles, cancer-fighting potential of, 267
Infections, chronic, 186–87, **416–17**
Infertility, Ayurveda for, 95, **418**
Inflammatory bowel disease (IBD). *See also*
    Crohn's disease; Ulcerative colitis
  allergy-type reactions in, 345
  Ayurveda for, 98
  chamomile for, 248
  diagnosing, 325
  dietary remedies for, **416–17**
  Specific Carbohydrate Diet for, 324, 326, 327
Inositol
  coffee consumption and, 219
  health claims for, 218, 231
Insomnia
  Ayurveda for, 94
  dietary remedies for, **420**
  herbal remedies for, 248–49
Insulin
  blood sugar and, 292
  dietary fat and, 296
  fat absorption and, 143
  production, refined or processed carbohydrates and, 152
  sugar consumption and, 130
  tryptophan and, 386–87

Interleukin-1, echinacea and, 241
Intermittent claudication, Pritikin Eating
    Plan for, 142
International Association of Hygienic
    Physicians, 179, 190
International Macrobiotic Directory, 56
INTERSALT, 380
Intestinal flora, fasting and, 257
Intestinal gas
    Ayurveda for, 93
    Beano for, 148, 207–8, 309
    preventing, 308–9
Iron
    absorption, vitamin C and, 17
    caffeine and, 333
    Daily Value for, 16
    deficiency, fatigue and, 332–33
    dietary sources of, 333
    in hunter-gatherer diet, 23
    from meat eating, 120
    for neurotransmitter function, 391
    supplements, for chronic fatigue
        syndrome, 290
    in vegetarian diet, 16–17
Irritable bowel syndrome (IBS)
    constipation in, 318–19
    dietary changes for, 316–17
    dietary remedies for, 421
    food sensitivity in, 319–21
    lifestyle changes for, 317
    symptoms of, 314–16, 325
Islam, dietary laws of, 76–77
Isoflavones, cancer-fighting potential of,
    267
L-isoleucine, health claims for, 195
Isothiocyanates, cancer-fighting potential
    of, 267
Italian restaurants, choices for Pritikin
    Eating Plan, 155

J

Japanese noodles, in macrobiotic diet,
    44
Japanese restaurants, choices for Pritikin
    Eating Plan, 155
Jet lag, melatonin for, 223–24, 420
Joint pain, in arthritis. See Arthritis
Judiasm, dietary laws of, 70, 74–76
Juices/juicing
    in fasting, 180
    in Ornish program, 130
    in raw foods diet, 175

K

Kale, in macrobiotic diet, 38
Kapha. See also Ayurveda
    balancing, eating for, 87, 89, 92
    characteristics of, 83, 85
    food recommendations for, 90–91
    menus, sample, 102
Karma, meat consumption and, 78–79
Ketogenesis, fasting and, 180
Ketosis, fasting and, 180
Kidney cancer, macrobiotic diet for, 51–52
Kidney failure, fish oil for, 215–16
Kidney stones
    Ayurveda for, 96–97
    dietary remedies for, 420, 421
Kombu
    in Chinese nutrition, 61
    in macrobiotic diet, 39
Kombucha, health claims for, 226–27
Koran, dietary laws in, 77
Kosher foods, 75–76, 343
Kosher laws, 70, 74–76
Kumquats, in Ornish Program, 129
Kushi Institute, 56

L

Lactaid, for lactose intolerance, 208, 313
Lactase, in lactose intolerance, 208, 313
Lactobacillus acidophilus, health claims for,
    219–20
Lactose, intestinal gas and, 308
Lactose-free diet, conditions helped by, 417,
    419, 421
Lactose intolerance
    acidophilus for, 220
    adults and, 24
    dietary control of, 312–13, 316
    dietary remedies for, 420–21
    vs. food allergy, 348
    genetic aspects of, 26
    lactase enzyme for, 208, 313
    symptoms of, 27
Lacto-vegetarian diet, 6, 11
Laryngitis, Ayurveda for, 95
LDL. See Low-density lipoproteins
Lecithin, health claims for, 221–22
Lectins, in cereal, 30
Legumes
    cancer-fighting potential of, 146
    in Chinese nutrition, 60, 64
    intestinal gas production and, 207

Morning breath, choline supplements and, 221
MSG, adverse effects of, 321, <u>346</u>, 347, 401
Multiple sclerosis
  Ayurveda for, 98
  dietary remedies for, **420–21**
  food allergies and, <u>403</u>
  Swank Diet for, 402–4
Mung beans, in Chinese nutrition, <u>60</u>
Mushroom extracts, health claims for, 224–27
Muslims, dietary rules for, 70, 75, 76–77, <u>77</u>

N

National Cancer Institute (NCI) dietary guidelines, 267–71
National Headache Foundation, <u>401</u>
National Osteoporosis Foundation, <u>407</u>
Natto, in macrobiotic diet, <u>39</u>
Nausea
  Ayurveda for, 93
  herbal remedies for, 249–50
NCI dietary guidelines 267–71
Nervous system, function of, 385
Neurotransmitters, nutrition and, 197, 385, 388, **391**. *See also specific neurotransmitters*
Nightshade-free diet, for arthritis pain, 262–64, <u>264</u>
Nitrates, adverse effects of, <u>346</u>
Nitrites, adverse effects of, <u>346</u>, 399–400
No-nightshade diet
  for arthritis, 262–64, <u>264</u>
  conditions helped by, **417, 419, 421**
Nonsteroidal anti-inflammatory drugs (NSAIDs), ulcers and, <u>320–21</u>
Nonstick cooking spray, for heart disease prevention, <u>370</u>
Noodles
  Japanese, in macrobiotic diet, <u>44</u>
  Hot Korean Vegetables and Noodles, <u>104</u>
Norepinephrine, energy and, <u>334</u>, 385, 387
Nori
  in Chinese nutrition, <u>61</u>
  in macrobiotic diet, <u>39</u>
No-trigger-food diet, conditions helped by, **417, 419, 421**
NSAIDs, ulcers and, <u>320–21</u>
NutraSweet, adverse effects of, <u>346</u>, <u>399</u>
Nutriceuticals, cancer prevention and, 267
Nutrients. *See specific nutrients*

Nutritional deficiencies, vegans and, 6
Nuts
  for cancer prevention, 277–78
  in Chinese nutrition, 64
  in hunter-gatherer diet, 22

O

OAS, foods as cause of, <u>342</u>
Oat bran
  in fiber supplements, 211
  for heart disease prevention, 366–67, <u>371</u>
Oats
  in macrobiotic diet, <u>38</u>
  sprouting method for, **174**
Oils. *See also specific oils*
  avoiding, for cancer prevention, 277
  monounsaturated, high-density lipoproteins and, <u>360</u>
  with polyunsaturated fats, 277
  Reversal Diet and, 122–23
  vegetable, 404
Old Testament, dietary laws in, 71–76
  kosher laws in, 74–76
Olive oil, 122–23, 275, <u>360</u>
  benefits for
    cancer prevention, 275
    heart disease prevention, <u>360</u>
  in Ornish program, 122–23, 275, <u>360</u>
Omega-3 fatty acids. *See also* Fish oil
  content in fish, **261**
  health claims for, 213–16
  high-density lipoproteins and, 26
  triglycerides and, 26
One Perfect World, <u>56</u>
Oral allergy syndrome (OAS), foods as cause of, <u>342</u>
Oral cancer
  dietary fat and, 269
  vegetarian diet for, 11
Oral contraceptives, heart disease risk and, <u>136</u>
Orange pekoe tea, cancer-fighting potential of, 238
Oregano, cancer-fighting potential of, 240
Organically grown foods, in raw foods diet, 175
Organosulfur compounds, cancer-fighting potential of, 267
Ornish program, 108, 114–16. *See also* Reversal Diet
  components of, <u>109</u>
  development of, 112–14

vegan diet during, vitamin B_{12}
supplements with, 18
vitamin B_{12} and, 173
Premature infants, inositol supplements for, 218
Premenstrual syndrome (PMS)
Chinese nutrition for, 68–69
chocolate and, 392
cravings and, 395
dietary remedies for, **420–21**
herbal remedies for, 250
symptoms of, 394–95
Preservatives, adverse effects of, 284, 346, 347
Pressure cookers, for macrobiotic cooking, 51
Pritikin Eating Plan
advocates of, 134–35, 140
benefits for
cancer prevention, 145–46
chest pain, 142
diabetes, 144–45
digestion, 146, 148
heart health, 138–42, 355
legs, 142
weight loss, 142–44
carbohydrates in, 151–53
complex carbohydrates and, 143
conditions helped by, **417, 419, 421**
development of, 135–37
ethnic restaurant choices for, 155
fiber in, **148**
food labels and, 149
fruits in, 146
Long Beach Study, 138
limiting fat intake in, 148–50
lunch, vs. fast-food lunch, **145**
motivation for, 154
recipes for, 141
salt and, 149, 150–51
servings in, 147
sugar and, 153–54
transition to, 140, 154
traveling and, 152–53
vegetables in, 146
Pritikin Longevity Center, 139
Propolis, health claims for, 200–201
Prostaglandins, arthritis pain and, 260, 261
Prostate cancer
dietary fat and, 8, 274
dietary recommendations for, 270
genistein and, 146
low-fat diet for, 266, 269

macrobiotics and, 50
phytoestrogens and, 9
preventing, dietary strategies for, **418–19**
recovery from, macrobiotic diet and, 47–48, 51
Reversal Diet and, 122
soybeans and, 278
Prostate gland enlargement
Ayurveda for, 94
fasting for, 189
Protease inhibitors, nutrient absorption and, 30
Protein. *See also* Amino acids
calcium loss and, 407
combining, 15
consumption
high, 11, 127
low, 11, **417, 419, 421**
reducing, for diabetes control, 294
Reversal Diet and, 126–27
sources, in raw foods diet, 173
in vegetarian diet, 13, 16
Protein-Carbohydrate Manipulation Diet, for depression, 389–91, **419, 421**
Prunes, for constipation, 306
Psoriasis
Ayurveda for, 96
dietary remedies for, **420**
evening primrose oil for, 209–10
shark cartilage for, 203–4
Psyllium, for digestive problems, 211–12, 310
Pumpkin seeds, sprouting method for, **174**
Pungent foods
in Ayurveda, 86
in Chinese nutrition, 63
Purines, foods high in, 256

Q

Quercetin, cancer-fighting potential of, 229, 372
Quinoa, in Ornish program, 127

R

Raffinose, for constipation, 308
Ramen noodles, in macrobiotic diet, 44
Raw foods diet
conditions helped by, **417, 419, 421**
fiber in, 173

Raw foods diet (*continued*)
  nutrient content of, 170–71, 172
  protein sources in, 173
  reasons for choosing, 171
  sprouting methods for, **174**
  transition to, 173, 175
  vitamin B$_{12}$ and, 173
Rectal cancer, low-fat, high-fiber diet for, 266, 269
Regularity, fiber for, 305, 310
Reishi mushrooms, health claims for, 225
Relaxation. *See* Stress, management
Religion-based diets
  Christianity, 71–74
  Buddhism, 79
  Hinduism, 78–79
  Islam, 76–77
  Judaism, 74–76
  vegetarianism as, 3
Reproductive system disorders. *See also specific disorders*
  Ayurveda for, 94–95
Respiratory system disorders. *See also specific disorders*
  Ayurveda for, 95–96
Restaurants
  ethnic, choices for Pritikin Eating Plan, 155
  selections, for heart disease prevention, 368
Re-stenosis, fish oil and, 214
Reversal Diet
  carbohydrates in, 128
  conditions helped by, **417**, **419**, **421**
  efficacy of, 114
  eggs and, 123, 126
  food pyramid for, 113
  grains in, 128
  health benefits of, 122
  low-fat dairy products and, 123, 126
  menus, sample, 124–26
  in Ornish program, 109, 111–12
  protein requirements and, 126–27
  shopping list for, 116–17
  sugar and, 130–31
  transition to, 119–20, 121
  vs. typical American diet, 120, 122
  vitamin/mineral supplements and, 133
  weight loss from, 115–19
Reversal theory, 113–14
Reye's syndrome, aspirin and, 199
Rheumatoid arthritis
  Ayurveda for, 99
  characteristics of, 255

diet and, 254–55
fasting and, 183–84
fish oil and, 215
gamma-linolenic acid for, 209
pain relief in, 256–57
shark cartilage for, 203–4
vegetarianism and, 12
Riboflavin, for neurotransmitter function, **391**
Rice
  in macrobiotic diet, 41, 152
  Nice Burgers, 107
  in Pritikin Eating Plan, 152
  rice balls, 41
  rice milk, 14, 313
  rice porridge, 41
  rice syrup, 41
Roasting, as low-fat cooking method, 118
Root vegetables, in macrobiotic diet, 38
Rosemary, cancer-fighting potential of, 240
Rotation diet, for food allergies and sensitivities, 349–53, **417, 419, 421**
Roughage. *See* Fiber, dietary
Royal jelly
  anaphylactic shock from, 231
  health claims for, 200, 230–31
Runner's high, endorphins and, 392

S

SAD, carbohydrate cravings and, 395–96
Saifun, in macrobiotic diet, 44
Salicin, in aspirin, 198
Salt
  consumption, blood pressure reduction and, 378–80
  intake
    osteoporosis and, 150–51, 408
    overweight and, 150
    reducing, 151, 408
  Pritikin Eating Plan and, 149, 150–51
  Reversal Diet and, 131, 131–32
  yin/yang and, 40
Salty foods
  in Ayurveda, 86
  in Chinese nutrition, 63
Saturated fat, cancer and, 8
Sea salt, in macrobiotic diet, 39
Seasonal affective disorder (SAD), carbohydrate cravings and, 395–96
Seasonal eating, Ayurveda and, 87–88
Seasonings. *See also specific seasonings*
  in macrobiotic diet, 39

Sea vegetables
  in Chinese nutrition, <u>61</u>
  in macrobiotic diet, <u>39</u>
Seaweed
  in Chinese nutrition, <u>61</u>, 65
  in macrobiotic diet, <u>39</u>
Seeds
  for cancer prevention, 277–78
  in Chinese nutrition, 64
  in hunter-gatherer diet, 22
Seitan, in macrobiotic diet, <u>38</u>
Selenium
  in Longevity Diet, 169
  for neurotransmitter function, **391**
Self-digestion, fasting and, 179
Senility, vegetarian diet for, 13
Serotonin
  chocolate craving and, <u>392</u>
  complex carbohydrates and, 393–94
  food sources, 385
  mood and, <u>334</u>, 386
  premenstrual syndrome and, 395
  seasonal affective disorder and, 395–96
  sugar and, 390
  tryptophan and, <u>196</u>, 386–88
Setpoint, weight and, <u>161</u>
Seventh-Day Adventists, vegetarian diet of,
    3, 13, 71–73, 75
Shark cartilage, health claims for, 202–4
Shiitake mushrooms, health claims for,
    225
Sinusitis
  Ayurveda for, 95–96
  dietary remedies for, **420**
  fasting for, 189
Skin cancer
  black tea and, 238
  dietary recommendations for, <u>270</u>
  green tea and, 237–38
  high-fat diets and, 145
Skin conditions. *See also specific conditions*
  Ayurveda for, 96
  fasting for, 189
Sleep
  patterns, migraines and, 400
  problems
    melatonin for, 223
    tryptophan for, 196
    valerian for, 248–49
Smoking
  with alcohol consumption, cancer and,
    269
  cessation, for osteoporosis, 409
  heart disease risk and, <u>136</u>

lung cancer risk, fruit and vegetable con-
    sumption and, 266
  vegetarians and, 9, 11
Snacks
  diabetes control and, 294–95
  high-fiber, 308
Soba, in macrobiotic diet, <u>44</u>
Soda pop, eliminating for digestive
    problems, 316
Sodium. *See also* Salt
  blood pressure reduction and, 150,
    378–80
  calcium excretion and, 29–30
  content, on food labels, 151
  diet low in, conditions helped by, **417**,
    419, 421
  restriction, 151
  vs. salt, 150
Solanine, in nightshades, 264
Somen, in macrobiotic diet, <u>44</u>
Sorbitol, adverse effects of, <u>309</u>, 319
Sour foods
Soybeans/soy products. *See also specific soy*
    products
  adding to diet, 279
  benefits for
    cancer prevention, 278–79
    heart disease prevention, <u>371</u>, 372–73
  diet high in, conditions helped by, **417**,
    419, 421
  low-density lipoproteins and, 372–73
  in macrobiotic diet, <u>39</u>, 272
  soy flour, <u>10</u>
  soy milk, <u>10</u>, 14, <u>60</u>, <u>313</u>, <u>371</u>
  in vegetarian diet, 9, <u>10</u>
Soy-free diet, for food allergies, 343
Specific Carbohydrate Diet
  conditions helped by, **417, 419, 421**
  for inflammatory bowel disease, 324,
    326, <u>327</u>
Spices. *See also specific spices*
  digestion and, <u>92</u>
  health claims for, 234
Spinach
  Tofu and Spinach Soup, <u>63</u>
Spirituality, dietary laws and, 73
Spirulina, health claims for, 231–33
Sports drinks, for diarrhea, 314
Sprouting methods, **174**, 175
Sprouts, in raw foods diet, 173
Starfruit, in Ornish Program, 129
Starvation diet, vs. fasting, <u>178</u>
Steaming, as low-fat cooking method, <u>118</u>
Stimulants, Ornish program and, 132–33

Stomach acid, heartburn and, <u>315</u>
Stomach cancer
    barbecued/smoked/pickled foods and, 269
    garlic consumption for, 236
Stomach emptying, acid reflux and, <u>315</u>
Stress
    body response to, 392–93
    complex carbohydrates for, 393–94
    eating habits and, 391–92
    free radical production and, 394
    ginkgo and, 217–18
    management
        dietary guidelines for, 393–94
        for irritable bowel syndrome, 317
        in Ornish program, <u>109</u>, 132
Stroganoff
    Vegetarian Stroganoff, <u>103</u>
Sugar, blood, <u>143</u>, 292
Sugar (food)
    chronic fatigue syndrome and, 285, 286
    colon cancer and, 272–73
    consumption, depression and, 389–90
    cravings for, 130–31
    diabetes control and, 294–95
    eating, effects of, 130
    fatigue and, 334–35
    in fruit juices, 130
    Pritikin Eating Plan and, 153–54
    Reversal Diet and, 130–31
Sulfites, adverse effects of, 345, <u>346</u>
Sulforaphan, cancer-fighting potential of, 267
Sunflower seeds, sprouting method for, **174**
Supplements. *See* Alternative supplements; *specific supplements*
Swank Dict, for multiple sclerosis, 402–4, **419**, **421**
Sweeteners, 319. *See also specific sweeteners*
Sweet foods
    in Ayurveda, 86
    in Chinese nutrition, 63
Sweets, Pritikin Eating Plan and, 153–54
Synephrine, migraines and, 399

T

Tartrazine, adverse effects of, <u>346</u>
Taste
    Ayurveda and, 86–87, 97
    Chinese nutrition and, 62–63

Tea. *See also specific teas*
    flavonoids in, 244
Tea mushroom, health claims for, 226–27
Tempeh
    in Chinese nutrition, <u>60</u>
    in macrobiotic diet, <u>39</u>
    in vegetarian diet, <u>10</u>
Textured vegetable protein (TVP), for heart disease prevention, 371, 373
Thiamin, for neurotransmitter function, **391**
Thinness, longevity and, <u>161</u>
Thromboxane, blood clotting and, 244
Thromboxane A_2, pregnancy-induced high blood pressure and, 216
Tinnitus
    fasting for, 189
    ginkgo for, 217
T-lymphocytes, fasting and, 186
Tobacco, 9, 11, 264. *See also* Smoking
Tofu
    in Chinese nutrition, <u>60</u>
    fat content of, 279
    for heart disease prevention, <u>371</u>
    in macrobiotic diet, <u>39</u>, <u>45</u>
    phytoestrogens in, 9
    Scrambled Tofu, <u>106</u>
    Tofu and Spinach Soup, <u>63</u>
    types of, <u>279</u>
    uses for, <u>10</u>, <u>45</u>
    Vegetarian Stroganoff, <u>103</u>
Tomatoes, arthritis pain and, 262–63
Torah, kosher laws in, 74–76
Trans-fatty acids, in margarine, <u>362</u>
Trifala, in Ayurveda, <u>92</u>
Triglycerides
    fish oil and, 213
    fruit juices and, 130
    lowering
        garlic for, 246
        royal jelly for, 231
    refined diets and, 152
Tryptophan
    carbohydrates and, 386–87
    seasonal affective disorder and, 395–96
    serotonin and, <u>196</u>, 386–88
Tumors
    benign, fasting and, 185
    fibroid, 185, 203–4
Turmeric
    cancer-fighting potential of, 239, 244
    for indigestion, 248
TVP, for heart disease prevention, <u>371</u>, 373
Tylenol, fasting and, <u>182</u>
Type I diabetes, 257, 292, 297

Type II diabetes
  fasting and, 187
  hunter-gatherer diet and, 28–29
  Pritikin Eating Plan and, 144–45
Tyramine, as migraine trigger, 399
Tyrosine, mood regulation and, 387, 388

U

Udon, in macrobiotic diet, <u>44</u>
Ulcerative colitis
  evening primrose oil for, 209–10
  fasting for, 187–88
Ulcers
  foods aggravating, <u>320–21</u>
  allergy-type reactions and, <u>345</u>
  Ayurveda for, 93
  dietary remedies for, **420**
  herbal remedies for, 250–51
  nonsteroidal anti-inflammatory drugs
    and, <u>320–21</u>
Umeboshi plums, in macrobiotic diet, <u>39</u>
Underweight, Ayurveda for, 93, **420**
Unsaturated fats, adverse effects of, 123
Uric acid, gout and, 255, 256
Urinary tract infections (UTIs)
  Ayurveda for, 96–97
  dietary remedies for, **420**
  herbal remedies for, 251
Uterine cancer, macrobiotic diet for, 51
UTIs. *See* Urinary tract infections

V

Valerian, for insomnia, 248–49
L-valine, health claims for, 195
Vata. *See also* Ayurveda
  balance, eating for, 87, 92
  characteristics of, 82–83, **84**
  food recommendations for, **90–91**
  menus, sample, 100
Vedas, 78
Vegan diet, 5–6
  calcium sources in, 17–18
  dietary suggestions, <u>14–15</u>
  vitamin B$_{12}$ and, 18
Vegetable(s). *See also specific vegetables*
  antioxidants in, 369–71
  benefits for
    cancer prevention, 9, 146, 266, 268,
      277
    cancer remission, 280

heart disease prevention, <u>370</u>, <u>371</u>
    multiple sclerosis, 404
  calcium in, 17, 29, 411–12
  canned, 129–30
  in Chinese nutrition, 64
  colors of, cancer prevention and, 268
  conditions helped by, **416**, **418**, **420**
  dietary fiber in, 9
  fiber content of, 309
  Fresh Dilled Eggplant, <u>106</u>
  frozen, 129
  gas-producing, <u>308</u>
  Hot Korean Vegetables and Noodles, <u>104</u>
  in hunter-gatherer diet, 22, 23
  juices, 130, 180
  nightshade, arthritis pain and, 262–64, <u>264</u>
  organically grown, 175
  Pasta Primavera, <u>105</u>
  in Pritikin Eating Plan, 146, <u>147</u>
  raw, diet of (*see* Raw foods diet)
  root, in macrobiotic diet, <u>38</u>
  sea, <u>39</u>, <u>61</u>
  Tofu and Spinach Soup, <u>63</u>
Vegetarian diet, 4, 122. *See also*
      Macrobiotic diet; Raw foods diet
  for arthritis, 257–60
  atherosclerosis and, 7
  Ayurveda and, 79
  benefits for
    blood pressure reduction, 377–78
    cancer, 8
    digestion, 12–13
    heart disease prevention, 6–8, 120, 355
    osteoporosis, 11–12
    regularity, 305
  conditions helped by, **417**, **419**, **421**
  cooking methods and, 20
  cost of, <u>5</u>
  duo-diet, <u>14–15</u>
  fiber intake and, 306, **307**
  food colors and, 20
  low-fat (*see* Reversal Diet)
  range/spectrum of, 4–6
  reasons for, 2–4
  transition to, 19–20
Veggie burgers
  for heart disease prevention, <u>371</u>
  Nice Burgers, <u>107</u>
  in vegetarian diet, 2, <u>3</u>
Vertigo
  fasting for, 189
  ginkgo for, 217
Very low density lipoproteins (VLDL), satu-
    rated fats and, 360

Vikriti, physical constitution and, 81
Vitamin A, for breast cancer, 266
Vitamin B$_6$, for neurotransmitter function, **391**
Vitamin B$_{12}$
  deficiency, 18
  macrobiotic diet and, 55, 56
  for neurotransmitter function, **391**
  raw foods diet and, 173
  supplements, 18–19
Vitamin C
  breast cancer risk and, 266
  in broccoli, 172
  cancer-fighting potential of, 9
  for chronic fatigue syndrome, 288
  for fatigue, 337
  food sources, 369, 394
  in fruits and vegetables, 146
  for heart disease prevention, 369, 371
  high-density lipoproteins and, 172
  in hunter-gatherer diet, 23
  iron absorption and, 17
  Longevity Diet and, 162, 169
  for neurotransmitter function, **391**
  Reversal Diet and, 133
  for stress management, 394
Vitamin D, for osteoporosis, 409, 412
Vitamin E
  cancer-fighting potential of, 9
  for cancer prevention, 277–78
  for chronic fatigue syndrome, 288
  for fatigue, 337
  food sources, 369, 394
  for heart disease prevention, 369, 371
  Longevity Diet and, 162, 169
  Reversal Diet and, 133
  for stress management, 394
  in wheat germ, 233
Vitamin K deficiency, gluten-free diet and, 328
Vitamins. *See also* Antioxidants; B-complex vitamins; *specific vitamins*
  benefits for
    arthritis, 262
    cancer prevention, 277
    energy, <u>336–37</u>
    heart disease prevention, <u>370–71</u>
  deficiency symptoms, 56
  Longevity Diet and, 169
  macrobiotic diet and, 55–56
  Reversal Diet and, 133
VLDL, saturated fats and, 360

W

Wakame
  in Chinese nutrition, <u>61</u>
  in macrobiotic diet, <u>39</u>, <u>61</u>
Water
  fasting and, 180
  intake
    dietary fiber and, 212, 301–2, 310
    for regularity, 310
  retention, 97, 250
Watercress, in macrobiotic diet, <u>38</u>
Weight loss
  benefits for
    arthritis pain, 255
    blood pressure control, 378
    diabetes control, 299
    gallstone prevention, 323
    heartburn, <u>315</u>
  by crash dieting, gallstones and, 323
  diets for, problems with, <u>115</u>
  from fasting, 189
  Ornish program and, 114–16
  Pritikin Eating Plan and, 142–44
  from Reversal Diet, 115–19
  yo-yo dieting, gallstones and, 323
Wheat
  in Chinese nutrition, <u>61</u>
  fatigue and, 337
  in macrobiotic cooking, <u>38</u>
  sprouting method for, **174**
  whole, for heart disease prevention, 371
Wheat bran
  for cholesterol reduction, 371
  as fiber supplement, 211
  in Ornish program, 128
  regularity and, <u>304</u>
Wheat-free diet, for digestive problems, <u>328</u>, 343
Wheat germ, health claims for, 233, <u>304</u>, 310
Whole foods. *See also* Grains, whole
  macrobiotic diet and, 41–42
  wheat, for heart disease prevention, <u>371</u>
Wild yams, <u>206</u>
Withdrawal symptoms, during fasting, 181

Y

Yang. *See* Yin/yang
Yeast-free diet
  for chronic fatigue syndrome, 285
  conditions helped by, **417**, **419**, **421**

Yeast infections
  acidophilus for, 219–20
  chronic fatigue and, 285
  dietary remedies for, **420–21**
  herbal remedies for, 251–52
Yin/yang
  cancer and, 49–50, 272
  Crohn's disease and, 57
  foods, identifying, 63–64
  heart disease and, 45–46
  macrobiotic diet and, 36, 37, <u>40</u>, 272
  macrobiotic healing theories and,
      44–45
  personality traits and, 58, **59**

Yogurt
  acidophilus cultures in, 219–20
  for heart disease prevention, <u>370</u>
  for lactose intolerance, <u>24</u>, <u>313</u>
  Yogurt Cheese, <u>141</u>
Yo-yo syndrome, weight loss and, <u>115</u>
Yuppie flu. *See* Chronic fatigue syndrome

Z

Zen macrobiotics, 36–37
Zinc, 17, 337
Zutphen Elderly Study, 244